Contents

(**Part 3**) **Self-assessment, 232**

Preface

Medicine is a mass of facts and complex science, which can be dull and indigestible. It is brought to life by patients with their individual stories, clinical mysteries and their need for help. Medicine is probably best learnt through clinical experience backed up by information and reflection. However in modern medical practice there is often too much to do and too little time for consideration.

This book is one of the first in a novel series that allows the reader to experience a virtual clinical attachment with enough time for reflection and teaching. Patients are described as they really present to hospital or general practice. The clinical reasoning required to explain symptoms and signs, order and interpret investigations and start management is demonstrated as the case develops. Relevant science is described in context to support understanding and patients are managed according to current guidelines. This format will allow the reader to develop knowledge and skills that are immediately useful for patient management, rather than to accumulate facts that need a lot more work to translate them into practice.

Twenty nine patients with respiratory disease are presented in the book, providing experience of the full breadth of adult respiratory medicine. We have chosen these cases as they are common problems that will be encountered at some point by all doctors in clinical practice, no matter what field they end up in. Many questions used to explore the cases are real questions posed by students during our teaching sessions and the answers are the end product of many attempts to answer these questions satisfactorily. As experienced examiners we have ensured that material covered in this book is sufficient for students to pass respiratory sections of undergraduate or general postgraduate exams. This book will also be a useful aid to practice for junior doctors and allied health professionals looking after patients with respiratory disease and as basic revision for doctors entering specialist respiratory training.

We have written the text book that we would have liked to use to learn respiratory medicine. If we were starting again we would begin with the patients, attempting to answer the questions posed throughout the cases alone or in groups before reading the written answers and relevant science. During relevant clinical attachments we would use the book to update clinical skills and practice OSCE checklists. In preparation for exams we would revise case summaries and key points and practice the self assessment questions. We hope you will enjoy using it and that it will help you understand respiratory medicine for the benefit of patients.

Emma H. Baker
Dilys Lai
2008

Acknowledgements

The authors gratefully acknowledge the help of the following:

Dr Belinda Brewer for invaluable comments on the manuscript; Dr Cathy Corbishley for generous donation of pathology slides from her personal collection; Mr Harry Young for his wonderful contribution to student education as a patient and for modelling for this book; Mark Evenden and staff of media services at St George's, University of London for endless production of fantastic illustrations; Sue Adie for tireless administrative support; and Dr Adrian Draper, Dr Yee Ean Ong, Dr Deirdre McGrath, Dr Laurie Hanna, Dr Sisa Grubnic, Dr Claire Wells, Dr Stephen Thomas, nursing staff on Marnham ward, Reg Ramai and Paula Mclean for provision of clinical material and other assistance.

How to use this book

Clinical Cases Uncovered (CCU) books are carefully designed to help supplement your clinical experience and assist with refreshing your memory when revising. Each book is divided into three sections: Part 1, Basics; Part 2, Cases; and Part 3, Self-Assessment.

Part 1 gives a quick reminder of the basic science, history and examination, and key diagnoses in the area. Part 2 contains many of the clinical presentations you would expect to see on the wards or crop up in exams, with questions and answers leading you through each case. New information, such as test results, is revealed as events unfold and each case concludes with a handy case summary explaining the key points. Part 3 allows you to test your learning with several question styles (MCQs, EMQs and SAQs), each with a strong clinical focus.

Whether reading individually or working as part of a group, we hope you will enjoy using your CCU book. If you have any recommendations on how we could improve the series, please do let us know by contacting us at: medstudentuk@oxon.blackwellpublishing.com.

Disclaimer
CCU patients are designed to reflect real life, with their own reports of symptoms and concerns. Please note that all names used are entirely fictitious and any similarity to patients, alive or dead, is coincidental.

Basic science

Anatomy and physiology

The primary function of the lungs is to take up oxygen from the air into the blood and excrete carbon dioxide. To achieve this, the following are required:
- Respiratory centre in the brain to control the process of breathing
- Respiratory muscles, chest wall and pleura to allow inflation and deflation of the lungs
- Airways to transmit air into and out of the lung
- Alveoli and capillaries to act as an interface for gas exchange
- Pulmonary circulation to carry deoxygenated blood into, and oxygenated blood out of, the lungs
- Host defence systems to protect the lung from inhaled foreign particles (e.g. organisms, allergens, pollutants) and maintain function

Control of breathing

The act of breathing requires the anatomical structures shown in Fig. 1. The following sequence of events occurs:
- The respiratory centre in the brainstem generates a signal to breathe
- This signal is transmitted via the:
  ○ spinal cord
  ○ anterior horn cells
  ○ motor nerves (phrenic and intercostal nerves)
  ○ neuromuscular junctions
- The signal stimulates contraction of respiratory muscles, which lowers intrathoracic pressure and sucks air into the lungs
- When the signal stops, the respiratory muscles relax and elastic recoil of the lungs and weight of the chest wall force air out of the lungs
- The next signal is generated from the respiratory centre and the cycle starts again

The respiratory centre

The respiratory centre is made up of groups of neurons in the medulla oblongata and pons of the brainstem.

The *dorsal group of neurons* in the respiratory centre is responsible for normal quiet breathing. These neurons automatically generate repetitive inspiratory signals. Each signal begins weakly and builds up over about 2 s, stimulating a smooth contraction of the respiratory muscles. After inspiration the signal ceases for about 3 s, allowing relaxation of the respiratory muscles and expiration before the inspiratory signal begins again. These signals continue from birth to death unless the respiratory centre is damaged. As each cycle takes about 5 s the normal respiratory rate is around 12 breaths/min.

The *chemosensitive area* in the brainstem detects changes in carbon dioxide concentrations and adjusts respiratory rate as follows:
- As CO_2 concentrations rise, H^+ ions are generated by interaction with water:

Henderson–Hasselbach equation

$$H^+ + HCO_3^- \rightleftarrows H_2CO_3 \rightleftarrows H_2O + CO_2$$

- H^+ ions stimulate chemosensitive neurons, which signal to other areas of the respiratory centre to increase the respiratory rate
- Increased ventilation blows off CO_2, lowering blood CO_2 concentrations back to normal
- H^+ ion concentrations in the brain decrease and this signals to the respiratory centre to slow the respiratory rate

Peripheral chemoreceptors are present in carotid and aortic bodies, where they are ideally placed to monitor arterial oxygen concentrations. When oxygen concentrations are normal, signalling from peripheral chemoreceptors is suppressed. However, when blood oxygen concentrations fall below normal, chemoreceptors send strong signals to the respiratory centre via the glossopharyngeal and vagal nerves, which drive an increase in respiratory rate. Signalling by peripheral chemoreceptors is also stimulated by an increase in H^+ ions, for example in renal failure or acidosis. Patients with acidosis appear

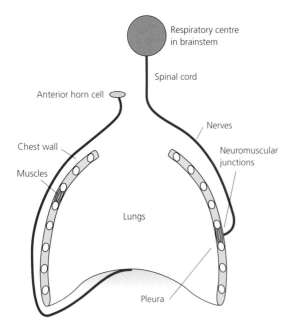

Respiratory centre in brainstem

Spinal cord

Anterior horn cell

Chest wall

Muscles

Nerves

Neuromuscular junctions

Lungs

Pleura

Figure 1 Structures required for the act of breathing.

breathless with deep sighing respiration (Kussmaul's respiration), which has been described as 'air hunger'.

Hierarchy of respiratory stimuli

The strongest drive to breathe is the repetitive inspiratory signal generated by the dorsal neurons:
• This signal is unstoppable, unless the respiratory centre is damaged
• However, ventilation driven by this signal may not be sufficient to maintain normal blood PaO_2 and $PaCO_2$
• Addition of other stimuli to this signal increases respiratory rate and depth as required

The next strongest drive to breathe is an increase in $PaCO_2$, detected by the chemosensitive area:
• This process is extremely sensitive. For example, a small increase in CO_2 of 0.13 kPa results in a 2–4 L/min increase in ventilation
• In patients with chronic hypercapnia, the chemosensitive area becomes less sensitive to changes in $PaCO_2$. As this central respiratory drive falls, the weaker drive from peripheral chemoreceptors takes over

The peripheral chemoreceptors generate the weakest respiratory stimulus. They are important in patients who have lost the chemosensitive drive to breathe because of chronic hypercapnia, or in patients with severe hypoxia or acidosis.

Respiratory muscles, chest wall and pleura
Respiratory muscles
Inspiratory muscles are:
• Diaphragm (quiet breathing)
• Intercostal muscles
• Neck muscles (accessory)

In inspiration, intrathoracic pressure is lowered by downwards movement of the diaphragm and upwards/outwards movement of the ribs, as a result of contraction of the intercostal muscles. This sucks air into the lungs. Neck and shoulder girdle muscles are recruited to help lower intrathoracic pressure when more vigorous inspiration is required (e.g. after exercise and during respiratory distress).

Expiration involves:
• Relaxation of inspiratory muscles
• Elastic recoil of lungs
• Abdominal muscles (accessory)

On expiration, the respiratory muscles relax and elastic recoil of the lungs and chest wall raise intrathoracic pressure. This process forces air out of the lungs. The abdominal muscles are accessory respiratory muscles that can be contracted to enhance expiration.

Chest wall and pleura
The chest wall comprises ribs and muscles, including internal and external intercostal, subcostal and *Transversus thoracis* muscles. The chest wall and diaphragm surround the thoracic cavity, which is lined by a membrane called the parietal pleura. The lungs are also covered by a pleural membrane called the visceral pleura, which is continuous with the parietal layer at the lung hila (Fig. 2). Parietal and visceral pleura are separated by a potential space, which contains a thin layer of fluid that allows the lungs to slide smoothly against the chest wall during inspiration and expiration. There is a negative pressure in the pleural space, thought to be generated by pumping of fluid out of the space by lymphatics. This negative pressure opposes the elastic recoil of the lungs, keeping them expanded and ensuring that they inflate and deflate with movement of the chest wall and diaphragm.

Airways
The airways comprise nose, pharynx, larynx, trachea, bronchi and bronchioles (Fig. 3).

Upper airways
Nose
The nasal cavity is divided into right and left sides by the nasal septum. As air enters the nose it passes over the turbinates, which are fleshy structures with a large blood

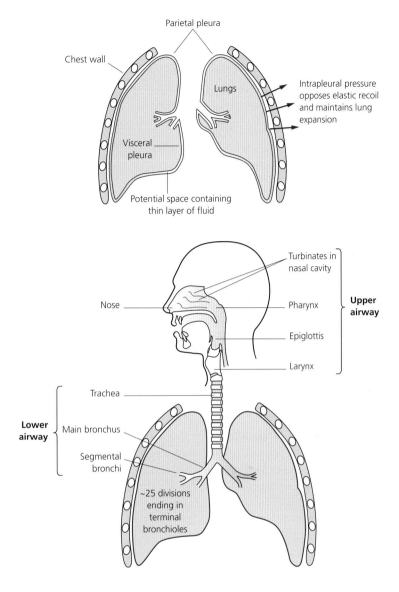

Figure 2 Anatomy of the pleura.

Figure 3 Anatomy of the airways.

supply that warm and humidify the air. High in the nasal cavity, air comes into contact with the olfactory nerve endings, generating the sensations of smell and taste. The nasal cavity is lined by ciliated epithelium with an overlying layer of mucus. This traps inhaled foreign particles, which can then be removed from the nose by mucociliary transport to the pharynx or by sneezing. The sinuses and lacrimal ducts drain into the nose and can become blocked in patients with nasal disease.

Pharynx

This is a muscular tube that extends behind the nasal and oral cavities and ends at the top of the oesophagus. Its purpose is to transmit air to the lower respiratory tract and food to the oesophagus. It contains lymphoid tissue (tonsils and adenoids) and mucus glands. The eustachian tubes enter the pharynx from the middle ear and can become blocked by swollen lymphoid tissue.

Larynx

This organ produces voice and protects the airways from aspiration of food and secretions. It is made up of cartilages (Box 1) held together by ligaments and moved by muscles. Inside the laryngeal cavity, connective tissue, muscles and ligaments make up the vocal folds or cords which are used to produce sound. At the top of the larynx

> **Box 1 Clinical reasons to know the anatomy of laryngeal cartilages**
>
> - Two laryngeal cartilages can be felt easily in the neck. The 'Adam's apple' is the laryngeal cartilage. Below that is a gap, then a smaller cartilage called the cricoid cartilage
> - In clinical medicine the distance between the cricoid cartilage and the sternal notch (cricosternal distance) is used to assess lung hyperinflation (see p. 26)
> - The cricothyroid membrane between the laryngeal and cricoid cartilages can be pierced (cricothyrotomy) in an emergency to allow a patient with severe upper airways obstruction to breathe

is the epiglottis, which is a leaf-shaped flap of tissue that is brought down to cover the laryngeal opening and prevent aspiration during swallowing.

Lower airways

The trachea is about 10–12 cm in length and divides at the carina into left and right main bronchi. These divide into lobar, then segmental and subsegmental bronchi. There are around 25 divisions between carina and alveoli.

Large airways

The trachea and first seven divisions of the bronchi have:
- Cartilage and smooth muscle in walls
- Submucosal mucus secreting glands
- Ciliated epithelium containing goblet cells
- Endocrine cells

Small airways

The next 16–18 divisions of bronchioles have:
- No cartilage and progressive thinning of muscle layer
- Single layer of ciliated cells and very few goblet cells
- Granulated Clara cells producing surfactant-like substance

Flow of air through the airways

Movement of air into and out of the lung depends on differences in air pressure between mouth and alveoli.
- On breathing in, contraction of respiratory muscles lowers intrathoracic pressure below atmospheric pressure, pulling air into the alveoli
- On breathing out, elastic recoil of the lung and chest wall raises intrathoracic pressure above atmospheric pressure, forcing air out of the alveoli

The rate at which air moves into and out of the lungs in response to these changes in pressure depends on the rate at which air can flow along the airways. This in turn depends on airway resistance and can be described by Ohm's law:

$$\text{Flow rate} = \frac{\text{Difference in pressure between mouth and alveoli}}{\text{Resistance to airflow in airways}}$$

Poiseuille's law describes the components of resistance to flow in more detail:

$$\text{Resistance} = \frac{8 \times \text{viscosity of air} \times \text{airway length}}{\pi r^4}$$

This is important as it shows that the radius of the tube is a very powerful determinant of airflow resistance. To test this, try breathing out through a tube with a large radius, such as the cardboard insert from kitchen roll. Flow will be rapid through this wide tube and you will be able to empty your lungs easily. Then try breathing out through a tube with a small radius, such as a drinking straw. Flow will be very slow through this narrow tube and it will take a long time to empty your lungs.

The radius of the lumen of airways in the respiratory tract depends on (Fig. 4):
- Smooth muscle tone
- Thickness of the epithelium and submucosa
- Luminal contents
- Pressure inside and outside the airways

Airflow obstruction

Disease causing airflow obstruction includes:
- Obstructive sleep apnoea (upper airways)
- Asthma (lower airways)
- Chronic obstructive pulmonary disease (COPD; lower airways)

In obstructive sleep apnoea, pressure outside the airway from neck soft tissues compresses the upper airway causing partial collapse with snoring, or complete collapse with cessation of breathing (apnoea). In asthma and COPD, smooth muscle spasm, mucosal oedema and increased airway secretions and sputum plugs obstruct the airway (Fig. 4).

Alveoli and capillaries

Alveoli

Alveoli are small air-filled sacs at the end of the smallest airways (terminal bronchioles). There are over 300 million in two lungs. The walls of the sacs include type I and II pneumocytes.

Type I pneumocytes
These cells form a single epithelial cell layer. They have extremely thin cytoplasm, which facilitates gas exchange

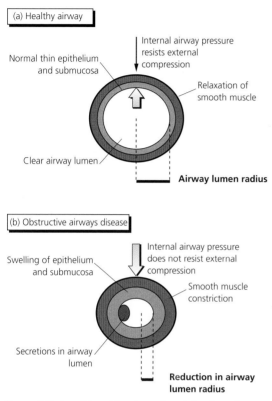

Figure 4 Factors determining the radius of the airway lumen.

and make up 90–95% of the surface area of the alveolar epithelium.

Type II pneumocytes
These cells make surfactant which lines the alveolar lumen. Surfactant reduces surface tension, preventing alveolar collapse and reducing the amount of work required for breathing.

Capillaries
Each single alveolus is surrounded by a dense network of around 1000 capillaries. The wall of the pulmonary capillaries comprises a single layer of endothelial cells, which facilitates gas exchange.

Alveolar–capillary membrane
The massive numbers of alveoli and capillaries in the lung result in around 50–100 m^2 of contact between these structures in a normal adult. The enormous alveolar–capillary interface is ideal for gas exchange. The barrier that respiratory gases must cross between air in the alveoli and red blood cells in the capillaries is called the alveolar–capillary membrane (Fig. 5). It has a thickness of approximately 0.6 μm. The alveoli, capillaries and intervening connective tissue are known collectively as the lung parenchyma.

Gas transport
O_2 and CO_2 move across the alveolar–capillary membrane by diffusion which depends on:
• The difference in partial pressure of each gas on either side of the membrane

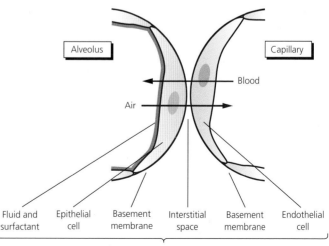

Figure 5 Components of the alveolar–capillary membrane.

- The ability of the gas to cross the membrane (diffusion coefficient)
- Membrane properties:
  - thickness
  - surface area

Oxygen transport

The partial pressure of O_2 (PaO_2) in atmospheric air is 21 kPa. When air is inhaled it mixes with air already in the lungs, so that the PaO_2 of air is around 13 kPa by the time it gets to the alveoli.

O_2 diffuses across the alveolar–capillary membrane from higher partial pressures in the air to lower partial pressures in the blood. When the lungs are functioning effectively they can elevate PaO_2 in arterial blood to similar levels to PaO_2 in alveolar air. Thus, normal arterial PaO_2 is 10–13.1 kPa.

The diffusion coefficient for O_2 is 20 times lower than that of CO_2, meaning that it crosses the membrane 20 times more slowly than CO_2.

In the blood, most of the O_2 taken up by the lungs is bound to haemoglobin and a small amount is dissolved in plasma.

Haemoglobin in blood leaving the lungs is 95–100% saturated with O_2. After delivery of O_2 to the tissues, haemoglobin in blood returning to the lungs is approximately 70% saturated with O_2. The relationship between PaO_2 and haemoglobin saturation with oxygen is shown in Fig. 6 and clinical relevance discussed in Box 2.

Carbon dioxide transport

CO_2 is generated by cells as a waste product. CO_2 is transported in the blood as:

- Bicarbonate (~70%), after interaction with water, catalysed by carbonic anhydrase (Henderson–Hasselbach equation)
- Carboxyhaemoglobin (15–25%), i.e. bound to haemoglobin
- Dissolved CO_2 in water

CO_2 is released in the lungs and diffuses rapidly across the alveolar–capillary membrane (high diffusion coefficient) down the partial pressure gradient from blood to air.

Ventilation removes CO_2 from alveolar air.

Respiratory failure

Respiratory failure is defined as arterial $PaO_2 < 8$ kPa (normal range 10–13.1 kPa).

Box 2 Clinical uses for the oxygen haemoglobin dissociation curve

The proportion of haemoglobin in blood that is deoxygenated determines its colour:
- Arterial blood is bright red because 95–100% haemoglobin is bound to oxygen
- Venous blood is dusky purple because it contains a larger proportion of deoxygenated haemoglobin (~25%)

Clinical detection of hypoxia

People normally look pink because most of the haemoglobin in blood below the skin is oxygenated

People look blue (cyanosis) when blood below the skin contains >5 g/dL deoxygenated haemoglobin.
- *Central cyanosis.* This is caused by failure of oxygenation of the blood (e.g. because of cardiac or respiratory failure). Patients look blue centrally (under the tongue) and peripherally (hands and feet)
- *Peripheral cyanosis.* This is caused by excess extraction of oxygen from blood when flow is slowed through peripheral tissues by vasoconstriction. Patients have blue peripheries but are pink centrally

Measurement of oxygen saturation

Oximetry is a non-invasive method of estimating the oxygen content of blood. A beam of red and infrared light is passed through a capillary bed, usually in a finger or ear lobe. Transmission of each wavelength of light through the capillary bed depends on the proportion of oxygenated haemoglobin in capillary blood. This is detected by a sensor and reported as percentage oxygen saturation of haemoglobin.

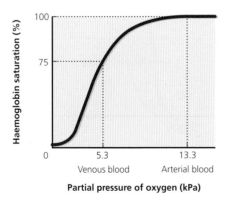

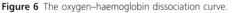

Figure 6 The oxygen–haemoglobin dissociation curve.

Box 3 Some causes of type I respiratory failure

Reduction in surface area of the alveolar–capillary interface

Reduced alveolar ventilation

- Obstructive airways disease – reduced airflow to alveoli, e.g.
  - asthma
  - COPD (chronic bronchitis)
- COPD (emphysema) – destruction of alveoli
- Pneumonia – pus replaces air in the alveoli
- Lung cancer – replacement of lung parenchyma with tumour or loss of air-filled alveoli because of associated lung collapse

Reduced capillary perfusion

- Pulmonary emboli – pulmonary arteries are obstructed by clots
- COPD (emphysema) – destruction of pulmonary capillaries

Increased thickness of the alveolar–capillary membrane

- Interstitial lung disease – increased connective tissue is deposited in the interstitial space
- Pulmonary oedema – the alveolar–capillary membrane is thickened by oedema fluid

Type I respiratory failure (Box 3)

- Defined as $PaO_2 < 8\,kPa$ without hypercapnia (PCO_2 low or normal)
- Caused by any disease that impairs gas transport across the alveolar–capillary membrane by:
  - reducing the surface area of the alveolar–capillary interface (loss of alveolar ventilation, capillary diffusion or both)
  - increasing the thickness of the alveolar–capillary membrane
- As the diffusion coefficient for O_2 is 20 times lower than for CO_2, mild or moderate impairment of gas transport across the alveolar–capillary membrane will cause hypoxia without altering blood $PaCO_2$ (type I respiratory failure). Severe impairment of gas transport across the alveolar–capillary membrane will impair CO_2 transport as well as O_2 transport and cause type II respiratory failure (see below)

Type II respiratory failure (Fig. 7)

- Defined as $PaO_2 < 8\,kPa$ *and* hypercapnia
- Caused by:
  - impaired ventilation, preventing exhalation of CO_2
  - any severe lung disease that causes sufficient impairment of gas transport across the alveolar–capillary

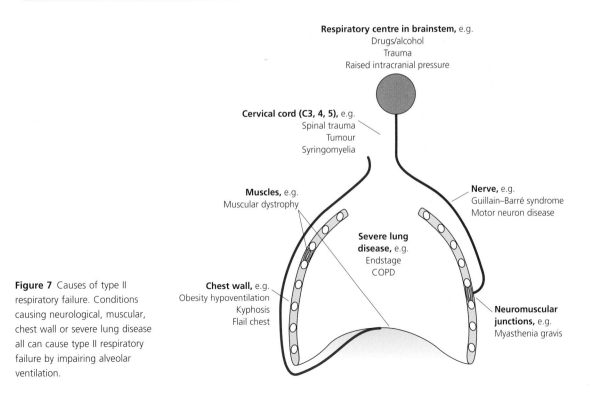

Figure 7 Causes of type II respiratory failure. Conditions causing neurological, muscular, chest wall or severe lung disease all can cause type II respiratory failure by impairing alveolar ventilation.

Respiratory centre in brainstem, e.g.
Drugs/alcohol
Trauma
Raised intracranial pressure

Cervical cord (C3, 4, 5), e.g.
Spinal trauma
Tumour
Syringomyelia

Muscles, e.g.
Muscular dystrophy

Nerve, e.g.
Guillain–Barré syndrome
Motor neuron disease

Severe lung disease, e.g.
Endstage COPD

Chest wall, e.g.
Obesity hypoventilation
Kyphosis
Flail chest

Neuromuscular junctions, e.g.
Myasthenia gravis

membrane to reduce both CO_2 and O_2 transport (e.g. advanced COPD, status asthmaticus, massive pulmonary embolus)

KEY POINT

Any lung disease that impairs oxygen transport can lead to type I respiratory failure. When the lung disease becomes more severe and carbon dioxide transport is also impaired, this leads to type II respiratory failure. For example, type I respiratory failure may be caused by exacerbations of mild to moderate COPD or by moderate to severe asthma exacerbations, but severe COPD or life-threatening asthma may cause type II respiratory failure.

Effects of respiratory failure

Respiratory failure may be life-threatening as both hypoxia (Box 4) and hypercapnia (Box 5) have serious detrimental effects on cells, tissues and organs.

Some cells are unable to tolerate hypoxia – e.g. neurons are damaged irreversibly after 4–6 min of hypoxia. Other cells (e.g. skeletal muscle cells) survive more prolonged hypoxia.

Pulmonary circulation (Fig. 8)
Circulation of deoxygenated blood
- Oxygen is removed from blood by tissues and organs
- Deoxygenated blood is returned to the right side of the

Box 4 Pathophysiological effects of hypoxia

Oxygen is essential for cell metabolism and lack of oxygen causes cell injury by:
- Adenosine triphosphate (ATP) depletion
- Intracellular acidosis
- Build-up of metabolic byproducts and free radicals
- Direct cell damage including to membranes and cytoskeleton
- Induction of inflammation

Box 5 Pathophysiological effects of hypercapnia

Hypercapnia has toxic effects, particularly on the brain and circulation

Brain
- Alterations in brain chemistry (glutamine, gamma-aminobutyric acid (GABA), glutamate and aspartate), contributing to depression of consciousness
- Increased cerebral blood flow
- Raised intracranial pressure

Circulation
- Depression of myocardial contractility
- Coronary and systemic artery vasodilatation, possibly mediated by vascular K^+ (ATP) channels

---

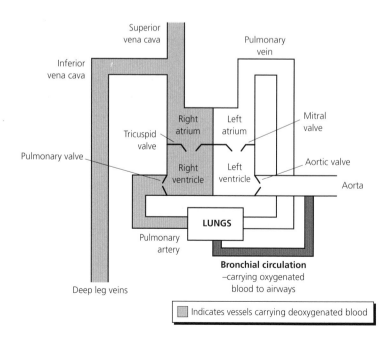

Figure 8 Diagram of pulmonary and systemic circulation.

heart by systemic veins, which feed into the superior and inferior vena cava
• The superior and inferior vena cava drain into the right atrium. Deoxygenated blood is pumped out of the right atrium through the tricuspid valve into the right ventricle
• Contraction of the right ventricle pumps deoxygenated blood through the pulmonary valve into the pulmonary artery
• Features of pulmonary arteries:
  ○ pulmonary arteries have thinner walls, less smooth muscle and greater internal diameters than systemic arteries
  ○ systolic and diastolic blood pressures in the main pulmonary arteries (~25/8 mmHg) are much lower than in systemic arteries (120/80 mmHg)
  ○ pulmonary arterial pressure is increased by hypoxia, hypercapnia and acidosis as well as by stimulation by the nervous system and inflammatory mediators
• The pulmonary arteries divide many times and these branches carry deoxygenated blood down into the network of 280 billion capillaries, where it is oxygenated

Circulation of oxygenated blood
• Blood oxygenated at the alveolar–capillary interface enters the pulmonary veins
• The pulmonary veins drain into the left atrium
• Blood in the left atrium is pumped through the mitral valve to the left ventricle
• Oxygenated blood in the left ventricle is pumped through the aortic valve into the aorta and circulates in the systemic arteries to carry oxygen to tissues and organs

Supply of oxygen to pulmonary tissues
The bronchial circulation is a second pulmonary blood supply which carries oxygenated blood to lung structures including trachea, bronchi down to the level of the terminal bronchioles, hilar lymph nodes and visceral pleura. Bronchial arteries arise from the aorta or from intercostal arteries and bronchial veins drain into the pulmonary vein. The lung parenchyma does not have a second blood supply as it receives oxygen directly from air in the alveoli.

Pulmonary defences (Fig. 9)
Inspired air may be contaminated with foreign particles, such as allergens, organisms and pollutants, with potential to injure the lung. Adults inhale around 10,000 L air each day, putting the lung at considerable risk of exposure to these damaging particles. The lung has an elaborate system of defences to trap and clear inhaled particles from the lung and additional mechanisms to deal with pathogens that evade removal from the lung.

Trapping of inhaled particles
• Large particles (>10–15 μmol) are trapped by nasal hairs
• Smaller particles (2–10 μmol) are trapped in mucus lining the upper and lower airways
• Tiny particles reach the alveoli, where they are deposited in alveolar fluid

Removal of trapped particles from the lung
Sneeze and cough
Receptors in the respiratory tract detect the presence of particles by mechanical or chemical means. This can trigger bronchospasm to prevent deeper penetration of particles into the lung. Stimulation of receptors also triggers a sneeze or cough reflex, generating explosive airflow that expels particles from upper and lower airways, respectively.

Mucociliary escalator
The upper and lower airways are lined with ciliated epithelium. Overlying the epithelium is a thin layer of liquid, called airway surface liquid, which has two components (Fig. 9). The watery liquid nearest the epithelial cell surface is called the 'sol' layer, and has a depth equivalent to the length of the cilia. This layer allows the cilia to extend fully and beat freely. Overlying the 'sol' layer is the gel layer, which contains mucus. This is the layer that traps inhaled particles. The beating of the cilia propels the 'gel' layer and trapped particles out of the airway into the pharynx, where mucus is expectorated or swallowed.

Alveolar macrophages
Inhaled particles that reach the alveoli are engulfed by alveolar macrophages. Potential outcomes of this are:
• Destruction of particles by macrophage lysosomes
• Removal of macrophages by the mucociliary escalator
• Clearance of macrophages by the lymphatic system
• Persistence of macrophages containing particles in the lung

Epithelial barrier
Airway epithelial cells are interspersed by tight junctions, forming a barrier that resists invasion of organisms or other particles into the body.

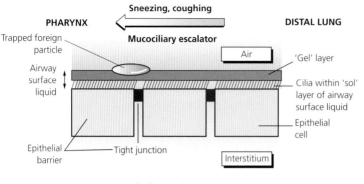

Innate and adaptive immune systems

Figure 9 Defence of the lung against inhaled foreign particles.

Immune system

Detection of foreign particles, such as organisms or allergens, in the lung triggers both innate and adaptive immune responses.

Innate immunity

- This is a non-specific front line immune system which broadly recognizes that a particle is foreign, but does not identify the particle
- When foreign particles are detected, innate immunity is activated rapidly and provides immediate defence
- The main action of the innate immune system is to dispose of foreign particles:
  - phagocytes such as neutrophils and macrophages engulf and destroy particles
  - lysozyme, lactoferrin, defensins and complement in airway surface liquid kill bacteria
  - surfactant molecules in airway surface liquid opsonize bacteria and particles, making them more susceptible to being engulfed by phagocytes
- The innate immune response changes little with age or exposure to infection and has no memory

Adaptive immunity

The adaptive immune system generates a specific response to individual pathogens that is much slower than the innate immune response (days rather than minutes–hours). The adaptive response destroys pathogens that evade the innate immune response and has a 'memory' that strengthens subsequent responses to the same infection.

Antigen-presenting cells. Antigen-presenting cells, such as dendritic cells, provide a link between innate and adaptive immune systems. Dendritic cells that have engulfed

pathogens migrate to the lymph nodes. During migration they process antigens from the pathogen and present them on their cell surface in association with a major histocompatibility complex (MHC), normally used for self-recognition. In the lymph nodes the MHC–antigen complex is recognized by and activates T lymphocytes.

CD4$^+$ cells (T helper cells). The role of CD4$^+$ T lymphocytes is to orchestrate the immune response. These cells do not directly destroy pathogens. Activated CD4$^+$ T lymphocytes generate cytokines and stimulate influx of phagocytes and cytotoxic cells. CD4$^+$ T lymphocytes can trigger two main responses to activation, mediated by different cytokines and leading to two different immune responses:

- *Th1 response.* Cytotoxic T cells are activated, activating cell-mediated immunity which is most effective against intracellular pathogens. CD8 cells (cytotoxic T cells) destroy infected cells by inducing apoptosis and releasing cytotoxic molecules, which lyse cells by punching holes in their membranes. Dead cells are cleared by phagocytes.
- *Th2 response.* B lymphocytes are activated by free antigen in combination with T helper (Th) cells. This stimulates them to differentiate into plasma cells that produce antibodies (IgM, IgG, IgA, IgE). Antibodies contribute to the immune response by binding to antigen, triggering phagocytosis and activating the complement cascade. They can also be directly cytotoxic. This response is called humoral immunity and is most effective against extracellular pathogens.

Immune memory. Some T and B cells activated during the adaptive immune response will become memory cells. If infection with the specific pathogen occurs again, memory cells allow the body to mount a strong response against infection. Immune memory occurs naturally after infection and can be induced artificially by vaccination.

Pathological processes affecting the lung
Inflammation

Inflammation is a process stimulated by tissue injury (Box 6), which has the physiological aims of eliminating the trigger and initiating healing and repair.

Acute inflammation

Initial exposure to an inflammatory trigger initiates an acute response including:
• Vascular changes. Capillary vasodilatation and increased permeability
• Release of chemical mediators
• Inflammatory infiltrate (innate and adaptive immune cells)

These responses account for the classic features of acute inflammation:
• *Rubor* – redness
• *Calor* – heat
• *Dolor* – pain
• *Tumor* – swelling
• *Laesio functae* – loss of function

The clinical features of lung inflammation depend on the part of the lung involved (Box 7). The Latin word for inflammation is *itis*, and addition of this term to an anatomical name implies inflammation of that part of the body. For example, rhinitis means nasal inflammation and bronchitis means bronchial inflammation.

Outcomes of acute inflammation

Acute inflammation brings phagocytes and lymphocytes to the site of tissue injury. These cells act to remove the inflammatory trigger and clear damaged or infected cells. The outcome of these processes may be:
• *Resolution.* Elimination of the trigger allows normal tissue architecture and function to be restored
• *Scarring.* After the trigger has been eliminated, damaged tissue is replaced with fibrosis. This reduces the

---

Box 6 Some triggers of inflammation in the lung

Infection
• Bacteria (e.g. *Streptococcus pneumoniae*)
• Viruses (e.g. influenza A)
• Fungi (e.g. *Pneumocystis jirovecii*, causes *Pneumocystis* pneumonia)

Allergens
• Plant (e.g. pollen)
• Animal (e.g. cat dander)
• Microorganisms (e.g. fungal spores, house dust mite)

Cigarette smoking
Pollutants
• Traffic fumes
• Smoke inhalation

Inorganic material
• Asbestos
• Silica
• Coal dust

Drugs
• Amiodarone
• Methotrexate

Box 7 Clinical features of acute inflammation in the lung

Upper airways (e.g. rhinitis, pharyngitis, laryngitis)
• *Tumor* – blocked nose, hoarse voice
• *Dolor/rubor* – sore/red throat
• Loss of function – difficulty breathing/swallowing/speaking
• Increased secretion – runny nose

Lower airways (e.g. bronchitis/ asthma)
• *Tumor* – airways obstruction, wheeze
• *Dolor* – cough
• Loss of function – respiratory failure
• Increased secretion – sputum production

Lung parenchyma (e.g. pneumonia/ infarction)
• *Tumor* – reduced air entry
• Loss of function – respiratory failure
• Increased secretion – sputum production

Pleura (pleurisy)
• *Dolor* – pleuritic chest pain
• Loss of function – difficulty taking a deep breath
• Increased capillary leak – pleural effusion

function of the affected organ to an extent depending on the amount of scarring

• *Persistence*. The trigger is not eliminated and drives chronic inflammation, leading to progressive tissue damage, scarring and loss of function. Chronic inflammation includes:

  ○ mononuclear cell infiltrate (macrophages, lymphocytes, plasma cells)
  ○ tissue destruction
  ○ production of granulation tissue containing fibroblasts and small blood vessels
  ○ fibrosis

• *Systemic spread*. One function of inflammation is to contain the inflammatory trigger to a local site. If this fails the problem may spread to the rest of the body

Respiratory examples of these processes are given in Box 8.

Hypersensitivity

Hypersensitivity is a heightened or excessive immune response to an antigen, that is pathological and has clinical consequences.

Type I hypersensitivity ('immediate' or 'anaphylactic')

Respiratory diseases caused by type I hypersensitivity reactions include asthma and allergic rhinitis, where the reaction causes mucosal oedema, increased volume of secretions and smooth muscle contraction, leading to airflow obstruction.

Exposure to an external allergen, such as pollen, animal dander or house dust mite, triggers production of immunoglobulin E (IgE) which becomes bound to mast cells. Subsequent exposure to the allergen causes bound IgE on mast cell surfaces to form cross-links, which results in degranulation of mast cells and release of:

• Histamine
• Leukotrienes
• Prostaglandins

These inflammatory mediators:

• Increase capillary permeability, causing mucosal oedema
• Attract inflammatory cells, including eosinophils, neutrophils and macrophages
• Cause bronchoconstriction

An *early phase* reaction occurs within 5–10 min of allergen exposure. Influx of inflammatory cells mediates a *late phase* response, which is maximal 4–6 h later.

> ### Box 8 Respiratory examples of outcomes of acute inflammation
>
> **Resolution**
> • Acute rhinitis (viral cold) and bronchitis recover completely when infection resolves
> • Acute anaphylaxis or asthma recover completely on removal of allergen
>
> **Scarring**
> • Bronchiectasis can be caused by single episode of whooping cough, measles or pneumonia
> • Acute lung injury (e.g. caused by aspiration, inhalation of toxic gases/smoke, trauma) may resolve with scarring
>
> **Persistence**
> • Respiratory disease caused by chronic exposure to inflammatory triggers leading to progressive disease includes:
>   ○ COPD – caused by tobacco smoking
>   ○ chronic asthma – e.g. caused by chronic allergen exposure
>   ○ pulmonary fibrosis – e.g. caused by ongoing connective tissue disease, chronic drug use (e.g. amiodarone) or unknown trigger
>   ○ pleural thickening brought about by persistence of asbestos fibres in the lung
>
> **Systemic spread**
> Diseases that spread from the respiratory tract to the rest of the body include:
> • Infections such as pneumonia, which may be complicated by septicaemia
> • Primary pulmonary tuberculosis, which can spread by blood and lymphatics to any site in the body, including lymph nodes, bone and kidneys

Type III hypersensitivity ('immune complex')

Respiratory disease caused by type III hypersensitivity includes extrinsic allergic alveolitis, where the immune reaction causes alveolar oedema and impairs gas exchange.

Antigen exposure leads to production of free circulating IgG antibodies. On re-exposure the antigen binds to these IgG antibodies, forming immune complexes. These complexes can cause some mast cell degranulation and release of inflammatory mediators, although much less than in type I reactions. The complexes are also deposited in target tissues where they stimulate an acute inflammatory response, with complement activation, neutrophil infiltration and lysosymal enzyme release with tissue destruction.

Type III reactions come on over 4–12 h following antigen exposure. Susceptibility to type III reactions is determined in part by genetic factors and also may be altered by environmental factors such as infection or cigarette smoking in conjunction with antigen exposure.

Type IV hypersensitivity ('delayed')

Respiratory disease caused by type IV hypersensitivity includes pulmonary tuberculosis, where the immune reaction causes progressive tissue destruction. This reaction is mediated by antigen-specific T cells and antibodies are not involved. The antigen driving the reaction is picked up by an antigen-presenting cell such as a tissue dendritic cell.

The antigen-presenting cell binds to type I or II MHC. Patrolling T lymphocytes (CD4 helper or CD8 cytotoxic cells) find the antigen in this context and become activated, releasing cytokines and chemokines. This attracts inflammatory cells and an infiltrate comprising mainly T cells and macrophages develops. These infiltrates may develop into granulomas.

Other types of hypersensitivity (II, V and VI) have been described but are not major contributors to lung disease.

Infection

Infection occurs when an organism enters a host, replicates and causes damage to the host during the process. The respiratory system is particularly vulnerable to infection as it is exposed to large volumes of inspired air which may contain microorganisms. Respiratory infection can be caused by a vast array of viruses, bacteria and fungi, which can come from human, animal or environmental sources (Box 9).

Evasion of respiratory defences by infecting organisms

An organism must overcome a series of immune hurdles (Fig. 9) before it can infect the respiratory tract.

Mucociliary clearance

This process traps inhaled organisms and clears them out of the respiratory tract. Some organisms evade this defence by adhering to the underlying epithelium, for example using molecules called adhesins or ligands that

---

> **Box 9 Sources of respiratory infection**
>
> **Humans**
> Most respiratory infection is spread between humans. Most organisms in the respiratory tract cause infection in their host, then are replicated and passed on in respiratory droplets, e.g.
> - Common cold (over 100 different viruses)
> - Influenza
> - Tuberculosis
>
>   Some organisms are 'carried' in the upper respiratory tract, but do not cause infection until they are passed on to a susceptible individual or until their host's immune defences are weakened (e.g. *Staphylococcus aureus*)
>
> **Birds and animals**
> Some microorganisms primarily infect birds or animals, but can infect humans who come into close contact with infected creatures, e.g.
> - *Coxiella burnetti* (from cattle/sheep)
> - *Chlamydia psittaci* (from parrots)
> - Influenza (from birds)
>
> **Environment**
> Some organisms normally live in water, soil or other places in the environment, but can infect the respiratory tract when they are aerosolized (e.g. as water droplets, dust), e.g.
> - *Legionella pneumophila*
> - *Pseudomonas aeruginosa*
> - *Aspergillus fumigatus*

---

recognize and stick to receptors on host cell surfaces. *Pseudomonas aeruginosa* has alternative strategies to promote adherence. These bacteria produce alginate, a thick substance that clogs up the mucociliary escalator, and pyocyanin, a compound that disrupts the beating of cilia.

Epithelial barrier

Epithelial cells interspersed with tight junctions form an intact barrier that resists invasion of organisms. Once adherence has occurred, organisms either can invade epithelial cells or disrupt the epithelial barrier and pass between the cells.

Innate and adaptive immunity

Organisms have a range of strategies to evade innate and adaptive immune responses. For example, *Streptococcus pneumoniae* and *Haemophilus influenzae* surround themselves with a glycocalyx to inhibit phagocytosis. *Staphylococcus aureus* and *Streptococcus pneumoniae* secrete a molecule, leucocidin, that kills leucocytes and macrophages.

Clinical impact of respiratory infection
The clinical features of respiratory infection are determined by properties of the organism, the strength of the host immune response and the interaction between them.

Organism virulence
Virulence or pathogenicity of an organism refers to its ability to cause disease.

Highly virulent organisms are capable of causing infection in anyone, irrespective of the strength of the immune response. Respiratory examples include:
• Viruses causing the common cold, which cause infection in 95% of people if they come into contact with the respiratory tract
• *Streptococcus pneumoniae*, which causes pneumonia in healthy people with normal immune systems

Organisms with low virulence do not cause respiratory infection in healthy individuals. However, if the immune response becomes suppressed they may cause opportunistic infection. Organisms causing opportunistic respiratory infection include:
• *Pseudomonas aeruginosa*
• *Pneumocystis jirovecii*
• *Aspergillus fumigatus*
• *Mycobacterium tuberculosis* – TB infection is contained in a primary focus, but may reactivate to cause post-primary infection if the host becomes immunosuppressed in later life

Immunosuppression
Opportunistic respiratory infections occur in patients with disruption of any aspect of the respiratory immune system.
• Loss of cough reflex leads to aspiration and respiratory infection, particularly with anaerobic organisms, e.g.
  ○ neurological disease
  ○ loss of consciousness
• Impaired mucociliary clearance leads to infection with Gram-negative bacteria such as *Pseudomonas aeruginosa*, e.g.

  ○ damage to ciliated epithelium (e.g. bronchiectasis, COPD)
  ○ increased viscosity of airway surface liquid (e.g. cystic fibrosis)
• Disruption of the epithelial barrier allows infection with *Staphylococcus aureus* and Gram-negative bacteria such as coliforms and *Pseudomonas aeruginosa*, e.g.
  ○ *Staphylococcus aureus* pneumonia following epithelial damage from influenza
  ○ secondary to cigarette smoking
• Impaired innate or adaptive immune responses:
  ○ human immunodeficiency virus (HIV) infection causes generalized suppression of the adaptive immune response allowing opportunistic infection (e.g. with *M. tuberculosis* and *Pneumocystis jirovecii*)
  ○ patients at the extremes of age have immature or failing immune systems and are predisposed to respiratory infection, particularly pneumonia
  ○ development of diabetes mellitus can impair immunity, leading to reactivation of *M. tuberculosis* in infected patients and predisposing patients to other respiratory infections
  ○ immunosuppressive drugs (e.g. cytotoxic chemotherapy, disease-modifying drugs for arthritis, prednisolone) increase the risk of all respiratory infections, including fungal infections with *Aspergillus*

Excessive host immune response
The immune response to infection can directly cause disease. For example, the cell-mediated immune response to infection with *M. tuberculosis* (type IV hypersensitivity) causes granuloma formation and destruction of lung tissue.

Site of infection
The clinical features of respiratory infection are also determined by the site of infection in the respiratory tract (Fig. 10) and whether the infection remains localized in the lung or spreads elsewhere in the body. Examples of effects of respiratory infection beyond the respiratory tract include:
• Viral infection:
  ○ systemic response to infection (e.g. fatigue, lethargy, myalgia)
  ○ involvement of other organs (e.g. Epstein–Barr virus infection may involve the liver and spleen)

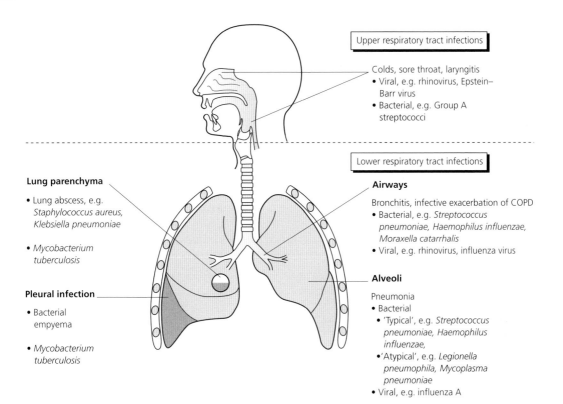

Upper respiratory tract infections

Colds, sore throat, laryngitis
- Viral, e.g. rhinovirus, Epstein–Barr virus
- Bacterial, e.g. Group A streptococci

Lower respiratory tract infections

Lung parenchyma
- Lung abscess, e.g. *Staphylococcus aureus, Klebsiella pneumoniae*
- *Mycobacterium tuberculosis*

Pleural infection
- Bacterial empyema
- *Mycobacterium tuberculosis*

Airways
Bronchitis, infective exacerbation of COPD
- Bacterial, e.g. *Streptococcus pneumoniae, Haemophilus influenzae, Moraxella catarrhalis*
- Viral, e.g. rhinovirus, influenza virus

Alveoli
Pneumonia
- Bacterial
  - 'Typical', e.g. *Streptococcus pneumoniae, Haemophilus influenzae,*
  - 'Atypical', e.g. *Legionella pneumophila, Mycoplasma pneumoniae*
- Viral, e.g. influenza A

Figure 10 Anatomy of respiratory infections.

- Bacterial infection:
  - bacteria may enter the blood stream (bacteraemia). If they cause adverse systemic effects including hypotension and multiorgan failure, this is called septicaemia
  - bacteria may spread from the lung to other tissues and organs where they cause infection. A good example is *M. tuberculosis* which spreads via blood and lymphatic system and causes infection elsewhere (e.g. in lymph nodes, bone and the kidney)

Neoplasia
Neoplasia or cancer is caused by a population of cells that become genetically altered so that they evade normal growth controls. Cancer cells:
- Grow and divide excessively
- Invade adjacent tissues and structures
- Spread to distant sites via blood and lymphatic systems
- Cause disease and death by destroying normal tissue and preventing normal function

Box 10 Carcinogens that increase the risk of respiratory cancers

- Tobacco smoke
- Marijuana and cocaine smoking
- Occupational carcinogens, including:
  - asbestos
  - arsenic
  - chromium
  - petroleum products and tar
- Environmental carcinogens
  - radon (gaseous decay product of uranium and radium that emits alpha particles, may accumulate in homes built above granite)

Genetic changes in cells that result in cancer may be caused by carcinogens (Box 10) or may be acquired randomly during cell division or by inheritance. Two main classes of genes are particularly important in the pathogenesis of cancer:

• *Oncogenes.* Genetic damage to normal genes (proto-oncogenes) activates oncogenes, increasing cell growth and division and altering differentiation. These new properties may allow cells to become cancerous

• *Tumour suppressor genes.* These genes are normally responsible for the control of cell division, DNA repair and programmed cell death. If they are damaged, loss of function can disrupt these processes, leading to cancer.

Cancers of the respiratory system are listed in Box 11. The sites of the primary cancers and their metastases determine the clinical features of the disease.

Box 11 Cancers of the respiratory system

• Nasopharyngeal carcinoma
• Mouth and tongue cancers
• Laryngeal carcinoma
• Bronchogenic carcinoma
• Bronchoalveolar cell carcinoma
• Mesothelioma

Approach to the patient

History

Most diagnoses are made from the patient's history and this should be taken carefully and thoroughly. At the start of the consultation you should always introduce yourself, giving your name and position, and ask for consent to take a history.

> **KEY POINT**
>
> Always introduce yourself and ask for consent for what you are going to do whenever working with patients.

Presenting complaint

The consultation should start with an open question to determine the presenting complaint. This question could be 'What is the main problem with your health at the moment?' or 'I understand that you are having problems with your chest, can you tell me about this in your own words.' You should then take a history of the presenting complaint to establish its cause and determine how it is affecting the patient's life.

Patients with respiratory disease most commonly present with breathlessness or cough.

Breathlessness

Breathlessness or shortness of breath describes the sensation of not being able to get enough air. The term dyspnoea means difficulty in breathing.

Breathlessness can be quantified using the Medical Research Council (MRC) dyspnoea score (Box 12). Repeat measurements are used to determine whether the patient is stable, improving or deteriorating.

An approach to taking a history from a patient presenting with breathlessness is shown in Fig. 11. The first step is to determine whether the breathlessness originates from respiratory, cardiac or other disease (Box 13). This allows the consultation to be structured towards a more specific differential diagnosis.

Respiratory and cardiac causes of breathlessness can be distinguished by asking about exacerbating factors, associated symptoms and risk factors.

Exacerbating factors
- Respiratory disease:
  - breathlessness caused by bronchospasm may be exacerbated by change in temperature, exercise or a smoky environment
- Cardiac disease:
  - breathlessness caused by pulmonary oedema is worse when lying down (orthopnoea)

Associated symptoms
- Respiratory disease:
  - pleuritic chest pain
  - cough
  - sputum
  - haemoptysis
  - wheeze
- Cardiac disease:
  - central chest pain/angina
  - palpitations
  - ankle oedema
  - other vascular disease (myocardial infarction, stroke, peripheral vascular disease)

Risk factors
- Respiratory disease:
  - smoking history, childhood illness, occupational exposure, home environment, family history, infectious contacts (see p. 19)
- Cardiac disease:
  - hypertension, diabetes, smoking, hypercholesterolaemia, obesity, lack of exercise, male gender, ethnic group, family history

Respiratory disease causing breathlessness
Once respiratory disease has been identified as the likely

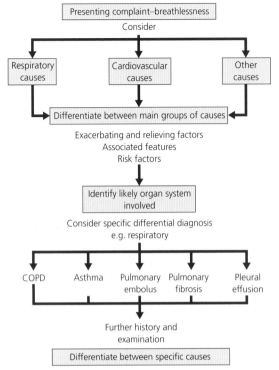

Figure 11 Mind map of a consultation with a breathless patient.

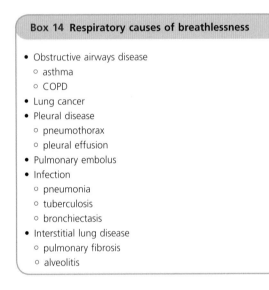

Box 13 Causes of breathlessness

- Respiratory, e.g.
  - obstructive airways disease, infection, cancer, pneumothorax, pleural effusion, thromboembolic disease, restrictive lung disease
- Cardiac, e.g.
  - Heart failure, arrhythmias, congenital heart disease
- Anaemia
- Renal failure
  - Kussmaul's respiration – acidosis
- Hyperthyroidism
- Deconditioning (lack of physical fitness)
- Anxiety

Box 14 Respiratory causes of breathlessness

- Obstructive airways disease
  - asthma
  - COPD
- Lung cancer
- Pleural disease
  - pneumothorax
  - pleural effusion
- Pulmonary embolus
- Infection
  - pneumonia
  - tuberculosis
  - bronchiectasis
- Interstitial lung disease
  - pulmonary fibrosis
  - alveolitis

Box 12 MRC dyspnoea score

1 Gets breathless with strenuous exercise
2 Gets short of breath when hurrying on the level or walking up a slight hill
3 Walks slower than people of the same age on the level because of breathlessness, or has to stop for breath when walking at own pace on the level
4 Stops for breath after walking about 100 yards or after a few minutes on the level
5 Too breathless to leave the house or breathless when dressing or undressing

cause of breathlessness, the next step is to construct a more specific differential diagnosis (Box 14). Demographic information, including age and gender (Box 15), may help to narrow down the differential diagnosis.

By this stage in the history-taking process you should be beginning to consider a differential diagnosis. Further enquiries as to the onset of breathlessness and respiratory risk factors may help you to narrow this down further.

Onset of breathlessness
- Sudden onset may indicate a sudden pathological process, e.g.
  - pulmonary embolus
  - pneumothorax
  - inhalation of a foreign body occluding an airway
- Onset over a few hours could indicate:
  - worsening inflammation in asthma
  - accumulation of fluid in the lungs in pulmonary oedema
- Onset over days or weeks could be caused by:
  - accumulation of pleural effusion

> **Box 15 Causes of breathlessness in different patient groups**
>
> **Age**
> *Older patients* are more likely to have degenerative or neoplastic disease, e.g.
> - Heart failure
> - COPD
> - Lung cancer
> - Anaemia (e.g. resulting from gastrointestinal bleeding)
>
> *Young adults* are less likely to present with breathlessness, but if they do it is often because of allergy, trauma or congenital abnormalities:
> - Asthma
> - Pneumothorax
> - Pulmonary embolus
> - Congenital heart disease
>
> **Gender**
> *Males* are more likely to:
> - Have a spontaneous pneumothorax
> - Smoke (although prevalence in women is increasing) and therefore develop COPD and lung cancer
> - Have heart disease at a younger age
>
> *Females* are more likely to:
> - Have connective tissue disease (e.g. rheumatoid arthritis, systemic lupus erythematosus)

> **Box 16 Calculation of pack year smoking history**
>
> Pack years smoked = (cigarettes per day smoked/20) × number of years smoked

○ growth of lung cancer with partial or complete airway occlusion
- Gradual onset over months or years could represent:
  ○ chronic obstructive pulmonary disease (COPD)
  ○ lung fibrosis
  ○ non-respiratory causes (e.g. anaemia, hyperthyroidism)

Risk factors for respiratory disease

A significant history of risk may point to a specific respiratory diagnosis. You should ask about:
- *Childhood respiratory illness:*
  ○ childhood infections such as whooping cough, measles or recurrent chest infections can cause bronchiectasis
  ○ asthma usually occurs first in childhood. Patients may 'grow out' of childhood symptoms only for asthma symptoms to recur many years later
- *Tobacco smoking.* Pack year smoking load should be calculated (Box 16). A 20-pack year history is widely accepted as significant risk for:

○ COPD
○ mouth, throat and lung cancer
- *Family history.* Diseases that run in families include:
  ○ asthma and atopy
  ○ emphysema (α_1-antitrypsin deficiency)
  ○ thromboembolic disease
- *Occupational and home environment:*
  ○ exposure to asbestos increases risk of lung fibrosis, pleural cancer (mesothelioma) and lung cancer
  ○ asthma can be provoked by dusty or damp accommodation or can be 'occupational' asthma (e.g. caused by exposure to flour in a bread-making factory)
- *Exposure to animals and birds:*
  ○ household pets (e.g. cats or dogs) may be a source of allergen (allergy-provoking factor) for asthma
  ○ regular contact with birds is a risk factor for extrinsic allergic alveolitis
- *Infectious contacts:*
  ○ a diagnosis of tuberculosis (TB) is much more likely if the patient has had contact with TB
- *Immunosuppression*
  ○ HIV, immunosuppressant drugs or diabetes mellitus can increase the risk of opportunistic lung infections

Effect of breathlessness on the patient's life

You should establish:
- The effect of breathlessness on activities of daily living (e.g. washing, dressing, cooking, eating)
- The available support network (e.g. family and carers)
- The patient's ability to take treatment

This information will help you decide on an investigation and treatment strategy with the patient and may also be used to initiate extra social support.

Cough

The British Thoracic Society defines cough as 'a forced expulsive manoeuvre, usually against a closed glottis and which is associated with a characteristic sound'. Cough has the important function of preventing foreign matter entering the lungs and is part of lung defence against infection (Box 17).

Box 17 The cough reflex

1 The cough reflex is initiated by stimulation of cough receptors in any of:
- upper and lower respiratory tract epithelium
- pericardium
- diaphragm
- oesophagus and stomach

2 An afferent impulse is sent from the receptors via the vagal nerve to the 'cough centre' in the medulla of the brain

3 The higher cortical centres are involved in the cough reflex, which to some extent is under voluntary control

4 Efferent fibres relay impulses to trigger:
- inhalation of around 2.5L air
- closure of the glottis and vocal cords
- forceful contraction of abdominal and intercostal muscles, generating a very high intrathoracic pressure
- sudden opening of the glottis and cords, allowing air to explode out of the lungs at speeds of up to 100 miles/h
- compression of the upper airways so that the air passes through slit-shaped airways

5 The rapidly moving air carries foreign matter out of the respiratory tract

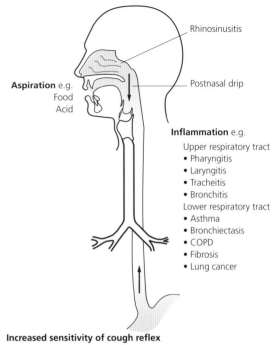

Increased sensitivity of cough reflex
Acid reflux stimulating vagal nerve

Figure 12 Causes of cough.

Taking a history from a patient with cough

The aims of history-taking are to establish the cause of the cough (Fig. 12) and the effect the cough is having on the patient's life.

Duration of the cough

The first step is to establish whether the cough is acute or chronic. British Thoracic Society definitions are:
- Acute cough:
  - <3 weeks
  - usually caused by viral infection
- Chronic cough:
  - >8 weeks
  - common causes are shown in Box 18

There is a grey area between 3 and 8 weeks where cough may be caused by recovering acute illness or developing chronic illness.

If the cough is chronic, the next step is to establish whether it is caused by pulmonary, nasal or oesophageal disease or drugs by asking about relevant associated features.

Pulmonary disease. Patients with lung disease may have associated symptoms of breathlessness or pleuritic chest

Box 18 Common causes of chronic cough

Pulmonary
- Asthma
- Smoking
- Any pulmonary disease

Nasal
- Rhinitis/sinusitis with postnasal drip

Oesophageal
- Gastro-oesophageal reflux

Drugs
- ACE inhibitors

pain. Sputum production, especially if purulent or blood-stained, points to a pulmonary cause.

Nasal or sinus disease. Patients with cough should be asked about symptoms of nasal (rhinitis) and sinus (sinusitis) inflammation, which may cause or merely be associated with a chronic cough. Symptoms of rhinitis include nasal blockage, sneezing and runny nose (rhinorrhoea). Sinus symptoms may include pain in the face and teeth or headaches. Patients may feel catarrh or slime running down the back of their throat (postnasal drip) and there may be a small amount of clear or purulent sputum. Rising from bed or other changes in head position may trigger cough by causing sinus drainage and increased postnasal drip.

Gastro-oesophageal reflux. If a cough is caused by reflux it may occur at times when the lower oesophageal sphincter is open, including after a meal or when talking or singing. Patients may have symptoms of choking during meals or of heartburn and acid or food refluxing into their mouths.

Other causes. It is essential to take a full drug history and ask about smoking habits.

Cough caused by lung disease

If the initial history indicates that the patient has lung disease as the cause of their cough, a detailed history establishing characteristics of the cough may point to a specific diagnosis.

Character of the cough
• A normal cough is explosive and percussive in character (Box 17)
• A whooping sound is usually caused by *Bordetella pertussis* infection (whooping cough)
• A bovine cough, which is breathy and has lost the percussive explosive character of a normal cough, is heard in patients with vocal cord paralysis. This may be caused by a lung cancer or enlarged lymph nodes impinging on the recurrent laryngeal nerves
• A wheezy cough may indicate turbulent airflow through narrowed airways as in the bronchoconstriction of asthma or COPD

Timing
The timing of when the cough occurs may be a clue to the underlying diagnosis:
• Nocturnal cough. This is classically caused by asthma which is worse at night. A cough occurring on lying flat may be also caused by pulmonary oedema or gastro-oesophageal reflux
• Seasonal cough in spring and summer may be caused by atopic asthma provoked by pollen. Cough occurring during the winter months may be caused by COPD or

chronic bronchitis, exacerbated by seasonal respiratory tract infections
• Cough on eating or drinking may indicate an inadequate swallow with aspiration of food into the respiratory tract (e.g. following a stroke)
• Cough on contact with allergens (e.g. household pets) indicates asthma
• Cough after exercise is usually indicative of asthma

Sputum
• A 'dry' cough indicates a lack of sputum production (e.g. seen in pulmonary fibrosis and as a side-effect of angiotensin-converting enzyme [ACE] inhibitors)
• A 'fruity' or 'rattly' cough indicates secretions which may or may not be coughed up (expectorated). Production of sputum usually indicates an infective or inflammatory process
If the cough is productive of sputum, further questions should be asked about sputum colour, consistency and volume:
• Colour:
  ○ clear or white phlegm (mucoid or mucus-like) is common in patients with COPD whose airways are chronically inflamed but not infected
  ○ yellow or green sputum (purulent) is caused by the presence of neutrophils or eosinophils which release myeloperoxidase, an enzyme that is green. Purulent sputum usually indicates infection, but may also be seen in uninfected patients with asthma caused by eosinophils
• Consistency:
  ○ firm plugs of sputum may be coughed up by patients with exacerbations of asthma
• Volume:
  ○ the daily volume of sputum expectorated can easily be quantified by the patient in terms of household measurements (e.g. teaspoonful/tablespoonful/teacupful)
  ○ expectoration of large daily volumes of sputum is characteristic of bronchiectasis
  ○ a cough productive of sputum on most days over at least a 3-month period for 2 or more consecutive years in a patient without other explanations for a cough may be termed 'chronic bronchitis'. Chronic bronchitis is usually seen in people who smoke and is part of COPD

Haemoptysis
Blood coughed up from the lungs (haemoptysis) can vary in amount from small streaks of blood to massive bleeding and should ring alarm bells as:

> ### Box 19 Causes of haemoptysis
>
> **Common and/or potentially life-threatening**
> - Lung cancer
> - Tuberculosis
> - Pulmonary embolus
> - Pneumonia
> - Bronchiectasis
> - Heart failure (sputum usually pink)
>   *Massive haemoptysis* may occur because of erosion of an airway blood vessel in patients with:
> - Bronchiectasis
> - Mycetoma (fungal ball)
>
> **Less common**
> - Idiopathic pulmonary haemosiderosis
> - Goodpasture's syndrome
> - Trauma
> - Blood disorders
> - Benign lung tumours

- Haemoptysis may indicate an underlying lung tumour or other life-threatening diagnosis (Box 19)
- The haemoptysis itself may be life-threatening:
  ○ large amounts of blood in the airway may asphyxiate the patient
  ○ torrential haemoptysis may cause hypovolaemia and shock

Haemoptysis should always be thoroughly investigated to identify or exclude serious underlying disease.

> ### !RED FLAG
>
> - A serious cause underlying a cough should particularly be considered in patients who have:
>   ○ haemoptysis
>   ○ weight loss
>   ○ night sweats
> - Patients with these symptoms require full investigation

Other associated features

- Sore throat and nasal congestion may indicate an upper respiratory tract infection
- Fevers are more indicative of a lower respiratory tract infection. Rigors and sweats may indicate pneumonia, whereas persistent night sweats may indicate TB
- Weight loss is a worrying or 'red flag' symptom and may be associated with:
  ○ malignancy
  ○ TB
  ○ other severe infection or lung abscess
- Wheezing occurs in asthma, COPD and other causes of airway obstruction
- Chest pain:
  ○ pleuritic pain (sharp, localized and worse on deep inspiration and coughing) is most commonly caused by pneumonia, pneumothorax, pulmonary embolus or viral pleurisy
  ○ pain occurring following vigorous coughing may be secondary to muscle strain or a fractured rib

Examination
Preparation
You should obtain informed consent before starting the examination and ensure that you consider the patient's wishes, comfort and feelings at all times. Examination of the respiratory system ideally requires positioning of the patient in the centre of a bed or couch, sitting up with their upper body at an angle of 45° to their legs. The chest should be exposed before examination and a blanket used to maintain patient dignity until it is time to examine the chest directly. Male doctors or students should consider use of an escort when examining female patients.

Routine
A thorough and professional respiratory examination is best carried out methodically in the following order.
- General inspection from the end of the bed
- Hands and arms
- Face
- Neck
- Chest front
- Chest back
- Lower limbs

At the end of the examination the findings should be presented in the same order so nothing is forgotten. This routine is outlined as an Objective Structured Clinical Examination (OSCE) checklist in Box 20.

General observation
General observations should initially be made from the end of the bed. In an exam situation this should take around 30 s and is valuable time that can be used to take a few deep breaths and look for diagnostic clues.

Around the patient
If available you should look at:

Box 20 OSCE checklist for respiratory examination (10 min station)

Preliminary

Introduces self (name and role)	1 mark
Explains procedure to patient	1 mark
Obtains consent to proceed	1 mark
Cleans hands	1 mark
Checks patient is at 45° angle and is comfortable	1 mark

General examination

Observes patient from end of bed	1 mark
Measures respiratory rate correctly	1 mark
Comments correctly on:	
Presence/absence of respiratory equipment around bed	1 mark
Use/no use of accessory muscles	1 mark
Shape of chest wall	1 mark
Presence or absence of thoracic scars	1 mark
Presence or absence of intercostal indrawing	1 mark

Hands

Examines patient correctly for presence or absence of:	
Nicotine staining	1 mark
Finger clubbing	1 mark
Cyanosis	1 mark
Asterixis	1 mark
Comments that would like to take the blood pressure	1 mark
Checks eyes for pallor	1 mark
Comments correctly on presence or absence of central cyanosis	1 mark

Checks JVP correctly	1 mark
Examines the neck for lymph nodes	1 mark
Determines the position of the trachea	1 mark
Correctly measures the cricosternal distance	1 mark
Comments on presence or absence of tracheal tug	1 mark

Chest

Checks expansion of upper and lower lung zones using correct technique	2 marks
Checks expansion front and back	1 mark
Comments appropriately on findings	1 mark
Percusses over both clavicles (0 if fails to warn patient)	1 mark
Percusses front and back of chest using correct technique	1 mark
Compares percussion note on right and left sides at each level	1 mark
Percusses over lateral chest bilaterally	1 mark
Comments appropriately on findings	1 mark
Auscultates over apices and lateral chest	2 marks
Over front and back of chest compares sides	2 marks
Comments correctly on findings	1 mark
Checks for vocal resonance or fremitus	1 mark
Comments correctly on findings	1 mark
Summarizes examination findings correctly	2 marks
Suggests a differential diagnosis	2 marks
Total	**44 marks**

- Sputum (in bedside pot) to determine amount produced and colour
- Medication (e.g. inhalers, nebulizers or oxygen)
- Other equipment and devices (e.g. intravenous cannula, urinary catheter, peak flow meter)

Patient affect

You should determine whether the patient is:
- Alert, drowsy, confused or cooperative
- In any pain

Breathing

- Measure the respiratory rate:
  - count the number of breaths taken over 15 s and multiply by 4 to arrive at respirations per minute. This is often best done when taking the patient's pulse, as respiratory rate is under voluntary control and

may change if the patient is conscious that you are counting
  - comment on whether this is normal (normal range 12–16 breaths/min)
- Look for difficulty in breathing or use of accessory muscles. This may be seen as contraction and prominence of the sternocleidomastoid muscles
- Describe the breathing pattern. Abnormalities include:
  - Kussmaul's respiration – deep sighing breaths seen in metabolic acidosis
  - Cheyne–Stokes respiration – alternate deep rapid breaths and shallow slow breaths with periods of apnoea occurring in cycles. This is caused by damage to the respiratory centre in the brainstem (e.g. caused by stroke or poor cardiac output in heart failure). It is enhanced by narcotic use

Chest wall
- Look for deformities including:
  ○ barrel-shaped chest (increased anteroposterior diameter) – caused by chronic hyperinflation in COPD patients
  ○ kyphosis and scoliosis (increased forward and lateral spinal curvature, respectively) – can impair chest wall movement and cause type II respiratory failure
  ○ funnel-shaped chest (*pectus excavatum*) – may be congenital
  ○ pigeon chest (*pectus carinatum*) – may occur if the patient had rickets as a child
- Look for unilateral thoracotomy scars indicating previous lung or heart surgery
- Look for intercostal indrawing – the muscle between the ribs is sucked inward as the patient breathes in. This is seen in patients with severe COPD

Breath sounds
- Listen for stridor. This is an inspiratory and/or expiratory sound caused by partial obstruction of the upper respiratory tract (e.g. caused by foreign body, tumour, oedema, laryngospasm or external compression)
- It is a medical emergency if the airway is compromised

Hands and arms
During respiratory examination four main signs should be looked for in the hands and arms, as follow.

Nicotine staining
Indicates ongoing cigarette smoking.

Finger clubbing (Fig. 13)
Finger clubbing is swelling of the soft tissue of the terminal phalanx. Characteristic features include:
- Loss of nail angle
- Increased bogginess of the nail bed
- Increased side-to-side and lengthwise curvature of the nail
- A drumstick appearance – where the distal ends of the fingers have a greater diameter than the proximal parts of the digits

Respiratory diseases causing finger clubbing are given in Box 21. These conditions appear to cause clubbing by triggering increased blood flow to the fingertips, causing oedema followed by expansion of the connective tissue. Clubbing may also be caused by cardiac and gastrointestinal disease, may be idiopathic or may run in families.

> **Box 21 Respiratory diseases causing finger clubbing**
>
> - Pulmonary fibrosis
> - Chronic pulmonary infection
>   ○ bronchiectasis, cystic fibrosis
>   ○ empyema
>   ○ lung abscess
>   ○ tuberculosis
> - Cancer
>   ○ bronchogenic carcinoma
>   ○ mesothelioma
>   ○ pulmonary metastases

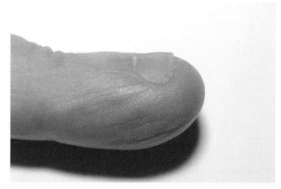

(a)

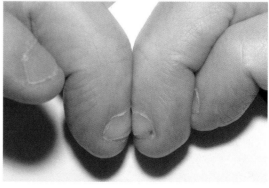

(b)

Figure 13 Finger clubbing. (a) Loss of nail angle characteristic of finger clubbing. (b) Shamroth's sign. When two nails are put back to back as shown you can normally see a diamond of daylight between them. In this picture the patient has finger clubbing so there is increased tissue in the nail bed with loss of angle and the diamond is lost.

Evidence of hypoxia

A blue discoloration of the nails (cyanosis) may be seen and is caused by increased deoxygenated haemoglobin in the blood in the fingers. It may be a result of central or peripheral causes.

Evidence of carbon dioxide retention

• *Asterixis.* This is looked for by asking the patient to extend their arms and hyperextend both hands at the wrist in a policeman 'stop' position. If CO_2 retention is present there may be a coarse low-frequency flapping tremor. This asterixis is caused by cerebral toxicity and may also be seen in patients with uraemia or hepatic encephalopathy. You should ask the patient to keep their hands in this position for 1 min to ensure asterixis is absent
• A bounding radial pulse and warm hands may indicate vasodilatation secondary to CO_2 retention

On the way up to the head, the upper arm should remind you to either take the blood pressure or in an exam to comment that you would like to take it.

Face
Eyes
Check for pallor of the conjunctivae, as an indication of anaemia as a cause of breathlessness.

Mouth
Ask the patient to touch the tip of their tongue to the roof of their mouth and look for cyanosis on the under surface of the tongue. Cyanosis indicates a mean capillary concentration of deoxygenated haemoglobin of around 5 g/dL.
• *Central cyanosis* occurs when the blood in the systemic circulation is not oxygenated completely because of cardiac or respiratory failure. Both the under surface of the tongue *and* the fingers will appear blue
• *Peripheral cyanosis* occurs when blood flow in the peripheries (fingers, toes, lips) is slow, allowing more oxygen than usual to be extracted from the peripheral blood. This can occur because of vasoconstriction on a cold day or because of vascular disease such as Raynaud's syndrome. Only the fingers will appear blue and the under surface of the tongue will be pink

Neck
Jugular venous pressure
Make sure that the patient is sitting with their upper body at a 45° angle. Ask them to rest their head back on the pillow to relax the neck muscles and turn their head to the left. Look for a pulsation along the course of the right internal jugular vein from between the sternal and clavicular heads of the right sternocleidomastoid up behind the angle of the jaw to the earlobe.

If a pulsation is seen, it is venous in origin if:
• The pulsation has two visible impulses per heart beat
• It is not palpable
• It is obliterated by compression of the vein below the pulse with a finger
• Pressure on the abdomen causes the pulsation to rise in the neck

Then estimate the level of the jugular venous pressure (JVP) by measuring the vertical height of the pulse (in cm) above the sternal angle.
• A raised JVP (>3 cm) may indicate right heart failure, which can be secondary to pulmonary disease (cor pulmonale)
• Engorged non-pulsating neck veins may indicate superior vena caval obstruction (e.g. caused by intrathoracic tumour or lymph node compression). This is usually accompanied by oedema of the head and neck

Lymphadenopathy
Cervical lymph nodes are most easily felt with the patient sitting forward and are usually palpated when the back of the chest is examined. Submental, submandibular, parotid, mastoid, occipital, anterior and posterior triangle node groups and supraclavicular nodes should be palpated. If enlarged lymph nodes are detected in the neck, nodes in the axillae and groins should also be palpated.

Trachea
• *Position.* Place your index and ring fingers on the clavicular heads and push your middle finger forward to feel the dome of the trachea. This should be immediately in front of your finger. Deviation to either side indicates displacement of the mediastinum (e.g. pulled towards pulmonary collapse or pushed away by tension pneumothorax or large pleural effusion)
• *Tug.* Ask the patient to take a deep breath in while palpating the trachea. A tracheal tug occurs if the trachea is felt to move downwards on inspiration. This is a sign of severe COPD, but its cause is unclear. It may be caused by downward displacement of the mediastinum because of high intrathoracic pressures generated during inspiration or by upwards movement of a barrel-shaped chest

• *Cricosternal distance.* You should be able to fit three fingers between the cricoid cartilage (Box 1) and the notch at the top of the sternum. A reduction of this 'cricosternal distance' indicates hyperinflation of the lungs

Chest

The front of the chest should be examined using the following routine, which should then be repeated at the back of the chest with the patient sitting forward.

Expansion

Expansion of the upper zones of the lungs (Fig. 14a) is assessed by placing your hands in the patient's axillae, bringing your thumbs together and asking the patient to breathe in. The degree of expansion is assessed by observing how far your thumbs are separated on inspiration. This manoeuvre should be repeated for the lower zones

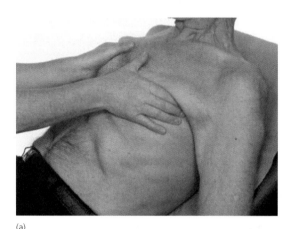

(a)

(b)

Figure 14 Examination of lung expansion. (a) Upper chest. (b) Lower chest.

of the lung (Fig. 14.b) and at the back of the chest. You should look for:
• Symmetry – do both lungs expand the same amount?
• Amount of expansion – is there any reduction in expansion?

Percussion

You should check the percussion note of upper, mid and lower lung zones systematically, comparing right and left sides. Percuss the apices by tapping the clavicles directly (Fig. 15a), but warn the patient before you do this that it may be slightly uncomfortable. Then percuss downwards through the zones (Fig. 15b), making sure that you compare the note on left and right sides at each level. Also percuss laterally over the lungs (Fig. 15c). Repeat percussion at the back of the chest. You should look for:
• Symmetry – is the percussion note the same on each side at all sites?
• Altered percussion note – is there dullness or hyper-resonance?

Auscultation

Ask the patient to take deep breaths in and out through their mouth and listen to the breath sounds over the lung apices with the bell of the stethoscope (used as it fits into the supraclavicular area better than the diaphragm). Then change to the diaphragm of the stethoscope and auscultate all zones of the lungs. Once again compare sides at each level and end laterally. Check the front and back of the chest. You should listen for:
• Breath sounds – are they present, reduced or absent?
• Characteristics of breath sounds:
   ○ vesicular breath sounds (normal) are heard longer on inspiration than expiration and there is a short quiet gap between them
   ○ bronchial breathing. These breath sounds are harsher. Inspiration and expiration are more equal in length and there is no gap between them
• Added sounds?
   ○ wheeze is caused by airflow obstruction
   ○ coarse crackles or crepitations are caused by secretions in large airways
   ○ fine inspiratory crepitations (like rustling a crisp packet) are caused by fluid or fibrosis in or around the alveoli

Vocal resonance

Ask the patient to say '99' repeatedly and listen to the sound this makes transmitted from the larynx to the chest wall. You should listen over the upper, mid and lower zones of the chest, front and back for:

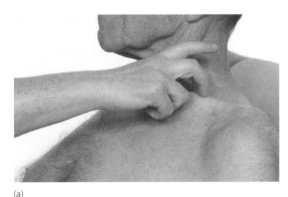

(a)

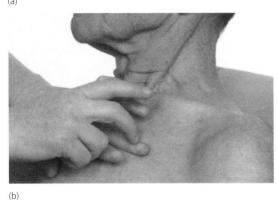

(b)

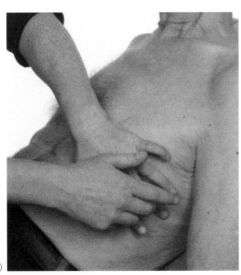

(c)

Figure 15 Percussion of the chest. (a) Lung apices. (b) Front of chest. (c) Lateral chest wall.

• Increased resonance – caused by fluid within the alveolar spaces (e.g. pus from pneumonia) which increases transmission of sound from the larynx
• Decreased resonance – caused by fluid or air in the pleural space (effusion or pneumothorax) which muffles transmission of sound from the larynx

Alternatively, transmission of sound can be sensed by touching your hand against the chest wall (vocal fremitus). It is not usually necessary to perform both vocal resonance and fremitus and you should choose which one you do depending on how easily you are able to detect abnormalities with each technique.

Legs

To complete respiratory examination you should check for

• Peripheral oedema, which may indicate right heart failure secondary to lung disease
• Unilateral leg swelling, which may indicate a deep vein thrombosis

Inspect the legs visually. Check for pitting oedema by pressing over the leg, removing your finger and looking for a dent. Pitting oedema may be immediately obvious, but can only be excluded if pressure is applied over the leg in one place for 1 min without causing denting.

On completion of the examination, thank the patient and help them back into their clothing if necessary.

Interpretation of examination findings

Once you have completed your examination decide whether the findings are symmetrical, affecting both lungs equally, or asymmetrical, affecting one lung more than the other (Tables 1 & 2).

Putting it all together

Some aims of taking a history and performing an examination are to:

• Make a provisional diagnosis
• Determine an investigation strategy
• Develop a treatment plan
• Form a therapeutic relationship with the patient
• Ascertain the patient's wishes regarding treatment
• Find out about social circumstances and comorbidities that may determine response to treatment
• Involve next of kin or other family and friends as necessary
• Establish the disease prognosis

Once the history and examination findings have been recorded, this information should be analysed and the deliberations documented as:

• *Differential diagnosis.* In straightforward cases a single diagnosis or a few possible diagnoses (differential diagnosis) may be apparent from the history and examination. This should be written in the notes under this heading

Table 1 Examination findings for diseases affecting both lungs.

	Asthma	COPD	Pulmonary fibrosis	Pulmonary oedema
Trachea	Central	Central Reduced cricosternal distance Tracheal tug	Central	Central
Expansion	Reduced bilaterally	Reduced bilaterally	Reduced bilaterally	Normal or reduced
Percussion	Normal	Normal	Normal	Normal unless associated effusions
Auscultation	Bilateral expiratory wheeze	Reduced air entry May be bilateral expiratory wheeze	Bibasal fine inspiratory crepitations. Fixed, do not clear on coughing	Bilateral inspiratory crepitations, may clear on coughing
Vocal resonance	Normal	Normal	Normal	Normal
Other features		Nicotine-stained fingers, intercostal indrawing, use of accessory muscles	Finger clubbing, associated connective tissue disease	Peripheral oedema, hepatomegaly if right heart failure

Table 2 Examination findings for diseases affecting one lung more than the other.

	Consolidation (pneumonia)	Collapse, e.g. tumour obstructing bronchus	Pleural effusion	Pneumothorax
Trachea	Not displaced	Displaced *towards* affected side	Small – not displaced Large – displaced *away from* affected side	Normal – not displaced Tension – displaced *away from* affected side
Expansion	Reduced on affected side	Reduced on affected side	Reduced on affected side	Reduced on affected side
Percussion	Dull on affected side	Dull on affected side	Stony dull on affected side	Hyper-resonant on affected side
Auscultation	Bronchial breathing Crackles	Reduced or absent air entry	Reduced or absent air entry	Reduced or absent air entry
Vocal resonance	Increased	Reduced	Reduced or absent	Reduced or absent
Associated features	Green/blood-stained/ rusty sputum, pyrexia	Associated features of malignancy, cachexia		

• *Problem list.* In more complicated patients (e.g. those with multiple illnesses and difficult social circumstances) there may not be a single diagnosis and a problem list should be written. This should include the new presenting problem, comorbidities and social complications. It can be helpful to document the patient's problems under this heading system by system so that no problems are missed out

Follow-up

Patients are often booked to return after a consultation or told to come back if they remain unwell. The primary purpose of follow-up is to review investigation results and ascertain response to treatment. In this situation it is helpful to record your thoughts as an 'Assessment', which both records the likely diagnosis and comments on change (e.g. whether the patient has improved or deteriorated). This is followed in the notes by a plan, detailing further investigations or treatment required.

> **KEY POINT**
>
> The focal point of patient notes should be the differential diagnosis, problem list or assessment. This directs patient care and helps communication between health professionals and with patients.

Investigations

Most diagnoses are made by taking a careful history, backed up by thorough examination. Roles of investigation therefore include:

- Confirmation of the clinical diagnosis
- Exclusion of possible differential diagnoses
- Identification of additional diagnoses (comorbidities) or unexpected diagnoses
- Assessment of fitness for treatment
- Monitoring of treatment response and adverse effects

All investigations have some potential to cause harm. Therefore, the decision to perform a test is made by weighing up the benefits and risks of the test and discussing these with the patient to ascertain their wishes. Excessive investigation should be avoided as this will delay investigations for other patients and waste resources that could have been used elsewhere for patient care.

Approach to investigation

It is usual practice to perform low-risk non-invasive tests first, then to use the results of these to direct further investigations as necessary.

Initial investigation

In patients with possible respiratory disease initial investigation usually includes:

- Chest radiograph (X-ray) to look for structural lung disease
- Peak flow recording and/or spirometry to look for airflow obstruction
- Oxygen saturations to assess gas exchange
- Blood tests (venous) including:

  ○ haemoglobin to look for anaemia
  ○ C-reactive protein (CRP) and white cell count to look for infection or inflammation
  ○ eosinophil count to look for allergy

Other investigations that may be useful at this stage include:

- electrocardiogram (ECG) to look for right heart abnormalities secondary to lung disease or an alternative cardiac diagnosis to explain symptoms
- Urea and electrolytes (U&E), bicarbonate, thyroid function tests, glucose to look for alternative causes of breathlessness
- Arterial blood gases to assess oxygenation, CO_2 excretion and pH

Chest X-ray

Procedure. A chest X-ray is normally performed with the patient standing and facing away from the X-ray tube, with breath held in deep inspiration. The X-ray beam thus passes through the patient's back (posterior) first, before passing through their front (anterior) to reach the recording plate. This 'PA' film is ideal because:

- A PA film does not exaggerate heart size
- Standing and full inspiration make sure the lungs are fully expanded and make abnormalities easier to detect

If a patient is unwell they may have their X-ray sitting or lying with the plate at their back and the beam passing from front to back. This is called an AP film and exaggerates the heart size.

Risk. The patient receives a radiation dose of 0.1 mSv, equivalent to 10 days of background radiation. In theory, any radiation dose carries a slight increased risk of cancer, but the risk from a chest X-ray is negligible.

Interpretation
- *Routine.* You should report chest X-rays using a set routine so that nothing is missed. This routine is outlined as an OSCE checklist in Box 22
- *Quality of X-ray.* You should comment on whether the film is:
  ○ PA or AP. If it is AP you should mention that it will be difficult to interpret heart size
  ○ the correct way round. The left/right marker should be on correct side. The correct position of the left marker is shown in Fig. 16
  ○ rotated. The ends of the clavicles (indicated as 'A' in Fig. 16) should be equal distances from the spinous

> **Box 22 Example OSCE checklist for chest X-ray interpretation**
>
> **Checks origin and quality of X-ray**
>
> | | |
> |---|---|
> | Checks patient's name | 1 mark |
> | Checks date of X-ray | 1 mark |
> | Checks side marker | 1 mark |
> | Checks whether PA/AP | 1 mark |
> | Checks rotation | 1 mark |
> | | |
> | Comments on (1 mark) and correctly describes (1 mark) major abnormality | 2 marks |
>
> **Correctly comments on**
>
> | | |
> |---|---|
> | Tracheal position | 1 mark |
> | Left heart border | 1 mark |
> | Right heart border | 1 mark |
> | Heart size | 1 mark |
> | Lung hila | 1 mark |
> | Right lung field | 1 mark |
> | Left lung field | 1 mark |
> | Height of diaphragms | 1 mark |
> | Clarity of diaphragms | 1 mark |
> | Costophrenic and cardiophrenic angles | 2 marks for both |
> | Adequate inspiratory effort/hyperinflated | 1 mark |
> | Breast shadows | 1 mark |
> | Bones | 1 mark |
>
> **Summary**
>
> | | |
> |---|---|
> | Correctly identifies abnormalities | 2 marks |
> | Suggests differential diagnosis | 2 marks |
> | **Total** | **25 marks** |

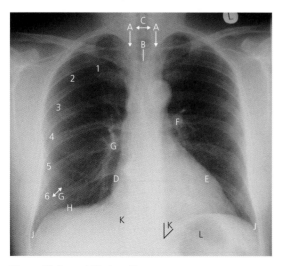

Figure 16 Normal PA chest X-ray.

processes (B). If they are not the film is rotated, which will distort the appearance of thoracic structures

• *Features of a normal chest X-ray* (Fig. 16). The appearance of a structure on a chest X-ray depends on its density and the extent to which it allows passage of X-rays. The least dense substance is air, which does not absorb X-rays and appears black on the X-ray. The densest substance is calcium, which absorbs X-rays well and appears white on the X-ray. In between are fat, which appears dark grey, and water, which appears light grey. Appearance of individual structures is also determined by their thickness, shape and relationship to adjacent structures (letters in brackets refer to Fig. 16):

○ the trachea contains air and appears black. It should be central and not deviated to left or right (C)

○ the heart contains tissue and fluid and appears very light grey. Its diameter should be less than half that of the total cardiothoracic diameter on a PA film. The heart borders (D, E) should be clearly outlined by the air in the adjacent lungs. Fuzziness may indicate fluid in the airspaces in adjacent lung

○ the left lung hilum (F) should be higher than the right hilum (G). The hila normally contain pulmonary vessels, main airways, lymphatics and nodes. Lymphadenopathy or pulmonary arterial hypertension may cause hilar enlargement

○ the lung fields should appear black and clearly delineated by adjacent structures. Lung markings comprising vessels (seen as small white streaks) should be seen extending all the way out to the chest wall

○ the right diaphragm should be higher than the left as it is pushed up by the liver. The top of the right diaphragm should be in the 5th intercostal space (G) anteriorly in the midclavicular line (H). Up to six ribs should be seen anteriorly above the diaphragm (numbered). More than this indicates lung hyperinflation

○ the costophrenic angles (J) between the rib cage and diaphragm, and the cardiophrenic angles (K), between the heart and the diaphragm, should be sharp. Blunting may indicate the presence of fluid (effusion) or fat

○ it is also helpful to look under the diaphragms at the gastric air bubble (L). Free gas under the domes of the diaphragm may indicate perforation of abdominal viscera

○ breast shadows should be present in female patients

◦ you should also look for abnormalities in the bones such as rib fractures (a break in the straight border of the rib) or black areas that might indicate metastases

The normal features of the chest X-ray should be kept in mind when looking at abnormal X-rays with the cases throughout the book.

Basic lung function

Peak expiratory flow rate recording

Procedure. Peak expiratory flow rate (PEFR) can be measured in most situations using a peak flow meter (Fig. 17). The patient stands or sits upright and inhales as deeply as possible. They then seal their lips around the disposable mouthpiece and make a short sharp expiration, as though attempting to 'blow out a candle'. The marker on the meter is displaced by the expiration and the distance achieved along the scale is noted and relates to a flow rate in litres per minute. This is carried out three times and the greatest flow rate noted (Box 23, p. 35).

Risk. There is a risk of cross-infection which can be countered by giving patients individual peak flow meters or by using disposable mouthpieces and cleaning the equipment between patients.

Interpretation. As flow through a tube is proportional to the radius of the tube to the power of 4 (flow $\propto r^4$), peak flow rate gives a crude estimate of airway calibre. Interpretation requires comparison of this with either the patient's known best values or with predicted values from normal range charts depending on gender, age and height. Peak flow can then be expressed as an absolute value in litres per minute and as a percentage of predicted or best. Reduction in peak flow indicates airflow obstruction resulting from asthma or COPD. The main use of peak flow recording is as serial measurements to look for or monitor variable airflow obstruction in asthma. It is not usually used to monitor COPD.

Spirometry

Procedure. To perform spirometry the patient is asked to stand or sit upright, to take a deep breath in and to blow out into the spirometer for as hard and as long as they can (up to 12 s). This differs from peak flow recording where a short sharp blow is required. The forced manoeuvre is used to standardize patient effort and flow of air out of the lungs.

Spirometry is recorded as a plot of volume of air blown out of the lungs in litres (y axis) over a period of time in seconds (x axis; Fig. 18). The slope of the line indicates flow (liters per second). Three measurements are derived from the spirometry curve:

- FEV_1 – forced expiratory volume in 1 s
- FVC – forced vital capacity, the total volume of air that is forcibly exhaled

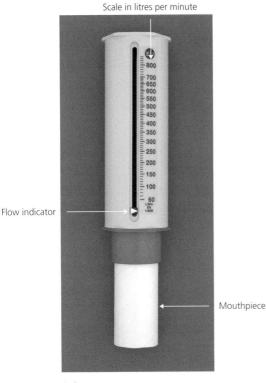

Scale in litres per minute

Flow indicator

Mouthpiece

Figure 17 Peak flow meter.

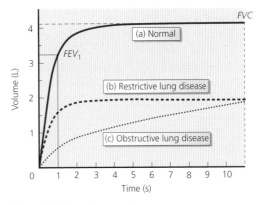

Figure 18 Spirometry recording.

- FEV_1/FVC ratio – this gives some measure of slope of the line and indicates whether there is airflow obstruction

Risk. There is a risk of cross-infection between patients with respiratory disease which can be countered by using disposable mouthpieces and regular cleaning of equipment. Patients may find this procedure makes them cough or feel breathless.

Interpretation. Normal lung function varies between individuals depending on age, gender and height. Standard tables are available to predict an individual's FEV_1 and FVC from these values. Values are normal if they are 80–120% of the predicted value. FEV_1 is also expressed as a percentage of FVC. If the airways are normal, then at least 70% of the total air in the lungs should have been blown out in the first second (i.e. FEV_1 should be ≥70% of FVC) (Fig. 18a).

FEV_1 and FVC can be reduced both by obstructive lung disease (e.g. asthma, COPD) and restrictive lung disease (e.g. lung fibrosis, sarcoidosis). An important difference between these groups of conditions is that obstructive lung disease reduces airflow, whereas restrictive lung disease does not affect the airways. The ratio of FEV_1/FVC can be used to determine airflow and distinguish between obstructive and restrictive lung disease:
- In obstructive lung disease, the proportion of the air in the lungs that can leave in 1 s is reduced, hence there is flattening of the slope of the spirometric curve and FEV_1 is <70% of FVC (Fig. 18c)
- In restrictive lung disease, the proportion of air in the lungs that can leave in 1 s is normal, the slope of the line is normal and FEV_1 is ≥70% of FVC (Fig. 18b)

Arterial blood gases

Procedure. Arterial blood is usually sampled from the radial or brachial artery into a heparinized syringe, to prevent blood clotting after sampling. The needle is inserted vertically through the arterial wall and the pressure of blood in the vessel forces blood into the syringe. The procedure can be painful and local anaesthesia can be used. However, this may obscure landmarks and make sampling more difficult. Once arterial blood has been obtained, blood gas analysis should be performed immediately or the sample should be kept on ice until tested to avoid changes in partial pressure of gases in the sample.

Risk. The main risks are of occlusion of the artery caused by spasm of the vessel wall or haematoma around the artery, which can cause distal ischaemia. Before sampling, the blood supply of the hand should be tested to ensure that it is receiving blood from both the radial and ulnar arteries:
- The patient is asked to make a fist to squeeze blood out of their hand
- The doctor presses on both sides of the wrist to compress radial and ulnar arteries
- The patient releases the fist. Their hand looks white
- The doctor releases the ulnar artery, but *not* the radial artery. Blood supply to the hand from the ulnar artery is proven if the hand goes pink
- The manoeuvre can be repeated, this time releasing the radial artery and not the ulnar artery to check its contribution to the hand blood supply
- Arterial blood gas sampling from the radial artery is safest if the hand has a dual blood supply from radial and ulnar arteries

After sampling, the puncture site should be compressed firmly for several minutes to ensure adequate haemostasis. This will take longer than haemostasis over a venepuncture site because the arterial blood is under higher pressure.

Interpretation. Values should be compared with normal ranges which will vary depending on the analyser used. Normal ranges used in this book are given below in brackets.

Start by looking at the PaO_2 (normal range 10–13.1 kPa). A reduction in PaO_2 indicates some problem with alveolar ventilation, pulmonary capillary perfusion or the matching of these processes, reducing gas exchange. PaO_2 <8 kPa is defined as respiratory failure.

Next, look at $PaCO_2$ (normal range 4.9–6.1 kPa). CO_2 excretion depends on its gradient from blood to alveoli, hence is determined by alveolar ventilation. A fall in CO_2 indicates increased alveolar ventilation; a rise indicates reduced ventilation. Respiratory failure can be classified further according to CO_2 levels:
- Type I respiratory failure – PaO_2 <8 kPa, $PaCO_2$ reduced or normal (Box 3)
- Type II respiratory failure – PaO_2 <8 kPa, $PaCO_2$ elevated (Fig. 7)

Determine from pH values (normal range 7.35–7.45) whether there is acidosis (low pH) or alkalosis (high pH). If there is acid–base disturbance you then need to decide whether this has a respiratory or metabolic cause using the following questions:

- Is PaO_2 abnormal? If yes this indicates a respiratory abnormality
- What is the relationship between pH and PCO_2?
  - in *respiratory* acid–base disturbance, changes in $PaCO_2$ drive changes in pH according to the Henderson–Hasselbach equation

$$H^+ + HCO_3^- \rightleftarrows H_2CO_3 \rightleftarrows H_2O + CO_2$$

A rise in $PaCO_2$ drives the equation to the left, increasing production of H^+ ions and causing a fall in pH (respiratory acidosis). A fall in $PaCO_2$ drives the equation to the right, decreasing production of H^+ ions and causing a rise in pH (respiratory alkalosis). Note that in respiratory acid–base disturbances $PaCO_2$ and pH changes occur in *opposite* directions
  - in *metabolic* acid–base disturbance, changes in pH drive changes in ventilation. A fall in pH (acidosis) stimulates an increase in respiratory rate with a fall in $PaCO_2$. A rise in pH stimulates a fall in respiratory rate with a rise in $PaCO_2$. Note that in metabolic acid–base disturbances $PaCO_2$ and pH changes occur in the *same* direction.
- Finally, look at the bicarbonate (normal range 22–28 mmol/L). In respiratory acidosis, this may be normal (acute) or raised (chronic) as renal compensation for acidosis. In metabolic acidosis (e.g. caused by renal failure, diabetic ketoacidosis or aspirin overdose), the bicarbonate is used up as a buffer to the excess acid and levels are low.

This routine should be used to interpret abnormal blood gases given with cases throughout the book.

Specialist respiratory investigations
Thoracic imaging
CT scanning
Procedure. Computerized tomography (CT) involves acquisition of multiple cross-sectional radiographic images that are reconstructed by a computer to give 3D images. The patient usually lies on their back (supine) and is asked to hold their breath to avoid any movement. The scanner then takes multiple images, either separately or in a continuous spiral.

- A standard thoracic CT scan images the thorax in 10 mm slices continually down the chest. This does not miss any part of the lung and is good for investigation of lung nodules and tumours for example. However, these thick slices do not obtain detailed images of lung parenchyma
- A high-resolution CT scan takes more detailed pictures of the lung in slices that are 1 mm thick. This scan is not continuous as images are taken at 10 mm intervals to minimize radiation dose. It is useful for imaging the lung parenchyma to see emphysema or fibrosis, but may miss small cancers
- CT pulmonary angiogram uses contrast to outline the pulmonary arteries and is used to look for pulmonary emboli
- CT scanning can also be used to guide biopsies of lung lesions

Risks. Radiation exposure from a thoracic CT scan is equivalent to 3 years of background radiation. The use of CT scanning should therefore be considered carefully particularly in young women, in whom breast exposure to radiation may be hazardous or who may be pregnant, and if repeated scanning is planned. The benefits of an accurate diagnosis should be weighed against the potential risks of CT scanning.

Other thoracic imaging includes
- *Ultrasound* – to evaluate and aspirate pleural effusions and guide sampling from nodes and soft tissue
- *Ventilation–perfusion scanning* – to investigate patients for pulmonary emboli
- *Magnetic resonance imaging* – sometimes used to clarify CT findings
- *Positron emission tomography* – used to assess metabolic activity of structural abnormalities (e.g. possible lung cancer) seen by other imaging

The use of these techniques is described where relevant in the cases.

Sampling for pathological diagnosis
A definitive diagnosis often requires sampling of lung secretions, fluid or tissue which is then sent to both microbiology and pathology laboratories for diagnostic analysis.

Sputum
Patients may expectorate sputum spontaneously or after inhaling nebulized saline (induced sputum).

Bronchoscopy
Procedure. Fibreoptic bronchoscopy is performed in patients with or without sedation. The patient is propped

in a sitting position and receives a lidocaine spray into their oropharynx to reduce their cough and gag reflexes. A thin endoscope is then inserted via the nose or mouth into the large airways, allowing inspection of the trachea, main and segmental bronchi.

Rigid bronchoscopy is performed under general anaesthesia and involves insertion of a much larger tube into the trachea. This is usually used where intervention is required to treat disease such as tumours obstructing the large airways or narrowing (stricture) of the trachea, although some centres can now perform such procedures using fibreoptic bronchoscopy.

Patients must give written informed consent before any type of bronchoscopy is performed and should be warned about the risk of complications.

Sampling that can be performed through the bronchoscope includes:
• *Bronchial aspirate.* Direct collection of bronchial secretions by suction into a sample pot
• *Bronchial washings.* Normal saline (10 mL) is syringed into the airways and removed into a sample pot. This takes samples from the large airways
• *Bronchoalveolar lavage.* The bronchoscope is pushed down in a chosen airway until it is wedged as far as it can go. A large volume (180–240 mL) of normal saline is syringed into the lung and removed by suction into a sample pot. This samples secretions from the distal lung
• *Bronchial brushings.* A fine brush can be used to collect cells from the epithelial surface
• *Endobronchial biopsy.* Forceps are used to take tissue samples directly from a large airway wall
• *Transbronchial biopsy.* Biopsy forceps are passed into the lung as deep as possible and biopsies are taken. This aims to take samples of the lung parenchyma
• *Transbronchial nodal aspiration.* A fine needle is inserted through the large airway wall into underlying enlarged lymph nodes and samples are aspirated into the needle. The site of the nodes is identified either by prior imaging or by ultrasound down the bronchoscope (endobronchial ultrasound)

Risks. Complications of fibreoptic bronchoscopy include:
• Bleeding
• Infection
• Respiratory compromise
• Pneumothorax
• Death (~0.01%)

Percutaneous procedures (Fig. 19)
Fine needle aspiration. A fine needle is inserted into the lesion, removed and the contents of the needle expelled onto a microscope slide for cytological or microbiological examination. This is particularly useful for sampling from cervical lymph nodes. The procedure causes minor discomfort and minimal risk of complications.

Biopsy. A long needle is inserted into the lesion, usually under radiological guidance, and a core of tissue removed for histological and microbiological examination. This is performed under local anaesthetic and may be complicated by bleeding or pneumothorax.

Other sampling
• *Percutaneous aspiration of effusion or pleural biopsy* – performed with or without radiological guidance to investigate pleural disease
• *Video-assisted thoracoscopy* – insertion of an endoscope through the chest wall to sample pleura and lung parenchyma
• *Open lung biopsy* – sampling of lung performed at open surgery

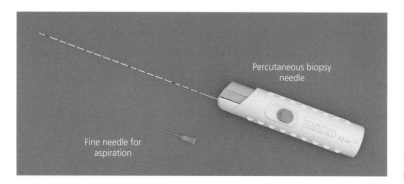

Percutaneous biopsy needle

Fine needle for aspiration

Figure 19 Sampling needles for percutaneous procedures.

The use of these techniques is described where relevant in the cases.

Other lung function testing

More detailed information about lung function can be obtained by measuring lung volumes and gas transfer.

> **Box 23 Example OSCE checklist for performing peak flow measurement**
>
> This is a rather brief procedure for a 5 min OSCE station and so is likely to be combined, e.g. with checking inhaler technique or giving advice
>
> Introduces self (name and role) — 1 mark
> Outlines procedure — 1 mark
> Obtains consent — 1 mark
>
> **Demonstration**
> Shows patient peak flow meter — 1 mark
> Explains principles of action — 1 mark
> Tells patient to make good seal with mouth around mouthpiece — 1 mark
> Explains that they should blow as hard as they can — 1 mark
> Asks patient not to put hand over flow indicator — 1 mark
> Demonstrates peak flow measurement correctly — 1 mark
>
> **Measurement**
> Changes mouthpiece — 1 mark
> Checks patient is standing or sitting upright — 1 mark
> Checks peak flow indicator is at zero — 1 mark
> Asks patient to perform manoeuvre — 1 mark
> Reads peak flow correctly — 1 mark
> Gives feedback to patient — 1 mark
> Asks them to repeat measurement twice more — 1 mark
> Thanks patient — 1 mark
>
> **Interpretation**
> Gives value as best measurement of the three performed — 1 mark
> Uses normal range charts to estimate value as percentage of predicted — 1 mark
> Interprets measurement — 1 mark
>
> **Simulated patient mark**
> Clear explanation — up to 2 marks
>
> **Total — 22 marks**

Lung volumes

Lung volumes are measured by asking the patient to breathe in and out of a known volume of air containing a known concentration of helium. Helium is not absorbed by the lung, so distributes throughout and is diluted by the air in the lung. The difference between the original and final helium concentrations allows the volume of air in the lung to be calculated. Values obtained include:

• *Total lung capacity.* Take a deep breath in until the lungs are full. The total volume of air inside them is now the total lung capacity, which may be:
  - increased in patients with emphysema who have reduced elastic recoil of the lung
  - reduced in patients with pulmonary fibrosis
• *Residual volume.* Breathe out as far as possible until the lungs appear empty. There is still some air left inside as the lungs are prevented from collapsing by negative intrapleural pressure. This is the residual volume which:
  - may be increased in patients with airflow obstruction (e.g. asthma, emphysema)
• *Vital capacity.* This is the volume of air exhaled (i.e. the difference between total lung capacity and residual volume). The vital capacity is reduced in both restrictive and obstructive lung disease

Gas transfer

The ease of diffusion of gases across the alveolar capillary membrane is tested using carbon monoxide. The patient breathes out then inhales a single breath of air containing 0.28% carbon monoxide. Their next exhalation is collected and the residual carbon monoxide concentration is measured. After correction of values for lung volumes measured by helium, initial and final carbon monoxide concentrations are compared. The difference indicates how much carbon monoxide was taken up and is expressed as a transfer factor.

Diseases of the lung parenchyma that interfere with transfer of gas across the alveolar–capillary membrane cause reduction in the transfer factor (e.g. emphysema, pulmonary fibrosis).

Treatment

General treatment principles are outlined in this section. Specific treatments for individual respiratory diseases are discussed under the relevant cases.

Approach to treatment of respiratory emergencies

Life-threatening emergencies affecting the respiratory system include:

- Respiratory arrest
- Life-threatening asthma
- Severe type II respiratory failure
- Massive pulmonary embolus
- Tension pneumothorax
- Anaphylaxis

In these situations the usual consultation order is reversed and the patient receives life-saving treatment before an attempt is made to make a diagnosis (Box 24).

The first three steps should always be basic life support:

A Ensure the **a**irway is patent and clear it if not

B Check if the patient is **b**reathing and support if not

C Check **c**irculation (pulse and blood pressure) and support if absent/inadequate

Once basic life support has been performed further assessment will determine action as described in the individual cases. In many cases patients will need respiratory support as well as disease-specific measures.

Respiratory support

Patients with respiratory failure have hypoxia with or without hypercapnia. These blood gas abnormalities cause cell and tissue damage (Boxes 4 & 5) and must be corrected.

Hypoxia

Hypoxia is treated by increasing the partial pressure of inspired oxygen. The patient wears nasal cannulae or a face mask (Fig. 20) which allows them to breathe a mixture of air (21% oxygen) and 100% oxygen (e.g. from a cylinder or piped supply). The final concentration of oxygen in inspired gas depends on the flow rate of the oxygen and the type of device used.

Nasal cannulae. These are convenient to wear and the patient receives continuous oxygen even when talking and eating. However, the oxygen concentration delivered is unpredictable (25–39% at oxygen flows 1–4 L/min) and insufficient for many patients.

Venturi mask. The attachments (A) shown in Fig. 21 are connected to the mask (E) and to the oxygen supply (D). Entry of oxygen into the attachment at the flow rate shown (C) draws air in through the side holes (B) and air and oxygen are mixed to a final fixed inspired oxygen concentration (C). These devices are particularly useful

---

> **Box 24 Priorities in managing the emergency patient**
>
> **1** Save life and minimize potential disability
> **2** Relieve distress
> **3** Make a diagnosis
> **4** Disease-specific treatment

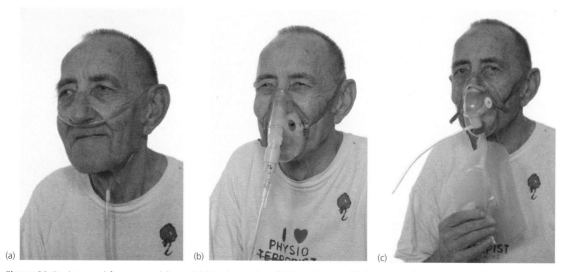

(a)   (b)   (c)

Figure 20 Devices used for oxygen delivery. (a) Nasal cannulae. (b) Venturi mask. (c) Oxygen mask and reservoir bag.

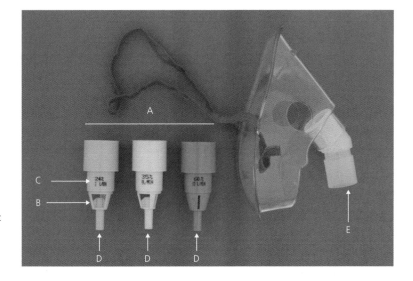

Figure 21 Venturi mask and attachments. (A) Attachments, (B) aperture allowing air entry, (C) required oxygen flow rate to achieve stated concentration of oxygen in inspired air, (D) attachment of tubing carrying 100% oxygen, (E) attachments (A) connect to mask here.

Box 25 Ventilation – definitions

Invasive versus non-invasive
Invasive. The patient is sedated and ventilated mechanically via an artificial airway such as endotracheal tube or tracheostomy
Non-invasive. The patient is awake and ventilated by face or nasal mask without artificial airway

Positive versus negative pressure ventilators
Positive pressure ventilators deliver gases into the airways using pressures above atmospheric to support the work of breathing
Negative pressure ventilators encase the chest and abdomen and generate negative extrathoracic pressure, 'sucking' the chest wall out and gases into the chest. Iron lungs used for polio in the 20th century were negative pressure ventilators

CPAP versus BiPAP
Non-invasive positive pressure ventilation is delivered by devices that generate:

Continuous positive airway pressure (CPAP) – at the same set level above atmospheric pressure throughout inhalation and exhalation. Used in the treatment of patients with heart failure and obstructive sleep apnoea
Bilevel positive airway pressure (BiPAP) – pressure is higher during inhalation and lower (but still above atmospheric pressure) during exhalation. Used in patients with type II respiratory failure caused by COPD

Spontaneous versus timed modes for bilevel ventilations (BiPAP)
In *spontaneous* mode, the ventilator detects the flow rate of the patient's breathing and changes the pressure to support their breathing cycle. High flow triggers high pressures to support inhalation and lower flow triggers lower pressures to allow exhalation
In *timed* mode, the ventilator alternates between high and low pressures at set time intervals irrespective of the patient's breathing cycle

---

in COPD where a fixed low inspired oxygen concentration (24–28%) is required (see Case 8).

Oxygen mask with reservoir bag. This device delivers high inspired oxygen concentrations (45–90% at oxygen flows 3–15 L/min). When the patient breathes out, oxygen fills the reservoir bag; when they breathe in, oxygen from the bag and from the supply source are inhaled with very little air, achieving high inspired oxygen concentrations. A valve prevents exhaled air from entering the bag.

Hypercapnia
Hypercapnia is treated by increasing ventilation by (Box 25):
• Invasive ventilation, delivered on an intensive care unit

• Non-invasive ventilation, delivered on an intensive care or high dependency unit or on an acute ward

Approach to treatment of respiratory disease

Respiratory medicine is a diverse specialty and patients present at all ages with a wide range of acute and chronic conditions. Treatment must therefore be tailored to the individual and can involve:

• Treatment of a single acute episode (e.g. upper or lower respiratory tract infection)

• Chronic disease management (e.g. asthma, COPD, cystic fibrosis)

• Treatment of terminal disease (e.g. lung cancer, pulmonary fibrosis)

Treatment options for patients with respiratory disease are (Box 26)

• Non-pharmacological

• Medical

• Invasive intervention/surgical

In practice, most patients are treated using a combination of approaches. For example, a patient with COPD may be treated with smoking cessation, physiotherapy and bronchodilators, whereas a patient with lung cancer may require psychological support, radiotherapy and bronchoscopic intervention. Close working of the multidisciplinary team is essential for effective treatment of respiratory disease (Box 27).

Principles of antibiotic treatment

Many respiratory diseases are caused by bacteria and require treatment with antibiotics. Factors influencing the choice of antibiotics include:

• Organism factors:
  ○ likely organisms (best guess)
  ○ local antibiotic resistance

• Patient factors:
  ○ allergies and side-effects
  ○ ability to take/absorb oral medication
  ○ immune competence or suppression

Box 26 Examples of treatment options for patients with respiratory disease

Non-pharmacological, e.g.

• Smoking cessation
• Physiotherapy
• Allergen avoidance
• Psychological support

Medical treatment, e.g.

• Bronchodilators for airflow obstruction (asthma, COPD)
• Immunosuppression for inflammatory disease (asthma, alveolitis)
• Antimicrobial drugs for infection
• Anticoagulation for pulmonary emboli
• Chemotherapy/radiotherapy for cancer
• Non-invasive ventilation for type II respiratory failure

Invasive intervention/surgery, e.g.

• Invasive ventilation
• Bronchoscopic intervention for large airways obstruction
• Pleural drainage of pneumothorax or effusion
• Video-assisted thoracoscopic procedures (e.g. pleurodesis)
• Lobectomy/pneumonectomy for lung cancer
• Lung transplant for end-stage respiratory failure

Box 27 Multidisciplinary team involved in care of patients with respiratory disease

Doctors

• Respiratory physicians
• General practitioners
• Intensive care doctors
• Cardiothoracic surgeons
• Infectious disease specialists
• Medical and clinical oncologists
• Microbiologists
• Pathologists

Nurses

• Specialist respiratory nurses in primary and secondary care:
  ○ asthma/COPD
  ○ TB
  ○ lung cancer
• Palliative care nurses

Physiotherapists

• Inpatient and outpatient

Other important team members

• Dietitians
• Pharmacists
• Occupational therapists
• Social workers
• Religious leaders
• Counsellors

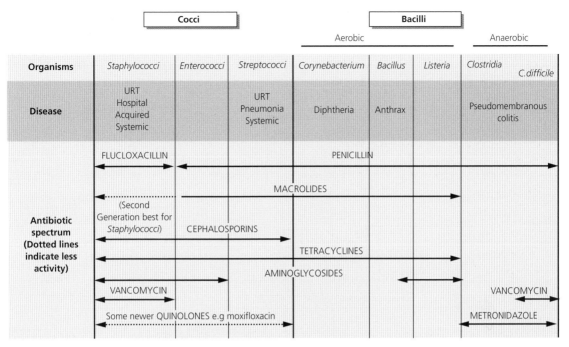

Figure 22 Spectrum of action of antibiotics against Gram-positive organisms causing respiratory infection. Dotted lines indicate less activity. URT, upper respiratory tract infection.

- Antibiotic factors:
  - broad or narrow spectrum
  - bacteriocidal or bacteriostatic
  - formulations available (enteral or parenteral)

Figures 22 and 23 show the spectrum of Gram-positive and Gram-negative bacteria causing respiratory infection, indicating the respiratory diseases caused by and the antibiotics effective against each organism. This chart is referred to throughout the book in consideration of antibiotic therapy for patients in relevant cases.

Prescribing antibiotics

Antibiotics are useful and effective drugs in the treatment of respiratory infection. However, they should be used with care as injudicious use may induce development of antibiotic-resistant organisms and cause side-effects. Good practice when prescribing antibiotics includes:
- Ensure antibiotics are really required
- Choose antibiotic(s) with as narrow a spectrum of action as possible to avoid killing commensal organisms (e.g. organisms in the gastrointestinal tract)
- Check the patient is not allergic to the chosen antibiotic(s) before prescribing
- State the duration of the course of treatment and ensure a stop date is given
- Ask the patient to complete the course of treatment
- If in doubt discuss choice with local microbiologist

Route of administration of antibiotics

If the patient can take oral medication and absorb it reliably, antibiotics should be given by mouth. Intravenous drugs are more expensive than oral drugs and injections can introduce infection. Intravenous antibiotics should be reserved for patients:
- Who are severely ill
- Who need high doses of antibiotics
- Who are vomiting or unable to swallow
- If the antibiotic is only available in injectable form (e.g. aminoglycosides)

If intravenous antibiotics are used initially, patients should be reviewed regularly and switched back to oral treatment:
- When temperature has been <38°C for 48 h or more
- Oral food/fluids are tolerated
- There is no unexplained tachycardia
- There is no contraindication to oral therapy (see above)

Palliative care

Palliative care is treatment intended to alleviate symptoms without improving or preventing progression of the

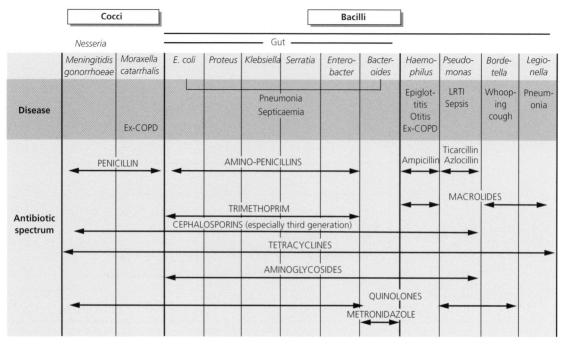

Figure 23 Spectrum of action of antibiotics against Gram-negative organisms causing respiratory infection. Ex-COPD, exacerbations of chronic obstructive pulmonary disease; LRTI, lower respiratory tract infection.

underlying disease. Palliative care may be provided for patients at home by a community team or at a hospice or hospital on an outpatient or inpatient basis. Major symptoms experienced by a patient with end-stage lung disease include breathlessness, cough, anxiety, depression and insomnia. Management of these includes the following.

Breathlessness
- Non-pharmacological approaches:
  - information and relaxation techniques to manage anxiety
  - physiotherapy to maintain mobility and avoid deconditioning
  - nutrition to maintain optimum body weight
  - alternative therapies such as acupuncture
- Pharmacological approaches:
  - oxygen
  - opiates

Cough
- Physiotherapy may help to clear secretions
- Opiates are also cough suppressants

Anxiety, depression and insomnia
- Non-pharmacological approaches:
  - psychological support and counselling
  - practical help (e.g. with finances)
- Pharmacological approaches:
  - benzodiazepines (e.g. sublingual lorazepam)
  - opiates
  - tricyclic antidepressants

Doctrine of double effect
Opiates and benzodiazepines can relieve symptoms in patients with end-stage lung disease. However, a side-effect of these drugs is respiratory depression, which could have the unintended result of hastening death. In general, it is considered ethically acceptable to administer these drugs as long as:
- The main intention is to do good (relieve symptoms)
- The adverse effect (hastening of death) is unintended
- The benefits of the good effect are considered to outweigh the risks of the adverse effect
- The good effect (symptom relief) is not caused by the adverse effect (death)

Case 1 A 64-year-old man with respiratory arrest

You are on the ward when you hear a shout and run over to see what has happened. A man has collapsed and is lying on the floor. His eyes are shut and his lips look blue.

What action should you take?

You are first on the scene so shout for help then assess the patient. Check it is safe to approach, then gently shake him by the shoulders, shouting in his ear 'Are you alright?' If he does not respond, you should next:

1 Check his **Airway** is clear of obstruction
2 Check whether he is **Breathing** by looking for chest movements, listening over his mouth and feeling for breath on your cheek (10 s)
3 Check his **Circulation** by feeling for a carotid pulse (10 s)

You find that he is not breathing but he has a weak pulse with a rate of 120 beats/min.

How do you interpret this information?

This is a respiratory arrest (for causes see Box 28). Untreated he will become increasingly hypoxic, leading to cardiac arrest and brain death.

What should you do now?
Open his airway

This should be performed as part of the initial assessment. Turn the patient onto his back, put your hand on his forehead and gently tilt his head back, then lift his chin with your fingertips. Look inside the mouth and remove foreign bodies, vomit or secretions with fingers, forceps or suction.

Support his breathing

The priority is to get oxygen into the patient, so you should do whatever you are trained to do that can be done most quickly.

Initial ventilation. Either:
• Perform mouth-to-mouth or mouth-to-mask ventilation using expired air from your lungs (~16% oxygen), or
• Use a bag, valve and face mask to ventilate the patient (Fig. 24). Use supplementary oxygen if possible, but air is better than nothing (21% oxygen).

The lungs should be ventilated 10 times per minute. Check the pulse every 10 breaths. If you cannot feel the pulse or are not sure if there is a pulse then full cardiopulmonary resuscitation with chest compressions should commence.

The patient's airway is clear and he is given mouth-to-mask ventilation until the resuscitation trolley arrives. As he is still not breathing spontaneously, a Guedel airway is inserted and he is ventilated using a bag, value and face mask and high flow oxygen. His oxygen saturations are 93% and on listening to his chest he has air entry bilaterally with no added sounds. A cardiac monitor is attached and shows a sinus tachycardia at 112 beats/min. His blood pressure is 100/60 mmHg. You are able to review his wristband and notes. His name is David Robson, he is 64 and was admitted for investigation of a transient ischaemic attack. He has hypertension, but no other significant past medical history.

What does this new information tell you about the cause of his respiratory arrest?

1 *Upper airway obstruction?* This was not the cause of Mr Robson's arrest as his airway was clear and he can now be ventilated successfully
2 *Underlying pulmonary disease?* This seems unlikely as he has no significant past medical history. An acute event such as massive pulmonary embolus or pulmonary oedema could have caused severe hypoxia and respiratory arrest
3 *Neuromuscular cause?* He has hypertension and a recent transient ischaemic attack and could have suffered

41

Box 28 Causes of respiratory arrest

Upper airway

Physical obstruction of the airway:

- Laryngeal oedema – anaphylaxis, infection, trauma
- Laryngeal spasm – post intubation
- Inhaled foreign body – (e.g. meat, chewing gum)
- Obstruction by tongue, palate, false teeth

Pulmonary

Severe disease causing hypoxia, which affects the brainstem causing respiratory arrest, e.g.

- Asthma
- COPD
- Massive pulmonary embolus
- Pneumonia
- Pulmonary oedema

Neuromuscular

Loss of respiratory drive or neuromuscular function:

- Raised intracranial pressure
- Cervical cord injury
- Neurological (e.g. Guillain–Barré syndrome)

Drugs

Central suppression of respiratory drive:

- Alcohol
- Opiates
- Benzodiazepines
- Anaesthetics

a stroke or intracranial haemorrhage that affected his respiratory centre directly (brainstem) or indirectly (raised intracranial pressure)

4 *Drugs?* This seems less likely, although a drug history is not given

What are your options for managing his airway?

The airway is normally kept patent by muscle tone, which prevents obstruction by the tongue, and by the cough reflex, which prevents inhalation of particulate matter such as food and vomit. Mr Robson is unconscious and unable to protect his own airway. Your options are as follows (Figs 25 & 26):

1 *Nasopharyngeal airway.* This airway is inserted through one nostril into the nasopharynx and top of the oropharynx. The safety pin shown in Fig. 26 is used to stop the airway slipping further into the nose and becoming difficult to remove. Nasal airways are used to keep the airway patent when oral airways cannot be used, but do not protect the patient from aspiration

2 *Oropharyngeal (Guedal) airway.* This airway is inserted via the mouth into the oropharynx and keeps the upper airway clear by keeping the tongue out of the way. It comes in a range of sizes and is easy to use with brief training. However, as it sits above the larynx it does not prevent aspiration of food into the lungs

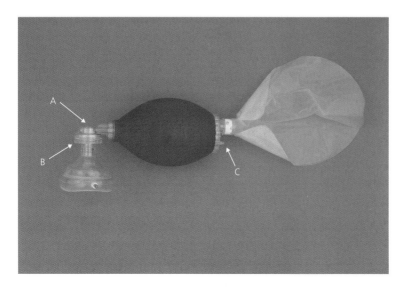

Figure 24 Bag, valve and mask for manual ventilation. (A) Attachment of bag to mask. The mask can be removed and the bag attached to an endotracheal tube. (B) One-way valve to prevent exhaled air from entering the bag. (C) Attachment for oxygen tubing.

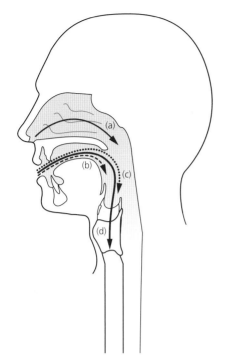

Figure 25 Depth and routes of insertion of equipment used to secure the airway. (a) Nasopharyngeal airway; (b) oropharyngeal airway (Guedal); (c) laryngeal mask; (d) cuffed endotracheal tube.

3 *Laryngeal mask.* This consists of a small inflatable mask and connecting tube which is inserted blindly into the pharynx and forms a low pressure seal around the larynx. The laryngeal mask is easier and quicker to place than the endotracheal tube and provides some protection against aspiration, although this is not as good as that provided by an endotracheal tube

4 *Endotracheal tube.* This tube is inserted through the larynx into the trachea. Once in place, a cuff around the tube can be inflated within the trachea to prevent aspiration. This is the best option to 'secure the airway'. However, insertion of entotracheal tubes requires specialized training. Problems with endotracheal tubes include incorrect placement, obstruction, cuff leak and tracheal damage.

The anaesthetist arrives and takes over the care of Mr Robson's airway and ventilation. She inserts an endotracheal tube and ventilates him via this tube using a bag, valve and face mask (Fig. 24) with entrained oxygen. After 10 min she stops ventilating him for a short period to see if he breathes spontaneously.

Why did the anaesthetist stop the ventilation?

If a patient is being ventilated rapidly this will increase carbon dioxide excretion. Carbon dioxide is an essential

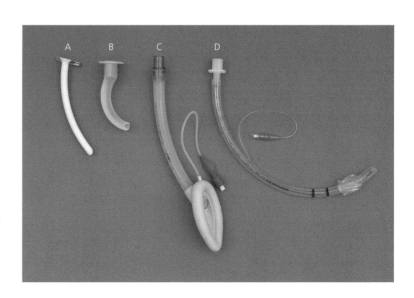

Figure 26 Equipment used to secure the airway. (A) Nasopharyngeal airway; (B) oropharyngeal airway (Guedal); (C) laryngeal mask; (D) cuffed endotracheal tube.

respiratory stimulant; hence the anaesthetist stops the ventilation to see if the increase in respiratory drive due to carbon dioxide accumulation stimulates spontaneous breathing.

> Mr Robson does not breathe spontaneously. Resuscitation has now been continuing for 30 min.

What should his management be now?

1 *Continued life support.* Ventilation should continue until further decisions are made about his management. Ventilation by hand using a bag and mask can continue on the ward, during patient transfer and during investigations. However, if ventilation is to be prolonged the patient should be moved to an intensive care unit, where a mechanical ventilator can be used to provide intermittent positive pressure ventilation (Box 25, p. 37).

2 *Diagnosis and prognosis.* Now that life support is secure and Mr Robson is temporarily stable it is essential to establish why he has had a respiratory arrest and determine whether he is likely to recover. This will allow the clinical team to decide on further treatment. If he is likely to recover he will require admission to intensive care for continued life support while treatment is instituted. If he is unlikely to recover then intensive care admission may not be appropriate.

Our previous analysis suggested that the most likely cause of his respiratory arrest was neurological. Hence, the most appropriate next investigation would be a computed tomography (CT) scan of his brain.

> Mr Robson's CT brain scan showed a massive intracranial haemorrhage with evidence of raised intracranial pressure.

Who decides what to do next?

This type of brain haemorrhage carries a poor prognosis, with a high likelihood of in-hospital death or severe disability if the patient survives. However, as Mr Robson is previously fit and relatively young he has some chance of recovery. In this situation, where Mr Robson is unable to say what he would like regarding treatment, decisions can be difficult.

In England, Wales and Northern Ireland, when a patient is unable to consent to treatment, doctors have the authority to act in the patient's best interest. These interests generally are determined by:

1 Likely outcome of any treatment
2 The patient's known or ascertainable wishes
3 The patient's human rights (Human Rights Act 1998), particularly rights to:
  ○ life
  ○ freedom from inhuman or degrading treatment
  ○ respect for privacy and family life
  ○ right to hold opinions and receive information
  ○ freedom from discrimination

Doctors are therefore generally advised to involve people close to the patient in the discussion about treatment as they may know the patient's previous wishes. However, although their views may be taken into account, relatives cannot insist on treatment or non-treatment for a patient.

> Outcome. The clinical team managed to contact Mr Robson's wife and daughter, who were extremely upset to hear of Mr Robson's sudden collapse. On arrival at the hospital they were adamant that Mr Robson would not have wanted to survive if there was any chance of disability. The doctors felt, in view of this and the grave prognosis, that it was in Mr Robson's interest that he be kept comfortable. The endotracheal tube was removed and he breathed spontaneously for 2 h, giving his family sufficient time to say goodbye before he died.

References

For more information about basic and advanced life support, see the Resuscitation Council UK website http://www.resus.org.uk/

CASE REVIEW

Mr Robson had a sudden respiratory arrest during hospital inpatient stay following a transient ischaemic attack. Basic life support was commenced immediately with mouth-to-mask ventilation then continued using a bag, value and face mask and high flow oxygen. The anaesthetist performed endotracheal intubation to secure his airway and continued manual ventilation until a CT scan demonstrated a massive intracranial haemorrhage with raised intracranial pressure. Mr Robson was assessed as having an extremely poor prognosis and after discussion with his family he received no further treatment and died peacefully.

KEY POINTS

- When approaching a person who has collapsed you should:
  - call for help
  - check it is safe to approach
  - see if the person is responsive
- If they are unresponsive you should:
  - **Airway** – check for obstruction and clear if necessary
  - **Breathing** – check for breathing and support if not
  - **Circulation** – check for pulse and commence cardiac massage if absent
- A respiratory arrest has occurred where the person has a cardiac output but is not breathing
- If untreated, a respiratory arrest will cause hypoxic cardiac arrest and brain death

- Ventilation should be started immediately by the most rapidly available means
- As equipment arrives the airway should be protected to assist ventilation and prevent aspiration
- Once resuscitation is established the cause of respiratory arrest should be identified and is likely to be one of:
  - upper airway obstruction
  - hypoxia
  - neuromuscular disease
  - drugs
- Further management of respiratory arrest will depend on the underlying cause and patient progress

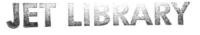

Case 2 A 19-year-old man with chest tightness

Giorgio Valente is a 19-year-old man who presents to his GP complaining of tightness in his chest and slight shortness of breath over the past 6 weeks. He particularly notices these sensations when he is running and on entering a smoky room. He also has a cough that wakes him up at night, although he is not producing any phlegm. He would like to start training for the marathon and asks his GP if these symptoms are just caused by lack of fitness.

How should the GP answer his question?

It is possible that his symptoms represent a lack of fitness. However, the combination of exercise- and irritant-induced chest tightness and night cough could be symptoms of asthma. His symptoms have come on relatively recently (6 weeks ago) so could also have been caused by a viral upper respiratory tract infection.

What questions should the GP ask to determine the likelihood of this being asthma?

• *Pattern of symptoms*. Are symptoms intermittent and variable, as is characteristic of asthma?
• *Triggers*. Do known asthma triggers make the symptoms worse? (Box 29)
• *Past history*. Has he had symptoms of asthma before? Adults with apparent new asthma often had symptoms of asthma in childhood that they seemed to grow out of
• *History of atopy*. Does he have a history of rhinitis or eczema that indicates he is atopic with a predisposition to asthma?
• *Family history of asthma or atopy*. Are family members affected? These conditions are more common in people with affected relatives

On further questioning, Mr Valente remembers having a blue inhaler at school. He had eczema as a child and hayfever when doing school exams. He is a non-smoker and does not have any pets. His mother has asthma which is well controlled. Examination is normal apart from bilateral expiratory wheeze over his lung fields.

How does this new information affect your assessment?

Wheeze is indicative of airflow obstruction (Box 30). Although there are other causes of airflow obstruction, asthma is the most likely diagnosis in Mr Valente's case as:

• He has a significant past and family history of asthma and atopy
• As a young non-smoker he is very unlikely to have chronic obstructive pulmonary disease (COPD) or heart failure

What causes asthma?

Asthma is a chronic inflammatory condition of the airways. The exact causes of asthma are still unclear; however, genetic and environmental factors both appear to play a part. A general summary of the processes leading to airways inflammation in asthma is shown in Fig. 27.

Early allergen exposure in susceptible individuals leads to generation of:
• Allergen-specific T cells (Th2 type)
• Allergen-specific immunoglobulin E (IgE), produced by B cells

Allergen-specific T cells move to the lung. Allergen-specific IgE coats mast cells and dendritic cells in the lung causing the person to become sensitized to that allergen.

On subsequent exposure allergen binds to:
• Sensitized mast cells – which degranulate and release inflammatory mediators, causing an immediate immune response (early phase reaction)
• Sensitized dendritic cells – which activate allergen-specific T cells to release inflammatory mediators and attract eosinophils. This perpetuates the immune response (late phase reaction). Ongoing inflammation leads to airway remodelling

Box 29 Asthma triggers

Factors that trigger asthma symptoms by increasing airway inflammation
- Allergens, e.g.
  - outdoors – grass and fungal pollens
  - indoors – house dust mites, pets
  - food – eggs, milk
  - occupational – animals, organic dusts (e.g. flour), textile dusts (e.g. cotton, hemp)
- Occupational irritants (e.g. chemical dusts and vapours)
- Other:
  - upper respiratory tract infections, mainly viral
  - drugs (e.g. aspirin, other non-steroidal anti-inflammatory drugs)

Factors that trigger symptoms by irritating inflamed airways
- Cold air
- Exercise
- Smoky atmospheres or strong perfumes
- Pollution

Other triggers
- Hormonal (e.g. premenstrual exacerbations)
- Emotion
- Drugs (e.g. β-blockers)

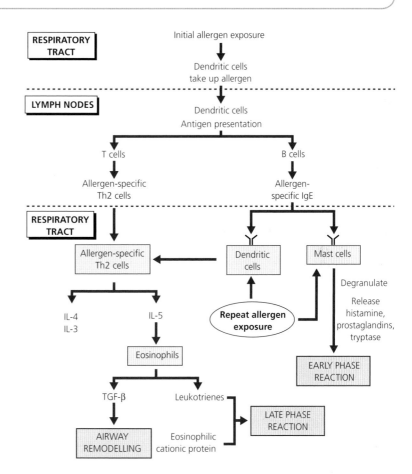

Figure 27 Pathogenesis of asthma.

Is asthma always caused by an allergic reaction?

- Asthma in children and adolescents is likely to be 'extrinsic' asthma, which is asthma associated with atopy and driven by allergen exposure. These patients have sys-temic IgE production with increased circulating IgE and a positive response to allergy testing. In this group asthma that persists into adulthood remains atopic
- Asthma arising *de novo* in adulthood is less frequently associated with atopy and may be termed 'intrinsic' or

> **Box 30 Wheeze**
>
> Wheeze is expiratory noise caused by airway narrowing
>
> **High pitched polyphonic ('many sounds') wheeze**
> Caused by disease affecting multiple small airways of different diameters, e.g.
> • Asthma
> • COPD
> • Heart failure (airways compressed by interstitial oedema)
>
> **Low pitched monophonic ('one sound') wheeze**
> Caused by disease blocking a single large airway, e.g.
> • Trachea blocked by stricture, swelling, tumour (stridor)
> • Bronchus blocked by tumour, foreign body

late-onset asthma. Many individuals with late-onset asthma appear to develop the condition following upper respiratory tract infections, usually viral in origin. These asthma patients do not have systemic IgE production, but may produce IgE locally at the bronchial mucosa, triggering similar pathological processes

How does the airways inflammation seen in asthma lead to airflow obstruction? (Fig. 4, p. 5)
Early phase reaction
Mast cell degranulation releases histamine, prostaglandins and leukotrienes which produce:
• Vasodilatation and increased vascular permeability, causing mucosal oedema
• Increased production of bronchial secretions
• Smooth muscle contraction, causing bronchospasm
These processes narrow the airway lumen immediately after allergen exposure.

Late phase reaction
Activated T cells attract eosinophils which release tissue-damaging proteins and leukotrienes, which perpetuate mucosal oedema, hypersecretion and bronchospasm.

Chronic asthma
Chronic inflammation results in:
• Airway epithelial damage
• Increased numbers of mucus-secreting goblet cells
• Basement membrane thickening
• Smooth muscle hyperplasia and hypertrophy

These processes can cause more permanent airflow obstruction in chronic asthma.

Why do patients with asthma wheeze?
Air flowing through narrowed airways makes a high-pitched noise, heard as a wheeze. The wheeze is 'polyphonic', which means it includes notes at different pitches, caused by narrowing of airways of different diameters.

Why is the wheeze worse on expiration?
During expiration the intrathoracic pressure is increased and compresses the airways. This does not impede airflow in normal lungs, but in asthmatic patients the inflamed airways are narrowed further and airflow obstruction is increased. Hence, wheeze is usually heard in expiration. As airflow is greater on inspiration than expiration in asthma, air can become trapped in the lungs, causing hyperinflation.

Why is asthma worse at night?
Airflow narrowing and symptoms in asthma are characteristically worse at night and early morning and better later in the day. Patients with unstable asthma often complain of nocturnal cough. The causes for this 'diurnal variation' probably include:
• Change in body temperature
• Change in intrinsic hormone levels (corticosteroids, catecholamines)
• Impaired mucociliary clearance during sleep
• Possible oesophageal reflux
• Diurnal variation in bronchomotor tone
• Increase exposure to allergens, particularly house dust mite in bedding

How could the GP investigate Mr Valente to make a diagnosis of asthma?
Asthma is a clinical diagnosis. There are no investigations that confirm the diagnosis; however, tests to look for atopy and variable airflow obstruction may help to support the clinical diagnosis.

Mr Valente has the following investigation results:

		Normal range
Hb	14.6 g/dL	(13–18 g/dL)
WCC	6.8×10^9/L	($4–11 \times 10^9$/L)
Platelets	230×10^9/L	($150–400 \times 10^9$/L)
Neutrophils	5.2×10^9/L	($3.5–7.5 \times 10^9$/L)
Eosinophils	1.0×10^9/L	($0.0–0.4 \times 10^9$/L)
Serum IgE	220 kU/L	(0–8 kU/L)

Home peak flow monitoring (Fig. 28)

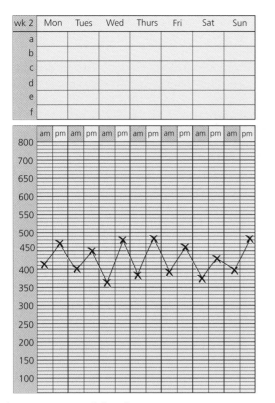

Figure 28 Home peak flow diary.

How do you interpret his investigations?

Mr Valente has a raised IgE and eosinophil count. These findings confirm that he is atopic, but are not diagnostic of asthma because:
- Not all people who are atopic develop asthma:
  - in the UK 40–50% children have symptoms of atopy but up to 20% develop asthma
- Not all people with asthma are atopic:
  - patients with 'instrinsic' or late-onset asthma are usually not atopic

However, his home peak flow monitoring is strongly indicative of asthma as there is evidence of variable airflow obstruction.

How is variable airflow obstruction assessed from peak flow measurements?

'Percentage' variability is determined by:
- Subtracting the lowest from the highest peak flow measurement
- Dividing the difference by the highest measurement
- Multiplying the result by 100

That is:

Percentage variability =

$$\frac{\text{highest measurement} - \text{lowest measurement}}{\text{highest measurement}} \times 100$$

In Mr Valente's case the highest measurement is 480 L/min and the lowest measurement is 360 L/min. The difference between the highest and lowest measurement is 120 L/min.
Percentage variability = 120/480 × 100 = 25%

This variability is considered to indicate asthma if it:
- Exceeds 60 L/min
- Exceeds 20% of the highest peak flow value
- Occurs on 3 days in any 2 weeks of a monitoring period

The GP makes a firm diagnosis of asthma based on Mr Valente's clinical features, the presence of atopy and evidence of variable airflow obstruction on peak flow monitoring. He sends Mr Valente for skin prick testing at the local hospital and commences him on beclometasone 100 µg 2 puffs twice daily and inhaled salbutamol for symptoms as required.

What is the purpose of skin prick testing?

Skin prick testing is performed to determine whether the patient has an allergic response to common allergens including house dust mite, cat dander and grass pollen. This determines whether the patient is atopic and identifies allergens that could be avoided to reduce symptoms.

How is skin prick testing performed?

Drops of aqueous extracts of relevant allergens, negative saline and positive histamine controls are placed on the skin and are each pricked gently into the epidermis with a fresh needle. The test results are read 15 min later. Histamine causes capillary permeability and leak in the epidermis, causing a swelling called a weal. This should be seen with the positive control, or other tests are unreliable. If the patient is allergic to an injected allergen, an early phase response will occur, with degranulation of mast cells and histamine release. The presence of a weal for any allergen that is 3 mm larger than the negative control is considered a positive reaction to that allergen.

Mr Valente's skin prick testing demonstrates a positive allergic response to house dust and grass pollen.

If Mr Valente avoids house dust and grass pollen will his symptoms improve?

A reduction in allergen exposure is worthwhile if possible as this can reduce the severity of allergic disease.

How can allergen exposure be reduced?

This depends on the allergen to be avoided and can be very difficult. Mr Valente is allergic to grass pollen and house dust mite and some tips for avoiding these are as follows.

Grass pollen

Exposure to this can be limited in pollen season by:
• Driving with windows shut
• Avoiding walking in the countryside
• Keeping bedroom windows shut at night
• Taking holidays by the coast
  Pollen forecasts now given with the weather forecast can help allergy patients to reduce exposure.

House dust mite

House dust mite faecal particles contain the allergen and are abundant throughout the house, particularly in soft furnishings. This allergen is particularly difficult to avoid but measures that can help if applied rigorously include:
• Removing soft furnishings – wooden floors and window blinds instead of carpets and curtains
• Complete coverage of mattress and pillows with suitable barrier
• Removal of soft toys from bed
• Wash bedding at high temperatures

Pets

Removal of household pets if an allergy is identified may improve symptoms, but remains controversial.

Outcome. Mr Valente did his best to implement allergen avoidance measures. He moved to a flat with wooden floors and no curtains and purchased a mattress cover. He used his steroid inhaler regularly twice a day and soon found that he only needed to use salbutamol once or twice a week. His peak flow diary no longer showed morning dipping and his chest tightness disappeared. He was able to continue his marathon training.

CASE REVIEW

Mr Valente presented to his GP with chest tightness and shortness of breath. Characteristic symptom patterns and expiratory wheeze on respiratory examination were sufficient to make a clinical diagnosis of asthma. This was confirmed by demonstration of variable airflow obstruction using a peak flow diary. Skin prick testing demonstrated allergy to house dust mite and grass pollen. Mr Valente's symptoms improved with low dose inhaled steroids and allergen avoidance measures and he was able to train for the marathon.

KEY POINTS

• Asthma is characterized by intermittent and variable airflow obstruction
• Asthma is a clinical diagnosis
• Clinical features pointing to a diagnosis of asthma include chest tightness, shortness of breath or cough that is worse:
  ○ on exercise
  ○ with a change in temperature
  ○ in smoky or irritant atmospheres
  ○ at night
• Atopy is a tendency to develop an allergic condition, including asthma, eczema and hayfever
• Atopy is *not* the same as asthma. Not all people with atopy develop asthma, not all people with asthma are atopic ('intrinsic' asthma)
• Asthmatic patients undergo investigation to:
  ○ confirm the presence of variable airflow obstruction
  ○ determine whether they are atopic and, if so, which allergens they react to
• After investigation treatment is:
  ○ non-pharmacological – allergen avoidance if appropriate
  ○ pharmacological – inhaled steroids to reduce airway inflammation and bronchodilators to reduce symptoms
• Patients with asthma can live an active life if their asthma is adequately treated

Case 3 — A 31-year-old woman with poorly-controlled asthma

Frances Johnson is a 31-year-old woman who presents to her GP with mild shortness of breath and a non-productive cough, worse at night. Her symptoms deteriorated slightly with a cold several weeks previously and have not improved. She also complains of itchy eyes, sneezing and persistent blockage of her nose.

She was diagnosed with asthma at the age of 12 and given a blue and a brown inhaler. She remembers undergoing skin prick testing, which was positive for house dust mite allergy. Her asthma was not a problem until the last few years when she restarted inhaled salbutamol. She now needs this 3–4 times per day to help her breathing. She does not measure her peak flow rates as she has lost her peak flow meter but remembers her best was around 400 L/min.

Summarize Miss Johnson's problems

• She has a past history of asthma as a child which has recurred as an adult

• Her symptoms appear to have worsened following a respiratory tract infection

• Her asthma symptoms are not controlled with 'as needed' use of a bronchodilator (salbutamol)

• Her persistent upper respiratory tract symptoms (itchy eyes, sneezing, nasal blockage) could indicate allergic rhinitis

How should you approach assessment of her asthma?

The key issues to be determined in this consultation are:

• Is she having an acute exacerbation of asthma severe enough to require oral steroid treatment or hospital referral?

• If not, how should her chronic asthma be managed?

What other information do you need to complete this assessment?

Criteria defining moderate, acute severe and life-threatening asthma exacerbations are given in Box 31.

Pulse rate, respiratory rate and peak flow measurement are required to complete the assessment.

On examination:
She is speaking in full sentences
Respiratory rate is 20 breaths/min
Pulse rate is 90 beats/min
Her peak expiratory flow rate (PEFR) is 320 L/min (best 400 L/min)
She has a mild expiratory wheeze to hear on auscultation of her chest

How does this new information alter your assessment?

She has no features of an acute severe asthma attack. As her peak flow is 80% of her previous best and her symptoms are slightly worse than usual but not increasing, she does not meet the criteria for a moderate asthma exacerbation. She can be treated as having poorly controlled chronic asthma.

What are the aims of asthma treatment?

The aims of treatment are to:
• Control symptoms
• Minimize exacerbations
• Achieve best possible lung function
• Minimize side-effects and inconvenience of treatment
  Asthma control is assessed against the standards given in Box 32.

What treatment will best achieve control of her asthma symptoms?

Asthma is a chronic inflammatory process of the airways (Fig. 4, p. 5 & Fig. 27, p. 47). Symptoms are caused by a combination of bronchospasm, mucosal oedema and mucus hypersecretion, causing airflow obstruction. The mainstay of treatment for asthma is **corticosteroids**, which reduce airway inflammation (Box 33) producing symptom control, preventing exacerbations and maintaining lung function.

Box 31 Levels of severity of acute asthma exacerbations in adults (British Thoracic Society Guidelines)

Moderate asthma exacerbation
- No features of acute severe asthma
- Increasing symptoms
- PEFR 50–75% predicted or best

Acute severe asthma
Any one of:
- Cannot complete sentences in one breath
- Tachypnoea ($\geq$25 breaths/min)
- Tachycardia ($\geq$110 beats/min)
- PEFR 33–50% of predicted or best

Life-threatening asthma
Any one of:
- Silent chest
- Cyanosis
- Feeble respiratory effort
- Bradycardia, dysrrhythmia or hypotension
- Exhaustion, confusion or coma
- PEFR <33% of predicted or best
- Arterial oxygen saturation <92%, PaO_2 <8 kPa

Near-fatal asthma
- Raised $PaCO_2$

Box 32 Features of well-controlled asthma

The British Thoracic Society Asthma Guidelines define good asthma control as:
- Minimal symptoms during day and night
- Minimal need for reliever medication
- No exacerbations
- No limitation of physical activity
- Normal lung function (in practical terms FEV_1 and/or PEFR >80% predicted or best)

KEY POINT

Treatment of symptomatic asthma must include the use of **corticosteroids** to control airway inflammation in all but the mildest cases.

Box 33 Pharmacology of corticosteroids

Mechanism of action
Inhibit inflammation by:
- Inhibiting influx of inflammatory cells
- Inhibiting release of inflammatory mediators from inflammatory cells
- Reducing microvascular leakage and oedema

Some of these actions are mediated by stimulating production of lipocortin which inhibits leukotriene and prostaglandin synthesis.

Uses
In respiratory medicine corticosteroids are used for diseases including asthma, COPD and interstitial lung diseases:
- In higher doses to treat inflammation
- In lower doses to prevent recurrence of inflammation

Pharmacokinetics
- Steroids can be given topically by inhaler (e.g. beclometasone, budesonide, fluticasone), which minimizes side-effects and maximizes activity in airways inflammation
- Higher doses given intravenously (hydrocortisone) or orally (prednisolone) may be required to treat severe inflammation, but should be given for as short a time as possible to minimize side-effects

Side-effects
Inhaled steroids
Local effects include sore mouth, oral thrush, hoarse voice

Systemic steroids
- Immune suppression – increased susceptibility to infection, especially organisms normally killed by cell-mediated immunity (e.g. *Candida*, TB, protozoa)
- Metabolic effects – e.g. osteoporosis, diabetes, hypertension, cushingoid features (moon face, buffalo hump), thin skin, easy bruising, suppress growth in children
- Adrenal suppression – hypoadrenalism if stop treatment quickly

How are corticosteroids given to asthmatic patients?

The administration of corticosteroids in asthma requires careful balancing of risks and benefits. In chronic asthma, inhaled steroids are usually sufficient to control asthma inflammation with minimal side-effects. In acute asthma, oral or intravenous corticosteroids are given as high treatment doses are required to control the asthma exacerbation and the benefits of treatment outweigh the risk of side-effects over the short treatment period required. The pharmacology of corticosteroids is discussed further in Box 33.

What corticosteroids should Miss Johnson receive?

Treatment should follow standard stepped guidelines for the management of chronic asthma (Box 34). Key features of this approach are:

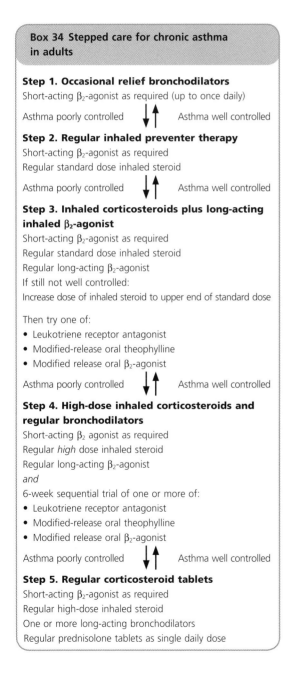

Box 34 Stepped care for chronic asthma in adults

Step 1. Occasional relief bronchodilators
Short-acting β$_2$-agonist as required (up to once daily)

Asthma poorly controlled ↓↑ Asthma well controlled

Step 2. Regular inhaled preventer therapy
Short-acting β$_2$-agonist as required
Regular standard dose inhaled steroid

Asthma poorly controlled ↓↑ Asthma well controlled

Step 3. Inhaled corticosteroids plus long-acting inhaled β$_2$-agonist
Short-acting β$_2$-agonist as required
Regular standard dose inhaled steroid
Regular long-acting β$_2$-agonist
If still not well controlled:
Increase dose of inhaled steroid to upper end of standard dose

Then try one of:
• Leukotriene receptor antagonist
• Modified-release oral theophylline
• Modified release oral β$_2$-agonist

Asthma poorly controlled ↓↑ Asthma well controlled

Step 4. High-dose inhaled corticosteroids and regular bronchodilators
Short-acting β$_2$ agonist as required
Regular *high* dose inhaled steroid
Regular long-acting β$_2$-agonist
and
6-week sequential trial of one or more of:
• Leukotriene receptor antagonist
• Modified-release oral theophylline
• Modified release oral β$_2$-agonist

Asthma poorly controlled ↓↑ Asthma well controlled

Step 5. Regular corticosteroid tablets
Short-acting β$_2$-agonist as required
Regular high-dose inhaled steroid
One or more long-acting bronchodilators
Regular prednisolone tablets as single daily dose

• The aim is to abolish symptoms and optimize peak flow as soon as possible
• The patient should be started on treatment on the stepped guideline at the level most likely to achieve this aim
• Once control of asthma is achieved treatment can be stepped down if control is good or stepped up for increasing symptoms

Miss Johnson's symptoms are not controlled by using 'as required' bronchodilators (step 1). A reasonable next step would therefore be to add in 'a regular standard dose inhaled corticosteroid' to her treatment (step 2).

Which inhaled steroid should the GP choose?

The main options are:
• Beclometasone
• Budesonide
• Fluticasone

Choice

In general, all of these drugs have similar efficacy and side-effects. Selection therefore comes down to patient choice of delivery device and cost. A reasonable first choice would be either beclometasone (metered dose inhaler; Fig. 29a) or budesonide (dry powder inhaler; Fig. 29d).

Dose

Beclometasone and budesonide have similar potency, therefore are used at a similar dose of 100–400 μg twice daily. However, fluticasone is more potent and provides equal clinical activity to beclometasone and budesonide at *half* the dosage. If used at step 2 it should therefore be given at 50–200 μg twice daily.

Miss Johnson's GP prescribes beclometasone 200 μg one puff morning and night and salbutamol 100 μg to use two puffs as required. The GP demonstrates use of the metered dose inhaler (MDI) and explains the difference between a reliever (bronchodilator) and a preventer (steroid) inhaler.

What is a metered dose inhaler and how is it used?

These inhalers comprise small canisters which contain the drug and a pressurized propellant gas. When the nozzle is compressed, a puff of drug is expelled from the canister. The difficult part for the patient is to coordinate a deep breath in with the puff of drug to ensure the medication reaches the lung. Patients should be advised to use their MDI as follows:

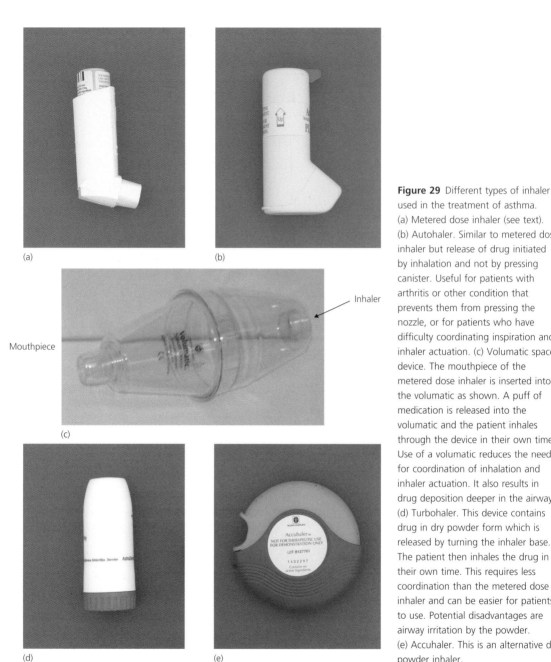

(a)

(b)

Mouthpiece

Inhaler

(c)

(d)

(e)

Figure 29 Different types of inhaler used in the treatment of asthma. (a) Metered dose inhaler (see text). (b) Autohaler. Similar to metered dose inhaler but release of drug initiated by inhalation and not by pressing canister. Useful for patients with arthritis or other condition that prevents them from pressing the nozzle, or for patients who have difficulty coordinating inspiration and inhaler actuation. (c) Volumatic spacer device. The mouthpiece of the metered dose inhaler is inserted into the volumatic as shown. A puff of medication is released into the volumatic and the patient inhales through the device in their own time. Use of a volumatic reduces the need for coordination of inhalation and inhaler actuation. It also results in drug deposition deeper in the airways. (d) Turbohaler. This device contains drug in dry powder form which is released by turning the inhaler base. The patient then inhales the drug in their own time. This requires less coordination than the metered dose inhaler and can be easier for patients to use. Potential disadvantages are airway irritation by the powder. (e) Accuhaler. This is an alternative dry powder inhaler.

- Remove the cap from the mouthpiece
- Shake the inhaler several times to mix the drug
- Breathe all the way out
- Put the inhaler in your mouth and seal your lips around the opening
- Simultaneously breathe in at a moderate and steady rate and depress the canister to release the aerosolized drug, optimizing drug delivery to the lungs
- Hold your breath for 10 s
- Breathe out, then repeat

How would you explain the difference between a reliever and a preventer inhaler to Miss Johnson?

It is important to explain that asthma symptoms are caused by swelling in the tubes carrying air into the lung. These

> **Box 35 Top tips – inhaler colours and appearance**
>
> If a patient with asthma is not sure what inhalers they are taking, the colour or appearance of the inhaler will often give the drug content away.
>
> | Inhaler | Colour/appearance |
> |---|---|
> | Short-acting β₂-agonist | Blue |
> | Short-acting antimuscarinic | Grey or clear with some green |
> | Long-acting β₂-agonist | Green |
> | Long-acting antimuscarinic | Oval container requiring insertion of a capsule |
> | Inhaled steroid | Brown/maroon |
> | | Orange (fluticasone) |
> | Combined steroid/long-acting β₂-agonist | Purple or red |

> **Box 36 Allergic rhinitis**
>
> Patients with atopy can develop nasal symptoms as a result of an allergic reaction in the nasal mucosa, similar to that seen in the lungs with asthma (Fig. 27).
>
> **Seasonal rhinitis**
> This is also known as hayfever and is the most common allergic disease with the highest prevalence in the second decade of life. Symptoms include:
> * Nasal blockage, watery discharge and sneezing
> * Itchy eyes, soft palate and ears
> * Watering eyes
>
> Seasonal rhinitis is limited to the part of the year when pollen and spore allergens are at high concentrations in the environment. Allergens causing seasonal rhinitis include:
> * Tree pollens – in April and May
> * Grass pollens – from June to August
> * Mould spores – from July to September
>
> **Perennial rhinitis**
> This is most common in the second and third decades of life. Symptoms are predominantly nasal blockage and discharge with loss of sense of smell and taste. Allergens causing perennial rhinitis include:
> * House dust mites
> * Domestic pets
> * Moulds
>
> Chronic rhinitis may lead to the development of *nasal polyps*, which are overgrowths of the nasal or sinus mucosa that remain attached to their origins by a thin stalk. These can obstruct the nasal passages, causing loss of sense of smell and taste and mouth breathing.

swollen tubes are very sensitive and can easily go into spasm. Both the swelling and the spasm narrow the air tubes, making it difficult to breathe and causing a cough. There are two types of treatment given to patients with asthma:

1 The 'preventer', or brown inhaler (steroid) (Box 35). This reduces swelling in the air tubes and, once the airways have recovered, prevents the swelling from coming back. The preventer inhaler must be taken every day to have its effects, even if the patient is feeling well
2 The 'reliever', or blue inhaler (β₂-agonist) (Box 35). This will not get rid of the underlying swelling of the air tubes, but it will relax muscle spasm and so can be used any time to make breathing easier or reduce cough. The patient does not need to take this inhaler if they feel well, but they should carry it with them to take if symptoms develop. The effects of this inhaler last about 2–4 h and repeat doses can be taken throughout the day

Frances Johnson returns for review after 2 weeks of step 2 treatment. She reports that she has noticed some improvement but she still has a non-productive cough. She is still using her short-acting bronchodilator 2–3 times per day and her steroid inhaler twice a day. Her PEFR is 350 L/min and her chest is now clear to auscultation. She comments that her blocked nose adds to her difficulty with breathing at night.

Should her asthma treatment be changed at this stage?

Her persistent cough, bronchodilator use and suboptimal PEFR indicate that her asthma is not well controlled (Box 32). She probably needs an increase in treatment to step 3. However, before this is carried out the GP should check that:

* Her inhaler technique is optimal
* She is adhering to the treatment regime
* Asthma triggers have been minimized

If these are satisfactory and her symptoms are still not controlled then her treatment should be increased to step 3 (Box 34).

How do you account for her nasal symptoms?

Nasal obstruction in patients with asthma may be caused by allergic rhinitis (Box 36) or nasal polyps. In her initial presentation Miss Johnson complained of itchy eyes and sneezing, making allergic rhinitis the likely diagnosis. Allergic rhinitis can be differentiated from infective rhinitis (the common cold) by persistence of symptoms for several weeks.

How would you confirm your provisional diagnosis of allergic rhinitis?

The diagnosis of allergic rhinitis is based on a detailed history of symptoms, atopy and nasal reactions to allergen exposure and removal. Nasal inspection should be performed to look for polyps. Investigations are not usually indicated but skin prick testing can be used to confirm allergic reactions to specific allergens that may guide allergen avoidance strategies.

How would you treat her rhinitis?

There is some evidence that treatment of rhinitis may improve asthma outcomes, as well as relieving nasal symptoms. Miss Johnson's GP should therefore consider treating her rhinitis in parallel with her asthma treatment. Treatment options for allergic rhinitis include antihistamines, decongestants and corticosteroids (Box 37).

The GP finds that Miss Johnson's asthma trigger factors have been addressed satisfactorily. She has no household pets, she does not smoke and she lives in a house with wooden floors and window blinds. She has mattress and pillow covers to reduce house dust mite exposure. Her inhaler technique is satisfactory and she is adamant that she is taking the prescribed treatment. Her GP escalates her treatment to step 3 by adding in salmeterol at a dosage of 50 µg twice a day. The inhaled steroid dosage is left at 400 µg/day. Miss Johnson is also prescribed mometasone nasal spray 50 µg (1 spray) to each nostril daily and cetirizine 10 mg in the morning for her rhinitis.

Are long-acting β_2-agonists effective and safe in asthma?

A large number of clinical trials have investigated the use of long-acting β_2-agonists in the treatment of patients with asthma and these have recently been summarized in a systematic Cochrane review (*Cochrane Database Systematic Review* 2007 Jan 24; 1: CD001385). The review found that there were benefits for patients of using long-acting β_2-agonists (Box 38):
- Improved lung function
- Significantly fewer symptoms

> **Box 37 Pharmacology of drugs used to treat allergic rhinitis**
>
> Drugs in each of these classes are available over-the-counter for self-medication.
>
> **Antihistamines**
> For example, chlorphenamine (Piriton), cetirizine:
> - *Mechanism of action*. Block histamine receptors, preventing the early phase reaction of the allergic response (Fig. 27)
> - *Uses*. Control symptoms in mild allergic rhinitis
> - *Pharmacokinetics*. Can be given orally or topically
> - *Side-effects*. Chlorphenamine causes drowsiness. Second-generation drugs (e.g. cetirizine) do not cross the blood–brain barrier and are therefore non-sedating
>
> **Decongestants**
> For example, ephedrine hydrochloride
> - *Mechanism of action*. Sympathomimetics cause constriction of mucosal blood vessels, reducing oedema of the nasal mucosa and relieving nasal obstruction
> - *Uses*. Short term to relieve congestion and allow penetration of nasal steroid
> - *Pharmacokinetics*. Can be given orally or topically
> - *Side-effects*. Once the use of decongestants is stopped there is secondary vasodilatation causing rebound nasal congestion and recurrence of symptoms. This is particularly problematic if decongestants are used for more than 7 days. Therefore, they should only be given as a short course
>
> **Corticosteroids**
> For example, beclometasone, mometasone
> - *Mechanism of action*. Anti-inflammatory (Box 33)
> - *Uses*. Treatment and prevention of allergic rhinitis
> - *Pharmacokinetics*. Used topically in allergic rhinitis as nasal drops or spray
> - *Side-effects*:
>   - worsening of untreated nasal infection
>   - dryness, irritation and bleeding of nasal mucosa
>   - raised intraocular pressure
>   - headache

- Less use of rescue medications
- Higher quality of life scores

However, the review also found that there were risks of treatment. The review estimated that for every 1250 patients with asthma treated with long-acting β_2-agonists

---

> **Box 38 Pharmacology of β₂-adrenoceptor agonists**
>
> **Mechanism of action**
> Act at β₂-adrenoceptors to stimulate bronchial smooth muscle relaxation through activation of adenyl cyclase
>
> **Uses**
> Relief of symptoms from airflow obstruction (asthma and COPD):
> - Short-acting β₂-agonists (salbutamol, terbutaline) are used for acute relief of bronchospasm or to prevent bronchospasm (e.g. before exercise or going out into cold air)
> - Long-acting β₂-agonists (salmeterol, formoterol) are used to maintain bronchodilatation and prevent symptoms over a 12-h period (e.g. overnight)
>
> **Pharmacokinetics**
> Duration of action:
> - Short-acting β₂-agonists (e.g. salbutamol, terbutaline) act immediately and have a biological half-life of 2–3 h
> - Long-acting β₂-agonists (e.g. salmeterol, formoterol) remain at the receptor longer and have a longer duration of action of up to 15 h. For example, salmeterol has a long lipophilic tail which binds to an exoreceptor near the β₂-adrenoceptors in airway smooth muscle
>
> Route of administration:
> - Inhaled directly into the lungs – maximizes efficacy and minimizes side-effects
> - Short-acting β₂-agonists can also be given:
>   ○ by nebulizer – higher dose and less coordination and respiratory effort required to take therapy
>   ○ orally – if inhalers cannot be used (e.g. small children)
>   ○ intravenously – emergency use where severe airflow obstruction prevents inhalation
>
> **Side-effects**
> Tremor, tachycardia, anxiety, hypokalaemia.

there was one extra asthma-related death. This was particularly seen in patients *not* taking inhaled corticosteroids.

Why might long-acting β₂-agonists increase the risk of asthma-related death?

The mechanisms are not fully understood. It is possible that long-acting β₂-agonists mask asthma symptoms and

delay patients from seeking medical care, which may result in a more severe or life-threatening asthma attack. Alternatively long-acting β₂-agonists may reduce the sensitivity of β₂-receptors, making short-acting β₂-agonists less effective during an acute attack.

What are the implications of these findings for patient care?

Long-acting β₂-agonists should *not* be used in patients with asthma without inhaled corticosteroids. However, they appear to have clinical benefit when used with inhaled corticosteroids as per stepped guidelines.

> **KEY POINT**
>
> Long-acting β₂-agonists should not be prescribed to patients with asthma without inhaled corticosteroids.

Miss Johnson returns for review 2 weeks later and has improved again. Her cough is much better and she has used her short-acting bronchodilator inhaler once in the last week. Her PEFR is now 380 L/min and her nasal symptoms are improving. Her GP refers her to the respiratory nurse for a self-management plan. Miss Johnson tells the nurse that she is not happy about taking inhaled steroids as she is worried she may put on weight and asks how serious it would be if she stopped taking them.

What is an asthma self-management plan?

This is a personalized action plan usually compiled by a respiratory nurse in consultation with the patient. It gives the patient instructions on how to increase treatment if their symptoms worsen or if the PEFR drops below a level identified as a percentage of their best PEFR. Similarly, if the patient's symptoms have been controlled and stable for suitable time period (e.g. 3 months), instructions are given about how to step down treatment. The patient is also given a reserve course of antibiotics and steroids so that prompt treatment can be started for an infective exacerbation. The management plan empowers the patient to manage their asthma themselves with the support of the respiratory nurse, who is usually contactable at short notice.

> **Box 39 Pharmacology of leukotriene receptor antagonists (montelukast, zafirlukast)**
>
> **Mechanism of action**
> The cysteinyl-leukotrienes (LTC_4 and LTD_4) are inflammatory mediators released by eosinophils and other inflammatory cells during the pathogenesis of asthma. They stimulate bronchoconstriction, mucus hypersecretion and mucosal oedema. Montelukast and zafirlukast block leukotriene receptors, inhibiting these inflammatory effects.
>
> **Uses**
> Step 3 or 4 treatment to control chronic asthma. Appear to be particularly effective in exercise- and aspirin-induced asthma and patients with associated rhinitis and/or nasal polyps.
>
> **Pharmacokinetics**
> Unlike most other asthma drugs they are taken orally once per day which may aid adherence to treatment.
>
> **Side-effects**
> These include gastrointestinal disturbances, headache, thirst and insomnia.

> **Box 40 Pharmacology of xanthines (theophylline, aminophylline)**
>
> **Mechanism of action**
> Xanthines inhibit phosphodiesterase enzymes which metabolize secondary messengers inside airway smooth muscle cells. Phosphodiesterase enzyme inhibition causes a build-up of cyclic adenosine monophosphate (cAMP) in airway smooth muscle cells and bronchodilatation.
>
> **Uses**
> Bronchodilatation in patients with severe acute asthma or stable COPD.
>
> **Pharmacokinetics**
> • Xanthines have a narrow therapeutic range; their lowest effective plasma concentration ($10\,\mu g/mL$) is close to their toxic concentration ($20\,\mu g/mL$).
> • Xanthines are metabolized in the liver by cytochrome p450 enzymes. If drugs that inhibit these enzymes are co-prescribed with xanthines, xanthine plasma levels may rise from therapeutic to toxic concentrations. Liver enzyme inhibitors include:
>   ○ erythromycin
>   ○ ciprofloxacin
>   ○ sodium valproate
> • Plasma levels of xanthines should be monitored routinely and the dose reduced if liver enzyme inhibitors are co-administered
>
> **Side-effects**
> More likely at toxic plasma concentrations:
> • Nausea and vomiting
> • Arrhythmias and convulsions

What therapeutic options could have been considered if Miss Johnson's asthma had not improved with step 3 treatment?

The next treatment options (Box 34) would have been to optimize step 3 treatment by increasing the dose of inhaled steroids and, if asthma was still not well controlled, to try a leukotriene antagonist (Box 39), theophylline (Box 40) or an oral β_2-agonist. If asthma still was not well controlled, step 4 options include high-dose inhaled corticosteroids and step 5 involves commencement of regular oral prednisolone.

How should the nurse answer Miss Johnson's question?

The nurse should explain that it is essential that Miss Johnson's asthma is adequately treated as if not:
• She may have an acute exacerbation which could be life-threatening
• Chronic inflammation can lead to airway remodelling with permanent narrowing and disabling breathlessness in the long term

The nurse can reassure Miss Johnson that very little of the inhaled steroids will be absorbed and she is extremely unlikely to put on weight. However, she should advise her that inhaled steroids can cause oral thrush and a hoarse voice. Miss Johnson can minimize the risk of these effects by rinsing her mouth and gargling with water after taking the inhaler. Miss Johnson can be reassured that it may be possible to reduce her inhaled steroids in the future if her symptoms are controlled.

Outcome. Miss Johnson took her inhaled steroids and salmeterol regularly for the next 3 months. Once her symptoms were well controlled she stopped the salmeterol and 6 weeks later reduced inhaled steroids from 400 to $200\,\mu g/day$. Six months later she was stable and opted to stop inhaled steroids altogether. She remained aware, using her self-management plan, that she would need to restart treatment and seek advice should her symptoms recur.

CASE REVIEW

Frances Johnson presents to her GP with symptoms of asthma recurring from childhood following a disease-free period in her twenties. Her GP finds no evidence of a moderate or severe exacerbation and decides to treat her as chronic poorly controlled asthma according to standard stepped asthma care guidelines. Miss Johnson requires escalation of asthma treatment to step 2 (addition of standard dose inhaled steroids), then step 3 (addition of long-acting β_2-agonist) to control her symptoms. She also receives nasal steroids and antihistamines for rhinitis and sees the respiratory nurse for a self-management plan. After her symptoms have been controlled for some months she is able to step her treatment down, but remains aware of the need to restart treatment and seek help early if her symptoms recur.

KEY POINTS

- The aims of asthma treatment are to control symptoms, minimize exacerbations and optimize lung function
- Features of poorly controlled asthma include:
  - daytime or nocturnal symptoms
  - regular use of reliever medication
  - falling PEFR
  - recent exacerbations
- In a patient presenting with poorly controlled asthma, the first step should be to determine whether this is a moderate or severe exacerbation requiring acute treatment
- If the poor asthma control is chronic, control should be improved using the stepped guidelines for chronic asthma management
- The mainstay of asthma treatment is **corticosteroids**
- In chronic asthma, corticosteroids are given as inhalers to optimize drug delivery to the affected airways and minimize side-effects
- After taking inhaled steroids patients should be advised to rinse their mouth and gargle to reduce the risk of oral thrush or a hoarse voice
- The stepped guidelines should be used both to increase treatment in patients with poorly controlled asthma and to reduce treatment in patients with well-controlled asthma. Treatment should be reviewed and adjusted approximately every 3 months
- Long-acting β_2-agonists can be used in the treatment of asthma, but should *only* be used with inhaled steroids as long-acting β_2-agonists are associated with an increased risk of asthma-related deaths if used alone
- Patients with asthma commonly have associated allergic rhinitis, which should be treated as this may improve symptoms and assist with asthma control
- Patients with asthma should see a nurse with appropriate expertise to develop a self-management plan and for support in management of their condition

Case 4 · A 22-year-old man with life-threatening shortness of breath

Chris Carter is a 22-year-old man who has been brought into accident and emergency by his girlfriend. He is unable to speak because of shortness of breath which came on suddenly 2 days ago. His observations are:
- *Respiratory rate 30/min*
- *Pulse 120 beats/min*
- *Blood pressure 110/70 mmHg*
- *Temperature 36.7°C*
- *Oxygen saturations 92% on room air*
- *Glasgow Coma Score 15*

What should you do first?
In an emergency always start by checking airway, breathing and circulation (ABC). On observation, Mr Carter has a patent airway, is breathing and has an adequate cardiac output.

What other assessment can you make from his initial observations?
Mr Carter is tachycardic, probably as part of a stress response to his acute illness, but is maintaining an adequate blood pressure. He is in respiratory distress but managing to raise his respiratory rate to maintain oxygen saturations at 92%. He is not compromised from a neurological point of view as he has a normal Glasgow Coma Score.

What are the priorities for his management?
In an emergency situation it is vital that you take measures to save life and minimize potential disability even before you make a full assessment (Box 24, p. 36). Mr Carter is potentially at risk of cell injury and death from his hypoxia, which will have greatest impact on his brain and his heart. Immediate measures for Mr Carter should therefore include:
- High concentration oxygen therapy, 15 L through a mask with a reservoir bag

- Insertion of an intravenous line to secure access for drug and fluid delivery
- Continuous monitoring:
  - oxygen saturation
  - cardiac rhythm
  - pulse
  - blood pressure

He then needs more detailed assessment to identify and treat the underlying cause of his hypoxia.

What is your differential diagnosis for his acute shortness of breath?
As he is a young man the most likely diagnoses are:
- Acute asthma attack
- Pneumothorax
- Inhaled foreign body
- Allergic reaction (anaphylaxis)
- Lung trauma

How would you assess him to distinguish between these causes?
Although Mr Carter is unable to speak he is conscious and his girlfriend is with him. You should therefore briefly (1–2 min) establish whether he has a past history of asthma, allergy or lung disease and ask about trauma or foreign body inhalation. He should then be examined quickly to look for clinical signs that could point to an underlying diagnosis.

Mr Carter has a past history of asthma but no known allergies. There is no history of trauma or foreign body inhalation. On examination he is holding the sides of the trolley, leaning forward and gasping for breath. Heart sounds are faint but normal and there are no signs of cardiac failure. On respiratory examination his trachea is midline, expansion is equal on both sides but appears reduced, percussion is resonant and he has widespread expiratory polyphonic wheeze throughout both lung fields.

Do these new findings help you to make a diagnosis?

Symmetrical findings on chest examination (Table 1, p. 28) and expiratory wheeze in a patient with a past history of asthma are most likely to be caused by an acute exacerbation of asthma. Anaphylaxis and large airway obstruction by an inhaled foreign body can also cause wheeze, but lack of relevant history makes these diagnoses less likely than asthma.

What does his posture signify?

Patients in respiratory distress may grip the sides of their hospital trolley to fix their upper limb girdle. This allows them to use accessory muscles, including their pectoral muscles, to support inspiration.

What treatment should you give him immediately?

He should be treated as an acute exacerbation of asthma with immediate β_2-agonists for bronchodilatation and steroids to reduce airway inflammation.

Mr Carter is commenced on 5 mg salbutamol, nebulized using high flow oxygen and given 200 mg hydrocortisone intravenously.

What is the pathology underlying an asthma attack?

The underlying pathology in asthma is airway inflammation, which leads to mucosal swelling, increased secretion of mucus into the airway lumen and spasm of the smooth muscle of the airway wall. The net effect of these processes is to narrow the airway lumen, making it more difficult for the patient to breathe.

How do bronchodilators help?

These relax smooth muscle spasm and open up the airways, making it easier to breathe and improving oxygenation.

How is salbutamol nebulized?

A liquid preparation of salbutamol is put into a chamber of a nebulizer mask (Fig. 30). A gas (usually oxygen or air) is bubbled through the liquid and this vaporizes the drug into small droplets that can be inhaled into the airways. Patients with asthma should receive salbutamol nebulized with high flow oxygen to prevent them from becoming hypoxic during nebulization. Antimuscarinics (ipratropium) and steroids (budesonide) can also be given by nebulizer.

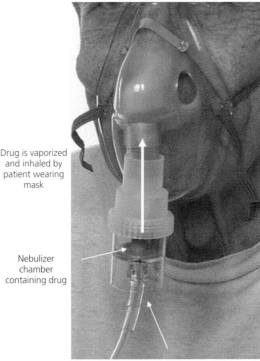

Drug is vaporized and inhaled by patient wearing mask

Nebulizer chamber containing drug

Oxygen or air input

Figure 30 Patient receiving nebulized bronchodilator.

Why is the nebulizer used instead of his normal inhaler?

A nebulizer allows delivery of high doses of β_2-agonists (i.e. 2.5–5 mg salbutamol over a few minutes compared to 100 μg salbutamol per single puff of an inhaler). It is also easier for a patient with acute asthma to inhale nebulized drug passively as they breathe, rather than to try to generate the active and coordinated deep breaths required to take an inhaler. However, if a nebulizer is not available high dose β_2-agonists can be delivered using 4–6 puffs of the inhaler through a volumatic device (Fig. 29, p. 54) taken every 10–20 min.

How quickly should the salbutamol act?

Bronchodilatation should commence immediately with rapid improvement of symptoms. Nebulizers should be repeated every 15–30 min in patients with acute exacerbations of asthma.

How do corticosteroids help?

These are anti-inflammatory and reduce mucosal oedema and secretions. Corticosteroids are crucial in asthma as they treat the underlying inflammation and the patient is unlikely to recover without steroids.

How quickly do you expect the steroids to act?

Corticosteroids exert most of their actions by binding to receptors and altering gene transcription. This process can take some time and corticosteroids are said not to have any effect for at least half an hour after the drug is given. However, studies have shown that the earlier corticosteroids are given in an asthma attack the better the outcome. The first dose of corticosteroids is usually given intravenously. This may be helpful in breathless patients who have difficulty swallowing and makes sure the patient receives the drug. However, oral steroids are just as effective in acute asthma as intravenous steroids.

Which investigations would you perform next (and why)?

• Peak expiratory flow rate (PEFR) to determine severity of asthma exacerbation
• Arterial blood gas to assess pH and $PaCO_2$ levels
• Chest X-ray to exclude other causes of breathlessness such as pneumothorax and underlying consolidation
• Full blood count and C-reactive protein (CRP) to look for evidence of infection
• Electrocardiogram (ECG) – to exclude cardiac disease as a cause or consequence of his condition

Initial investigation results are as follows:

		Normal range
PEFR	210 L/min	(Predicted 590 L/min)
Chest X-ray see Fig. 31		
Blood tests:		
Haemoglobin	14 g/dL	(12.5–17 g/dL)
White cells	12 × 10⁹/L	(4.0–11.0 × 10⁹/L)
Platelets	220 × 10⁹/L	(120–400 × 10⁹/L)
CRP	2 mg/L	(<4 mg/L)
ECG	Sinus tachycardia	

How do you interpret these results?

• His peak flow is 35% predicted, which is a feature of acute severe asthma (Box 31, p. 52)

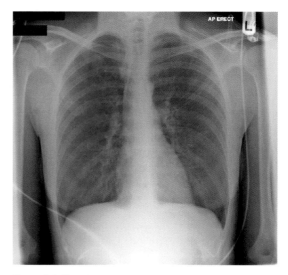

Figure 31 Chest X-ray.

• There is no evidence of pneumothorax or pneumonia on his chest X-ray. Evidence of more than six ribs anteriorly seen above flattened diaphragms indicates that his lungs are hyperinflated
• He has a mildly elevated white cell count. This could indicate underlying infection or be part of the inflammatory process of asthma. His CRP is normal, making infection less likely
• The ECG reassures you that there is no cardiovascular problem, either as a cause or consequence of his breathlessness. Tachycardia is a normal response to hypoxia and the physiological stress of an asthma attack

His arterial blood gases on air show:

		Normal range
pH	7.58	(7.35–7.45)
PaO₂	8.5 kPa	(10–13.1 kPa)
PaCO₂	4.1 kPa	(4.9–6.1 kPa)
HCO₃⁻	23 mmol/L	(22–28 mmol/L)

How do you interpret his arterial blood gases?

• PaO_2 is low, indicating reduction of alveolar ventilation secondary to airflow obstruction. He is hypoxic but is not in respiratory failure, which is defined as $PaO_2 < 8$ kPa
• $PaCO_2$ is low, indicating increased ventilation to compensate for hypoxia
• pH is raised (alkalosis). When $PaCO_2$ is reduced [1], this drives the Henderson–Hasselbach equation to the right [2], reducing hydrogen ion concentration [3] and

causing an alkalosis. As the respiratory problem is the primary abnormality, this is called a respiratory alkalosis

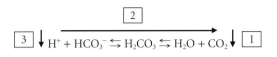

How do you decide how severe his asthma attack is?

Mr Carter meets the criteria for a severe asthma attack (Box 31, p. 52). His peak flow is <50% predicted (35%), he has a respiratory rate of >25/min (30/min), is tachycardic (120 beats/min) and is unable to complete full sentences. He does not have any features of life-threatening asthma. It is important to make this assessment as this determines how and where he should be treated. Patients with severe attacks should usually be admitted to hospital for intensive therapy. Patients with life-threatening or near-fatal asthma will need intensive care monitoring.

After Mr Carter has received three 5 mg salbutamol nebulizers and 200 mg hydrocortisone he is reviewed. His observations now are:
- *Respiratory rate 32/min*
- *Pulse 132 beats/min*
- *Blood pressure 124/82 mmHg*
- *Oxygen saturations 96% on high inhaled oxygen concentrations*
- *PEFR 170 L/min*

How do you assess his progress?

Mr Carter has shown no signs of improvement on treatment. He remains tachycardic and tachypnoeic. If anything his asthma has deteriorated as his PEFR has fallen from 210 L/min (35% predicted) to 170 L/min (28% predicted) and his exacerbation is now classified as life-threatening (Box 31, p. 52). His increasing tachycardia could be a side-effect of salbutamol.

As he has not responded to initial treatment, what would you do next?

He needs additional bronchodilator treatment and referral to intensive care should be considered. He should continue with repeated nebulized salbutamol 2.5–5 mg every 15–30 min or continuously if possible. Other bronchodilators can be added to this treatment.

Nebulized ipratropium bromide (Box 41)

This should be given at the dose of 0.5 mg every 4–6 h and should produce significantly greater bronchodilatation than salbutamol alone. It is only used in acute severe or life-threatening asthma or patients who are not responding to β_2-agonists.

Intravenous magnesium sulphate

A single infusion of 1.2–2 g should be given over 20 min. Clinical trials have shown an improvement in PEFR and FEV_1 measurements in patients with acute severe asthma exacerbations treated with intravenous magnesium sulphate compared to placebo (Box 42).

Other options include the use of intravenous β_2-agonists or intravenous theophylline. However, there is less evidence to support the use of these treatments.

Box 41 Pharmacology of antimuscarinic bronchodilators

Mechanism of action
- Cholinergic nerves maintain resting tone in the bronchi and stimulate mucus secretion. Antimuscarinic drugs block these effects, resulting in bronchodilatation and reduced mucus secretion

Uses
- Acute severe or life-threatening asthma with salbutamol to increase bronchodilatation. *Not* part of stepped guidelines for chronic asthma
- Chronic obstructive pulmonary disease (COPD). Antimuscarinic drugs are particularly useful in COPD patients who have increased resting bronchial tone and increased mucus secretion

Pharmacokinetics
- Duration of action
  - short-acting (e.g. ipratropium bromide) causes bronchodilatation for up to 5 h, therefore given four times daily
  - long-acting (e.g. tiotropium bromide) causes bronchodilatation for 24 h, therefore given once daily
- Route of administration
  - Inhaler (all) or nebulizer (short-acting only)

Main side-effects
- Dry mouth, urinary retention, constipation

> **Box 42 Pharmacology of intravenous magnesium**
>
> **Mechanism of action**
> Magnesium sulphate causes bronchodilatation. The mechanism is unclear but may include:
> - Relaxation of bronchial smooth muscle by altering intracellular calcium concentrations
> - Reduction of neurotransmitter release at motor nerve terminals, reducing excitability of smooth muscle membranes
> - Facilitating activation of adenyl cyclase by β_2-agonists
> - Anti-inflammatory effects, reducing production of superoxide by neutrophils
>
> **Uses**
> - Single infusion for bronchodilatation in acute severe or life-threatening asthma exacerbations
>
> **Pharmacokinetics**
> - Administered intravenously. Causes diarrhoea if given orally
>
> **Main side-effects**
> - Transient flushing, lightheadedness, lethargy, nausea or burning at the IV site
> - Hypermagnesaemia could cause muscle weakness and respiratory failure if excessive doses are given

Mr Carter receives nebulized 0.5 mg ipratropium and intravenous 2 g magnesium sulphate and continues with nebulized salbutamol. He remains tachypnoeic and his blood gases are repeated on high oxygen concentrations:

		Normal range
pH	*7.36*	*(7.35–7.45)*
PaO$_2$	*11.7 kPa*	*(10–13.1 kPa)*
PaCO$_2$	*6.3 kPa*	*(4.9–6.1 kPa)*
HCO$_3^-$	*26 mmol/L*	*(22–28 mmol/L)*

How have his blood gases changed?

The most concerning change is an increase in $PaCO_2$ levels and fall in pH. At first sight his PaO_2 appears normal, but in fact he is requiring high inspired oxygen concentrations to maintain oxygenation.

What is the significance of the new findings?

A rising $PaCO_2$ now puts him into the category of near-fatal asthma. He requires urgent intensive care input with possible ventilatory support.

What might have caused this deterioration?

- Mr Carter may be tiring with decreased respiratory effort leading to a $PaCO_2$ rise
- Patients with asthma can develop a secondary pneumothorax during exacerbation and this should always be considered if there is a sudden deterioration or failure to improve

Mr Carter is transferred to the intensive care unit for monitoring, treatment and consideration of invasive ventilation. A chest X-ray shows no evidence of pneumothorax. His condition is optimized with continuous nebulized salbutamol and intravenous theophylline. Over the next 30 min there is a gradual improvement in Mr Carter's condition until he is able to say a few words. He is considered not to require invasive ventilation. After 48 h his condition has improved sufficiently for him to continue his recovery on a general medical ward.

How should his asthma be monitored on the general ward?

Ongoing assessment is important to evaluate response to treatment and recovery. Observations should include respiratory rate and O_2 saturations.

Peak flow chart

Peak expiratory flow rate should be measured morning and evening, before and after nebulizers. During an asthma attack PEFR will be reduced, lower in the morning than in the evening and increased by nebulizer treatment (bronchodilator reversibility). A rise in peak flow to normal values with disappearance of morning dipping and reduction in bronchodilator reversibility indicates recovery.

As his asthma improves, how should his treatment be modified?
Corticosteroids

- British Thoracic Society guidelines state that patients with acute asthma should receive 40–50 mg oral prednisolone for at least 5 days or until recovery

• He should commence inhaled steroids as soon as possible during admission. The main reason for this is to ensure that he is taking inhaled steroids on discharge to form part of his chronic asthma management plan to prevent further exacerbations. Patients who have had an exacerbation in the past 2 years requiring steroids or nebulized bronchodilator should be taking inhaled steroids as per the stepped asthma guidelines (see Case 3).

Bronchodilatators

He should have nebulized bronchodilators until:
• His symptoms have resolved
• PEFR morning dipping has decreased to less than 20% of PEFR

Bronchodilators should then be switched to inhaled therapy.

Suggested treatment regime on discharge

A reasonable approach to treatment on discharge after an asthma exacerbation would be to give patients:
• A steroid inhaler at standard or high dose twice daily
• A long-acting β_2-agonist twice daily

• A short-acting β_2-agonist inhaler initially to use regularly (e.g. 4 times per day) and then to use when needed (p.r.n.)

Patients with asthma will thus leave hospital following an exacerbation on step 3 or 4 treatment (depending on inhaled steroid dose) of the asthma guidelines, with a view to stepping down treatment in outpatients when their asthma is stable.

When is it safe to discharge Mr Carter from hospital?

A reasonable approach is to allow patients to go home when:
• They are able to mobilize around the ward without shortness of breath
• They are not breathless or troubled by severe cough at night
• They have been stable for 24 h after switching from nebulized to inhaled bronchodilators
• There is no significant morning dipping (<20% of maximum) on PEFR chart and values have risen to >75% best or predicted values

| Mr Carter's peak flow chart is shown in Fig. 32.

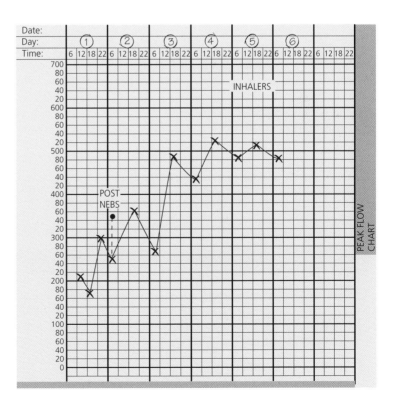

Figure 32 Inpatient peak flow chart.

PART 2: CASES

How do you interpret this chart?

Initially, Mr Carter's PEFR recordings are low, there is morning dipping and a pre-nebulizer reading is lower than the post-nebulizer reading. As he improves, his peak flow rises and morning dipping is reduced. By day 4, his morning dipping is less than 20% and his peak flow is 530 L/min (90% predicted best of 590 L/min). He is therefore switched to inhaled therapy and remains stable on this for a further 24 h, at which stage he is ready for discharge.

What should be done before he leaves hospital to reduce the chance of further exacerbations?

Mr Carter should receive education about his asthma and how to prevent further attacks, preferably from a specialist respiratory nurse or other trained staff. This education should include:

- Correct inhaler technique
- Making and recording home peak flow measurements
- Explanation of the purpose of different inhalers prescribed and the importance of taking them
- Self-management plan, including advice about early management of future exacerbations and when to seek help

Some of this will need to be carried out or continued as an outpatient and so an appointment should be given for follow-up in the respiratory clinic.

Why is education and follow-up so important?

Asthma can kill. There are around 1400 deaths annually in the UK from asthma according to national statistics. Factors associated with death include:

- Severe asthma
- Inadequate treatment or monitoring of asthma
- Adverse behavioural or psychosocial features leading to inadequate asthma management

Most severe acute asthma exacerbations develop over 6 h or more, so there should be time for patients to receive appropriate help. Prompt action at the onset of an exacerbation may prevent hospitalization and death. Education and follow-up can be used to advise patients when and how to seek timely help.

Education should also address asthma triggers (Box 29, p. 47) and measures that can be taken to avoid exacerbations. Patients with severe asthma or recent hospital admission should be advised to have vaccination against influenza.

Reference

Further advice and information for patients with asthma is provided by Asthma UK and can be found at www.asthma.org.uk/index.html

---

Outcome. Mr Carter is seen by the respiratory nurse specialist. His inhaler technique is corrected and he receives a self-management plan and a number to contact if he has questions. He is discharged taking:

40 mg prednisolone orally for 5 more days

250 μg beclometasone per dose, 2 puffs twice daily

25 μg salmeterol per dose, 2 puffs twice daily

Salbutamol metered dose inhaler (100 μg per dose), 2 puffs as required

In outpatients 4 weeks later his symptoms have resolved. His PEFR is 580 L/min. His treatment is gradually stepped down over several months until he is maintained on 200 μg beclometasone twice daily and salbutamol p.r.n.

CASE REVIEW

Mr Carter presents to accident and emergency with a severe asthma exacerbation. He does not respond to initial treatment with nebulized salbutamol and intravenous hydrocortisone, so ipratropium nebulizers and intravenous magnesium are given. He tires and his $PaCO_2$ starts to rise, which puts him into the category of 'near-fatal asthma'. The intensive care team are called and manage to avoid intubation and mechanical ventilation by optimizing medical treatment. Mr Carter is monitored on intensive care for 48 h, and then transferred to the ward to complete his recovery. Prior to discharge, asthma triggers, inhaler technique and self-management issues are addressed by the respiratory nurse specialist to reduce the risk of exacerbation recurrence and he is followed-up in the chest clinic.

KEY POINTS

- Asthma kills around 1400 people annually in the UK
- Recognition and prompt treatment of asthma exacerbations is essential to reduce asthma-related deaths
- At presentation, clinical features and basic investigations should be used to determine the severity of the asthma exacerbation
- Corticosteroids *must* be given to patients with asthma exacerbations as soon as possible to treat underlying inflammation
- 2.5–5 mg nebulized salbutamol every 15–30 min should be used to improve symptoms and respiratory function in severe asthma while the anti-inflammatory effects of corticosteroids are taking effect
- If patients respond poorly to nebulized salbutamol other bronchodilators recommended for use are:
  - nebulized ipratropium
  - intravenous magnesium
- Intravenous theophylline or salbutamol can also be tried by respiratory clinicians
- Failure to respond or deterioration in a patient with acute asthma can be caused by:
  - intractable disease
  - tiring/exhaustion
  - secondary pneumothorax
- Intensive care should be considered early for patients with life-threatening or near-fatal asthma
- Recovery from asthma exacerbation can be judged by improvement in symptoms and peak flow recordings
- Patients can usually be discharged safely when they have minimal symptoms and PEFR >75% best or predicted with <20% morning dipping after 24 h on inhalers
- Prior to discharge, patients should receive education from trained staff to reduce the risk of further exacerbations
- Patients should be followed-up by a respiratory specialist after hospitalization for an asthma exacerbation

Case 5 · A 65-year-old man with worsening shortness of breath

Mr Newman is a 65-year-old man who attends the chest clinic with the following letter from his general practitioner:
Dear Doctor,
Thank you for seeing this 65-year-old man who complains of worsening shortness of breath. He first presented to our practice 2 years ago with mild shortness of breath on exercise and was started on inhaled salbutamol. This helped initially but he is now more breathless. I would be grateful for your assistance in establishing the cause of his breathlessness and advising on further treatment as appropriate.
Yours faithfully,
Dr Clarkson

How will the specialist approach the consultation?

Mr Newman has been referred to hospital for a specialist opinion. Dr Clarkson's letter is helpful as it clearly states why the patient has been referred and what is required of the specialist. Thus, the focus of the consultation will be the diagnosis and treatment of breathlessness. Mr Newman may have other health concerns which can be raised, but if unrelated to his breathlessness may be referred back to his GP.

How would you approach taking Mr Newman's history?

An approach to a consultation with a breathless patient is outlined in Part 1B. You should start with an open question, quantify his shortness of breath, then attempt to determine if the cause of his shortness of breath is respiratory, cardiac or from another source (Fig. 11, p. 18), before constructing a more specific differential diagnosis.

Mr Newman describes his problem in his own words. 'I'm an active man but my breathing won't keep up with me. I now walk more slowly than my wife if we go out together and have to stop to get my breath if I am carrying shopping or going uphill'.

How would you quantify his breathlessness?

Breathlessness can be quantified using the MRC dyspnoea score (Box 12, p. 18). From the information given Mr Newman appears to have a score of 3 as he has to walk more slowly than his wife.

On further questioning Mr Newman states that his breathing is comfortable at rest, he sleeps on one pillow and does not wake up breathless at night. His breathlessness is worse following a cold or during humid weather. He has had a persistent cough for the past 2 years and brings up clear or grey sputum on most mornings. He has never coughed up blood, had chest pain or experienced palpitations. His weight is stable.

He is a current cigarette smoker and has smoked 20 cigarettes daily since the age of 19. He works as a builder, although he recently moved into the office to do lighter work because of his breathlessness. His job has always been dusty and he probably was exposed to asbestos in the past. His father died of emphysema.

Do you think his breathlessness is caused by respiratory or cardiac disease?

His history is very suggestive of respiratory disease. Particular features that point to a respiratory diagnosis are:
• Chronic productive cough consistent with chronic bronchitis
• Symptoms exacerbated by respiratory infection and change in the weather
• Extensive respiratory risk factors including cigarette smoking (46 pack years; Box 16, p. 19), dust and asbestos exposure and family history

Lack of orthopnoea, chest pain or palpitations make cardiac disease less likely. However, smoking is a risk factor for cardiac as well as respiratory disease.

How does this direct the consultation?

It would now be reasonable to consider a respiratory differential diagnosis and direct questions towards this. However, cardiac disease should remain at the back of your mind and be reconsidered if respiratory lines of enquiry draw a blank.

Give a respiratory differential diagnosis for Mr Newman

• New symptoms in older patients are usually caused by degenerative or neoplastic disease (Box 15, p. 19), so chronic obstructive pulmonary disease (COPD) and lung cancer are strong possibilities. Pulmonary fibrosis should also be considered
• Mr Newman's breathlessness has come on gradually over 2 years. This is more consistent with degenerative disease such as COPD or pulmonary fibrosis, rather than lung cancer which usually causes more rapid deterioration
• Mr Newman has not noticed haemoptysis, weight loss or other systemic features. This does not exclude lung cancer but makes it less likely
• The diagnosis is therefore most likely to be COPD. Other diagnoses still to be excluded include lung cancer, lung fibrosis, cardiac disease and anaemia

If Mr Newman has COPD, how can this diagnosis be confirmed?

The definition of COPD is given in Box 43. Mr Newman has a history of tobacco smoking and symptoms of chronic bronchitis, both of which are strongly indicative

---

> **Box 43 Definition of chronic obstructive pulmonary disease (COPD)**
>
> A disease characterized by airflow obstruction that is:
> • Usually caused (in the UK) by tobacco smoking
> • Not fully reversible
> • Does not change markedly over several months
> • Is progressive
>   COPD includes diseases previously defined as chronic bronchitis and emphysema:
> • *Chronic bronchitis*. This term refers to the clinical symptoms of a daily cough productive of sputum for 3 months in 2 consecutive years
> • *Emphysema*. This term refers to a pathological process seen on histology or by computed tomography (CT) scanning. There is an abnormal increase in airspace size because of irreversible expansion of the alveoli or destruction of alveolar walls

---

of COPD. A firm diagnosis of COPD requires objective evidence of airflow obstruction. Examination and investigation are therefore required to confirm the diagnosis and exclude the main differentials and unexpected causes of breathlessness.

> *On examination Mr Newman has:*
> *No finger clubbing, no lymphadenopathy*
> *Nicotine-stained fingers*
> *Pulse 84 beats/min regular, jugular venous pressure (JVP) not elevated, blood pressure 110/70 mmHg*
> *Heart sounds normal, nil added, no pitting ankle oedema*
> *Trachea – midline, cricosternal distance two finger breadths*
> *Expansion – reduced bilaterally*
> *Percussion – resonant bilaterally, loss of cardiac dullness*
> *Breath sounds – vesicular with bilateral expiratory wheeze*

How do you interpret his examination findings?

• He has symmetrical lung disease (Table 1, p. 28) with hyperinflation (reduced cricosternal distance, loss of cardiac dullness) and expiratory wheeze. These findings are consistent with obstructive airways disease
• Nicotine-stained fingers indicate active cigarette smoking
• Absence of finger clubbing and lymphadenopathy is reassuring, as these can be features of malignant disease
• He has no clinical evidence of heart failure or arrhythmias

How would you investigate Mr Newman?

Initially, the diagnosis of COPD should be confirmed with spirometry and other diagnoses excluded with a chest X-ray and full blood count.

> *Mr Newman's spirometry is compared with predicted values in a graph in Fig. 33.*

From the graph what are Mr Newman's spirometry measurements?

• FEV_1 – he has exhaled 1.3 L after 1 s
• FVC – he exhales 3.4 L by the end of the test
• FEV_1/FVC ratio is $(1.3/3.0) \times 100 = 43\%$

How do Mr Newman's actual measurements compare with his predicted values?

• His measured FEV_1 (1.3 L) is 41% of his predicted value (3.2 L), i.e. is reduced

• His measured *FVC* (3.0 L) is 73% of his predicted value (4.1 L), i.e. is reduced
• *FEV*$_1$/*FVC* ratio is 43%, i.e. is less than 70%. The reduction in *FEV*$_1$ is therefore a result of airways obstruction (see p. 31)

Is airways obstruction always a result of COPD?

Airways obstruction is usually caused by COPD or asthma. Less commonly, airways obstruction is caused by other pathologies of large or small airways (Box 44).

How can you distinguish between COPD and asthma?

Airflow obstruction caused by COPD is characteristically not fully reversible and does not change markedly over several months. By contrast, airflow obstruction caused by asthma is usually fully reversible, unless chronic scar-

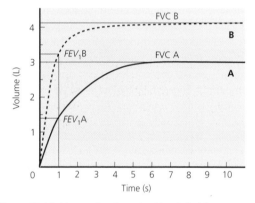

Figure 33 Mr Newman's spirometry. Line A (bold) represents Mr Newman's spirometry recorded in clinic. Line B (dotted) is his predicted spirometric curve for comparison.

ring (remodelling) has occurred, and is variable. COPD and asthma can be distinguished by:
• *Clinical features.* A useful table for distinguishing between COPD and asthma is given in national clinical guidelines and reproduced in Table 3
• *Spirometry.* If there is doubt about the diagnosis, reversibility testing can be performed. Spirometry is measured before and after inhalation of a short-acting bronchodilator (e.g. salbutamol). Significant reversibility is usually taken as an improvement in *FEV*$_1$ of ≥15% baseline value or 400 mL (NICE guidelines) and indicates asthma rather than COPD

Mr Newman is a smoker with symptoms developing in his sixties who has a chronic productive cough and progressive breathlessness. He clearly has COPD and does not need reversibility testing.

How does COPD cause airflow obstruction?

COPD is a combination of airway inflammation (bronchitis) and loss of alveoli and lung parenchyma

---

Box 44 Causes of airways obstruction other than asthma or COPD

Large airways – trachea or main bronchus
• Stricture
• Tumour
• Compression

Small airways
• Obliterative bronchiolitis
• Pulmonary oedema, compressing small airways

Table 3 Clinical features differentiating COPD and asthma. [From COPD National Clinical Guidelines. *Thorax* 2004; **59** (Suppl I): 33.]

	COPD	Asthma
Smoker or ex-smoker	Nearly all	Possibly
Symptoms under age 35	Rare	Often
Chronic productive cough	Common	Uncommon
Breathlessness	Persistent and progressive	Variable
Night-time waking with breathlessness or wheeze	Uncommon	Common
Significant diurnal or day-to-day variability of symptoms	Uncommon	Common

---

Box 45 Pathophysiology of airflow obstruction in COPD

Bronchitis

In COPD the airways are inflamed and scarred and the respiratory epithelium is partly replaced by mucus-producing goblet cells. A combination of thickened airway walls, increased luminal secretions and smooth muscle spasm narrows the airway lumen, reducing airflow (Fig. 4, p. 5).

Emphysema

The lung parenchyma is destroyed, partly because of digestion of the lung by proteolytic enzymes released by neutrophils. Figure 34 shows a lung resected from a patient with emphysema at postmortem. The lung has black staining caused by carbon from cigarettes and air pollution and contains multiple small holes resulting from loss of lung parenchyma. Figure 35 compares slices from high-resolution CT scans from a patient with normal lungs and a patient with emphysema. The emphysematous lung has multiple black holes where there should be heterogeneous grey lung parenchyma. The very large black holes are called bullae.

Emphysematous destruction of the lung parenchyma causes loss of lung elasticity and elastic recoil, which leads to airflow obstruction (Fig. 36).

Role of elastic recoil in normal respiration

- In normal lungs, the elastic recoil acts to collapse the lung and is opposed by negative intrapleural pressure which maintains lung expansion
- At rest, when intrapleural pressure (−5 kPa) equals elastic recoil (+5 kPa), no air moves into or out of the lungs (Fig. 36a)
- When the respiratory muscles contract, the intrathoracic pressure becomes more negative, overcoming elastic recoil and sucking air into the lungs
- When the respiratory muscles relax, the chest wall and diaphragm return to their resting positions, making the intrathoracic pressure more positive and pushing air out of the lungs

- Positive intrathoracic pressure has different effects on alveoli and airways:
  o the pressure forces air out of the 'spherical' alveoli into the bronchioles
  o the pressure compresses the cylindrical airways, causing them to collapse
  o during normal expiration the pressure in the airway lumen generated by air moving from the alveoli is greater than the pressure outside the airways and compression is prevented. The airways remain open throughout expiration
  o if expiration is forced the intrathoracic pressure becomes more positive (Fig. 36b) so that external pressure exceeds luminal pressure and the airways partially collapse. This can be demonstrated by comparing what happens if you breathe out quietly and when you force your breath out. On gentle expiration, your breathing will sound quiet. On forced expiration, you will hear wheezing caused by compression of your large airways

Loss of elastic recoil causes airflow obstruction

- Elastic recoil contributes to positive intrathoracic pressure required to force air out of the alveoli and maintain pressure in the airway lumen. As elastic recoil is reduced in emphysema, airway luminal pressure is reduced (Fig. 36c) and falls below external pressure during normal expiration, resulting in airway collapse
- Patients with emphysema thus find it harder to breathe out than breathe in and air gets trapped in the alveoli, causing hyperinflation
- Emphysematous patients often purse their lips to narrow the exit from their airways. This increases the pressure in the airway lumen, preventing airways collapse and making it easier (although slower) to breathe out

---

(emphysema) that causes airflow obstruction by the mechanisms discussed in Box 45.

How severe is Mr Newman's airflow obstruction?

Severity of COPD is classified according to the degree of reduction in FEV_1 as a percentage of the predicted value (Box 46).

Mr Newman's FEV_1 (1.3 L) is 41% of his predicted value (3.2 L). Thus, he has moderate airflow obstruction.

Mr Newman's chest X-ray is shown in Fig. 37.

His haemoglobin (Hb) was 14.2 g/dL (normal range 13–18 g/dL).

Oxygen saturations were 96%.

How do you interpret these results?

On the chest X-ray the top of the liver should be in the 5th intercostal space in the midclavicular line and 5–6 ribs should be visible anteriorly. On Mr Newman's chest X-ray, 9 anterior ribs are visible (numbered) and the diaphragms are flattened (arrow), indicating hyperinflated lungs. There is no evidence of lung cancer.

Mr Newman's Hb is normal, ruling out anaemia as a cause of his breathlessness.

Oximetry was normal, indicating that his COPD is not causing hypoxia.

How should his COPD be managed?

The major aims of COPD management are:
• To minimize progression, thus preventing or delaying disability and prolonging life
• To relieve symptoms

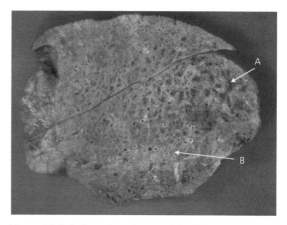

Figure 34 Pathology of emphysema. (A) Carbon stained lung from cigarette smoking. (B) Multiple small 'holes' in the lung caused by loss of lung parenchyma.

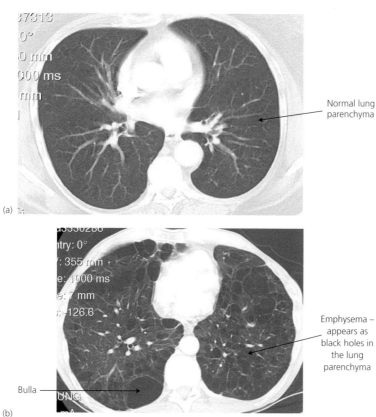

Normal lung parenchyma

(a)

Emphysema – appears as black holes in the lung parenchyma

Bulla

(b)

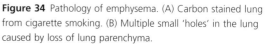

Figure 35 Computed tomography (CT) scans showing radiology of emphysema. (a) Normal lung. (b) Emphysema.

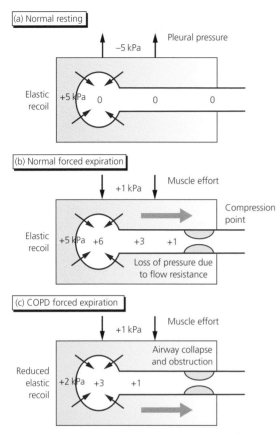

Figure 36 Mechanism underlying development of airflow obstruction in patients with emphysema. (a) Normal resting. (b) Normal forced expiration. (c) COPD forced expiration.

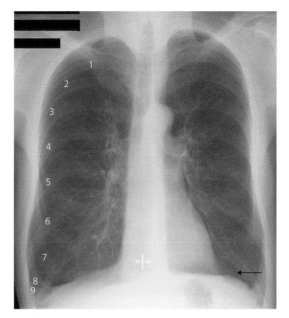

Figure 37 Chest X-ray.

What treatment will minimize COPD progression?

The most important thing Mr Newman can do is to stop smoking. This will slow his lung decline to the rate of a non-smoker.

What treatment relieves COPD symptoms?

The most useful treatments for patients with COPD are smoking cessation and pulmonary rehabilitation. Pharmacological therapy of airways disease also has some benefits.

Pulmonary rehabilitation

This is a 6–12 week programme of physical exercise, disease education, psychological and social interventions, usually provided in secondary care. The programme is run by multidisciplinary teams, primarily physiotherapists and nurses. The benefits of pulmonary rehabilitation include:

• Reduced breathlessness
• Increased exercise capacity
• Improvements in health-related quality of life

Drug treatment

The drugs used to relieve symptoms and improve health status in COPD are similar to those used for asthma. However, these drugs are used slightly differently in patients with COPD.

Mild COPD

Patients should be started on 'as required' short-acting bronchodilators to relieve breathlessness and prevent symptoms by use before exercise. Although airflow obstruction in COPD is mostly irreversible, bronchodilatators produce some symptomatic relief, possibly by partial relief of airways obstruction and by reducing air trapping and hyperinflation. In COPD, short-acting antimuscarinics (e.g. ipratropium; Box 41, p. 63) may be used in preference to β_2-agonists (Box 38, p. 57) as they reduce mucus hypersecretion as well as causing bronchodilatation.

Moderate and severe COPD

• If 'as required' short-acting bronchodilators do not control COPD symptoms, **long-acting bronchodilators** are added to treatment. Options are:

○ long-acting β$_2$-agonists (LABA; e.g. salmeterol, eformoterol; Box 38)

○ long-acting antimuscarinics (e.g. tiotropium; Box 41) – if this is started ipratropium should be stopped

In patients with asthma, use of LABA alone is associated with increased risk of asthma-related death. It is not clear whether COPD patients using LABA alone are also at increased risk of death, but until further information becomes available LABA are usually prescribed with inhaled steroids.

• **Inhaled corticosteroids** (Box 33, p. 52) are the mainstay of treatment for asthma patients but only have a small effect in COPD. In COPD, high dose inhaled steroids slightly improve FEV_1 by about 0.07 L and reduce exacerbation rate slightly. Thus, they are reserved for COPD patients with FEV_1 ≤50% predicted who are having two or more exacerbations per year

• **Xanthines** (e.g. theophylline; Box 40, p. 58) have been shown in clinical trials in COPD patients to increase lung function, improve blood gases and possibly reduce exacerbations, although it is less clear whether they improve patient symptoms. A therapeutic trial may be worthwhile in patients with COPD symptoms unresponsive to inhalers

• **Nebulizers.** Patients with severe symptoms despite optimal inhaled therapy (e.g. combination of LABA, long-acting antimuscarinic, high dose inhaled steroid and as required short-acting β$_2$-agonist) may benefit from higher dose regular nebulized short-acting β$_2$-agonist/antimuscarinic

---

Outcome. Mr Newman made a concerted effort to stop smoking using nicotine replacement therapy with the support of his local practice nurse. He underwent pulmonary rehabilitation and by the end of the programme was able to walk further. He joined a 'breathe easy' support group at his local gym to keep up his exercise regime. He was already taking inhaled salbutamol, so 50 μg salmeterol b.d. and 500 μg fluticasone b.d. were added to his treatment. He noticed partial reduction in his symptoms, which were improved further when he started 18 μg tiotropium o.d.

CASE REVIEW

Mr Newman presents to the chest clinic with a 2 year history of worsening shortness of breath on exercise. A chronic cough, extensive smoking history and lack of cardiac features point to a diagnosis of COPD. The diagnosis of COPD is confirmed by demonstration of airflow obstruction of moderate severity on spirometry. Mr Newman is treated with smoking cessation and pulmonary rehabilitation. Inhaled long-acting bronchodilators and steroids are used to improve his symptoms and reduce the risk of exacerbations.

KEY POINTS

• COPD is defined as progressive airflow obstruction that is not fully reversible
• COPD is usually caused by tobacco smoking
• Common COPD symptoms include progressive shortness of breath on exertion and a chronic productive cough
• Common examination findings indicating COPD include:
  ○ face – purse lip breathing
  ○ hands – nicotine-stained fingers
  ○ hyperinflation – reduced cricosternal distance, loss of cardiac dullness
  ○ increased respiratory effort – use of accessory muscles, intercostal indrawing
  ○ airflow obstruction – expiratory wheeze on auscultation
• The diagnosis of COPD is confirmed by spirometry if:
  ○ FEV_1 <80% predicted value
  ○ FEV_1 <70% FVC
  ○ the changes are consistent and irreversible
• The most effective treatments for COPD are smoking cessation and pulmonary rehabilitation
• Inhaled bronchodilators and steroids can be used to improve symptoms and reduce exacerbation rate

Case 6   A worried 56-year-old man

Mr McPherson is a 56-year-old man who presents to his GP with a cough, productive of yellow sputum and slight shortness of breath. He is concerned that this is the fourth time he has had these symptoms this year. He denies coughing up blood or weight loss.

He works as a sales representative and travels long distances each week. He has smoked 40 cigarettes per day since age 18. He has three grandchildren aged 1, 2 and 4 whom he sees most weekends. Mr McPherson comments that his father died of lung cancer aged 61 years and wonders whether this could be causing his own symptoms.

What is the differential diagnosis for Mr McPherson's current symptoms?

His symptoms are suggestive of bronchitis (inflamed bronchi). This could be caused by:
- Chronic obstructive pulmonary disease (COPD)
- Recurrent upper respiratory tract infections. Young children get frequent respiratory infections as they are exposed to many different organisms and have naïve immune systems – they often pass these on to their carers
- Lung cancer can cause recurrent chest infections if the tumour obstructs the bronchi, causing distal infection

How would you answer Mr McPherson's question?

- Currently, there are several possible explanations for his symptoms, including chest infections or chronic bronchitis caused by smoking
- Lung cancer does occur in people who smoke heavily and there is some increased risk of lung cancer in people who have a close relative with the disease
- Lung cancer does not seem to be the most likely diagnosis in Mr McPherson's case as he does not have other suggestive symptoms such as haemoptysis or weight loss. However, his doctor will arrange some tests for him to make sure he does not have cancer

What tests would you arrange?

- Chest X-ray to look for:
  - lung shadows, suggestive of lung cancer
  - consolidation/lung collapse, suggestive of central airways obstruction by tumour
- Spirometry to look for evidence of COPD
- Sputum culture to look for respiratory infection
- As a heavy smoker in a sedentary occupation Mr McPherson is at risk of cardiovascular as well as respiratory complications of smoking. This is a good opportunity for a general health screen, checking full blood count, renal function, cholesterol and glucose

How many 'pack years' has Mr McPherson smoked?

Mr McPherson has smoked 40 cigarettes per day from age 18 to 56 which equates to 76 pack years (Box 16, p. 19).

Does this help you with your diagnosis?

The risk of lung cancer is proportional to the total lifetime consumption of cigarettes:
- In people who do not smoke, the lifetime risk of lung cancer is less than 1%
- In lifelong heavy smokers, the cumulative lifetime risk of lung cancer may be as much as 30%
- One study showed that there was a 70% increase in risk of lung cancer for every 10 pack years smoked

As a heavy smoker, Mr McPherson is at risk of lung cancer.

There is also a strong 'dose–response' relationship between cigarettes smoked and the risk and severity of and mortality from COPD. In the UK, where cigarette smoking is the main cause of COPD, it is unusual to have COPD without having smoked around 20 pack years. Mr McPherson is therefore also at risk of COPD.

What other diseases are caused by tobacco smoking?

- Worldwide, tobacco kills 1 in 10 people
- In the UK, tobacco causes 120,000 deaths per year (330 per day)

- Smokers die 3–12 years earlier and have more health problems than non-smokers
- Diseases caused by tobacco are shown in Box 47

Box 47 Detrimental effects of tobacco

Tobacco use (usually smoking) increases the risk of many health problems including the following.

Respiratory
- COPD
- Lung cancer
- Laryngeal cancer

Cardiovascular
- Ischaemic heart disease
- Cerebrovascular disease (stroke)
- Peripheral vascular disease
- Thromboembolic disease

Gastrointestinal
- Peptic ulcers (more common and heal less well)
- Cancers of:
  - mouth (esp. tobacco chewers)
  - oesophagus
  - stomach
  - pancreas

Genitourinary
- Decreased fertility in men and women
- Carcinoma of cervix
- Bladder cancer

Musculoskeletal
- Osteoporosis, fractures

Skin
- Ageing, wrinkles
- Delayed ulcer healing

Pregnancy
- Low birth weight babies
- Miscarriages and placental abruptions

Passive smoking
- Spouses of smokers have an increased risk of lung cancer and deaths from myocardial infarction
- Children of smokers have increased risk of:
  - sudden infant death syndrome
  - asthma
  - respiratory tract/ear infections

What else should be done as part of the consultation?

This is an ideal opportunity to advise Mr McPherson to quit smoking. Brief advice from a health care practitioner alone causes 2% smokers receiving it to stop smoking for at least 6 months in addition to those who would have stopped smoking anyway. If this does not seem many, consider that around 25% of adults smoke and there are many millions of health care encounters each year. Thousands of people would stop smoking if we all remembered to advise smoking cessation at every consultation (Box 48).

Dr Morrison used the 5 As model to perform a brief quit smoking intervention for Mr McPherson.

   Ask. *She recorded Mr McPherson's 76 pack year smoking history in his notes.*

   Advise. *She reassured Mr McPherson that he probably did not have lung cancer but suggested that his symptoms*

Box 48 The '5 As' model for discussing smoking cessation

Ask
- Ask all patients whether they smoke
- Record smoking history in their notes

Advise
- Advise them to stop smoking in a clear, strong but non-judgmental manner

Assess
- Find out if they are willing to quit
- Discuss factors that prevent them from quitting (e.g. habit, enjoyment)
- Discuss previous quit attempts and why these might have failed

Assist
- Personalize assistance for individual patients including:
  - self-help strategies
  - support from family and friends
  - referral for quit smoking support, counselling (many GP surgeries provide this)
  - nicotine replacement or other drug therapy

Arrange
- Follow-up and support

were a warning to him to stop smoking and strongly advised him to do so.

*   **Assess.** Mr McPherson felt that he had not previously stopped smoking because smoking helped him concentrate when driving long distances for work. However, this illness had given him a fright and he was now keen to stop.*

*   **Assist.** Dr Morrison gave Mr McPherson a leaflet that had basic advice on how to stop smoking and a contact number which he could call to access quit smoking services. They discussed possible changes he might make to his job to reduce driving and the use of chewing gum instead of cigarettes to aid concentration. As he was such a heavy smoker she prescribed him 15 mg nicotine patches to be worn during the day and taken off at night.*

*   **Arrange.** Dr Morrison arranged to see Mr McPherson in 2 weeks to see how he was getting on with his smoking and to give him the results of his investigations.*

What basic tips might help someone to stop smoking?

*   Set a quit date and stick to it
*   Prepare by:
    *   telling family and friends and asking for support
    *   getting nicotine replacement or other treatment
*   On the day and after:
    *   throw away left over cigarettes and ashtrays
    *   change your routine to avoid times and places you used to smoke
    *   ask people not to smoke around you
    *   never buy, hold or light cigarettes for others or have even one puff
    *   do something active when the urge to smoke hits
    *   keep going, getting used to being without cigarettes will take a while

What quit smoking services are available?

Many GP surgeries provide smoking cessation clinics.

Patients can ring the NHS stop smoking helpline **0800 169 0169**. This number gives them access to:

*   Information packs
*   Registration for the 'Together programme', where participants choose to receive motivation and support by phone, text or email
*   Telephone support from specialist smoking cessation advisers
*   Phone numbers for their local smoking cessation services, through which they can receive face-to-face support either in groups or on a one-to-one basis

Why did Dr Morrison prescribe nicotine?

Tobacco smoke contains nicotine, which is addictive and drives the smoking habit (Box 49). Nicotine addiction has a chemical basis and withdrawal creates unpleasant symptoms (Box 50). Nicotine replacement reduces withdrawal symptoms and helps smokers quit:

*   Nicotine replacement leads to 5–12% of patients receiving it to stop smoking for at least 6 months in addition to those who would have stopped anyway
*   Nicotine plus behavioural support from quit smoking services is even better (13–19% extra stop)
*   Very heavy smokers such as Mr McPherson are unlikely to stop smoking without nicotine replacement or other pharmacological support

---

Box 49 Constituents of tobacco smoke

Tobacco smoke contains over 4000 compounds, 60 of which are carcinogenic. It comprises two phases.

Gas phase
This includes carbon monoxide, acetaldehyde, ammonia, nitrosamines and hydrogen cyanide.

Particulate phase
An aerosol of tar and nicotine which is well absorbed in the lungs:

*   Nicotine is an addictive psychoactive stimulant, which drives the smoking habit and has some cardiovascular effects
*   Tar is a carcinogenic mix of polycyclic aromatic hydrocarbons and some radioactive elements including polonium. These components of tobacco smoke are the main cause of smoking-related disease

---

Box 50 Nicotine

Nicotine addiction
Nicotine appears to activate dopaminergic pathways in the mesocorticolimbic system that are involved in positive brain reward which drives addictive disorders. Other neurotransmitters including glutamate and serotonin may be involved in learning and sensitization to drug use.

Withdrawal symptoms

0–7 days	Dizziness, tiredness, sleep disturbance
2–4 weeks or longer	Irritability, poor concentration, strong cravings, anxiety
Months	Weight gain 2–3 kg

Why did she prescribe nicotine in patch form?

Nicotine is available in six forms:

1 Transdermal patch
2 Chewing gum
3 Lozenge
4 Inhalator
5 Nasal spray
6 Sublingual tablet

There was no difference in quit smoking success or withdrawal discomfort in studies where the different forms were compared. Choice is therefore based largely on common sense and patient preference:
• Transdermal patches release nicotine throughout the day and are good for background irritability and cravings. Patients take them off at night to avoid nightmares
• All the other forms give the patient something to do (i.e. chew, sniff, puff or suck nicotine) when they crave a cigarette which may help them beat the urge. They also give an acute dose of nicotine which can replicate or exceed the physical 'buzz' of having a cigarette
• Different nicotine therapies can be used in combination (e.g. nicotine patches reduce background withdrawal and other forms control acute cravings)

Mr McPherson attends for follow-up 2 weeks later. He has enrolled for group support through the local smoking cessation programme and has set a quit smoking date for 1 week's time. In the meantime he has cut down to 10 cigarettes per day with the help of nicotine patches, but has noticed redness and blistering when he takes the patches off.

His investigation results are as follows:
Chest X-ray – hyperinflated lung fields, no other abnormality.
Spirometry:
• *FEV_1 1.8 L (55% predicted)*
• *FVC 3.04 L (76% predicted)*
• *FEV_1/FVC 59%*
Cholesterol and glucose were normal

How do you interpret his investigations?

• His chest X-ray shows no evidence of lung cancer
• His spirometry shows mild airflow obstruction, which in combination with his hyperinflated chest X-ray and smoking history would be consistent with a diagnosis of COPD

• COPD could account for his persistent productive cough and slight breathlessness

What has happened to his skin?

Skin reactions can occur as a side-effect of the nicotine patches and if severe require discontinuation of treatment.

Does nicotine replacement therapy have any other side-effects?

Nicotine treatment can cause nausea, dizziness and flu-like symptoms. It also stimulates the sympathetic nervous system and has been reported to cause chest pain and blood pressure changes. It is thus contraindicated in severe heart disease and immediately after a stroke. However, even in these situations, using nicotine at low doses may be preferable to continuing to smoke.

Are there any alternatives to nicotine replacement?

• Bupropion (amfebutamone) is an antidepressant which, when given with intensive behavioural support, caused 9% of patients receiving it to stop smoking for at least 6 months in addition to those who would have stopped anyway
• It is given initially for 4 weeks, with a repeat prescription if the quit attempt is continuing
• Common side-effects are dry mouth and insomnia

> **KEY POINT**
>
> Bupropion can trigger seizures and is contraindicated in patients with a history of or predisposition to seizures.

Does he need any treatment for his COPD?

Stopping smoking is the single most important intervention for his COPD. It slows the decline in FEV_1, delaying progression of symptoms and prolonging survival. His symptoms may resolve when he stops smoking. If not he may benefit from bronchodilatators (see Case 5).

Outcome. Mr McPherson was delighted that he did not have lung cancer. The fright was sufficient to motivate him to stop smoking with the assistance of group support and bupropion. During his first few weeks as an ex-smoker he found his cough was worse, but this slowly improved and his mucus production reduced. He found that an ipratropium inhaler reduced his breathlessness and he increased his exercise in an attempt to 'get fit'. Twelve months later he remained an ex-smoker.

CASE REVIEW

Mr McPherson attended his GP with recurrent respiratory symptoms, concerned that he might have lung cancer. He had a 76 pack year smoking history and agreed a smoking cessation plan with his GP. He initially managed to cut down from 40 to 10 cigarettes per day using nicotine patches, but developed skin hypersensitivity to the patches. He was able to stop smoking completely using bupropion and group support and remained a non-smoker 12 months later.

KEY POINTS

- Around 25% of adults in the UK smoke tobacco
- Lifetime smoking load is calculated as pack years, where 1 pack year is equivalent to having smoked 20 cigarettes per day for 1 year
- Tobacco smoking increases the risk of lung disease, particularly COPD and lung cancer. There is a strong dose–response relationship between lifetime smoking load and the risk of these diseases
- Brief advice from a health practitioner causes 2% smokers receiving it to stop smoking for at least 6 months in addition to those who would have stopped smoking anyway

- Brief quit smoking intervention by health professionals should include:
  - ask
  - advise
  - assess
  - assist
  - arrange
- Interventions that increase the chance of a successful quit smoking attempt include:
  - support and counselling
  - nicotine replacement, to reduce withdrawal symptoms
  - bupropion

Case 7 An 81-year-old man with acute shortness of breath

Mr Ronald Harrison is an 81-year-old man who lives in sheltered accommodation. This morning his warden found him to be acutely short of breath and summoned his GP, who sent him into hospital. On arrival, emergency assessment was:

- *Airway – patent*
- *Breathing – respiratory rate 26 breaths/min, oxygen saturations 89%*
- *Circulation – pulse 104 beats/min, blood pressure 126/76 mmHg*

How do you evaluate these results?

He is hypoxic with an increased respiratory rate and tachycardia.

What should be done to stabilize him before further assessment?

Hypoxia is the abnormality that could cause death or disability and therefore should be corrected as soon as possible. It is not yet known whether he has type I or II respiratory failure and whether he is at risk of carbon dioxide retention. A reasonable first approach therefore would be to:

- Give 28% oxygen by mask
- Monitor oxygen saturations, aiming for >92%
- Check blood gases to assess $PaCO_2$ and pH as soon as possible

He should also have a cannula inserted to secure intravenous access and cardiac monitoring to exclude arrhythmias.

Mr Harrison is commenced on 28% oxygen and his oxygen saturations improve to 93%. A cardiac monitor shows sinus rhythm. He gives a brief history in broken sentences.

He is normally able to walk a few hundred yards to collect his paper, stopping once or twice because of breathlessness. He has not been out for the last 3–4 days because of worsening shortness of breath. He has slept in a chair for 3 nights because he was too breathless to lie down.

He usually has a daily cough, productive of grey sputum. His sputum is currently a dark green colour.

He has smoked 20 cigarettes per day from his teens, but has cut down to 5 per day in the last year after advice from his doctor. In the last few years he has had frequent chest infections in the winter, requiring antibiotics 3–4 times each year.

What is the most likely diagnosis?

This appears to be an acute exacerbation of chronic obstructive pulmonary disease (COPD).

What features in the history point to this diagnosis?

- He is a life-long smoker, which puts him at risk of COPD
- He had chronic shortness of breath with limited exercise tolerance before this episode, indicating underlying chronic respiratory disease
- A persistent daily productive cough indicates underlying chronic bronchitis
- Worsening breathlessness with a change in sputum colour are features of exacerbation of underlying COPD (Box 51)

What is the differential diagnosis?

This includes:
- Pneumonia
- Bronchogenic carcinoma
- Heart failure

Why should these diagnoses be considered?

- Green sputum indicates infection, which could be in the airways (acute exacerbation of COPD) or alveoli (pneumonia) (Fig. 10, p. 15; Table 4)
- Mr Harrison has an extensive smoking history and so other smoking-related diseases including lung cancer and heart disease should be considered:

Table 4 Differences between infective exacerbations of chronic obstructive pulmonary disease (COPD) and pneumonia.

	COPD exacerbations	Pneumonia
Underlying COPD	Always	Sometimes
Site of infection (Fig. 10)	Airways	Alveoli
Chest X-ray changes	Clear lung fields	Consolidation, may be lobar
Systemic upset	Mild	Varies from mild to severe including septic shock
Respiratory failure	Destabilization of compromised lungs, often type II respiratory failure	Effect of consolidation, often type I respiratory failure
Mortality of hospitalized patients	About 15%	22–30% in severe cases
		Assessed by CURB-65 score (see Case 17)
Most common organisms	*H. influenzae*	*S. pneumoniae*
	M. catarrhalis	*H. influenzae*
	S. pneumonia	Viruses
	Viruses	Atypical organisms
First choice antibiotic	Usually can be given orally	Given intravenously if severely ill
	Aminopenicillin or macrolide or tetracycline	Aminopenicillin + macrolide if severe (atypical organism likely)
Oral steroids	Yes	No

Box 51 Definition of acute exacerbation of COPD

A sustained worsening of symptoms from the stable state, e.g:
• Increased cough, breathlessness, sputum production
• Change in sputum colour
which is:
• More than usual day-to-day variations
• Acute in onset
• May require a change in treatment

○ his symptoms are too acute to be caused directly by lung cancer, although an underlying tumour could obstruct the large airways leading to infection
○ heart failure is possible, although this does not cause green sputum

On examination Mr Harrison looks short of breath sitting upright and is using accessory muscles of respiration. His temperature is 37.6°C. His fingers are nicotine-stained, he has no asterixis and he has peripheral, but not central cyanosis while wearing the oxygen mask. His trachea is central, the cricosternal distance is one finger breadth and there is a tracheal tug. He has poor chest expansion with intercostal indrawing. There is symmetrical hyper-resonance on chest percussion with loss of cardiac dullness. He has bilateral expiratory wheeze and normal vocal resonance.

How do you interpret these examination findings?

• Use of accessory muscles during inspiration (neck and shoulder girdle muscles) and expiration (abdominal muscles) indicates respiratory distress
• His mild pyrexia would fit with a diagnosis of infection
• Nicotine-stained fingers are a sign of current smoking (also look for yellowed hair if grey/white and smell of smoke)
• Lack of central cyanosis indicates that he is not severely hypoxic and absence of asterixis (coarse flap of out-

stretched hands) suggests that there is no clinical evidence of CO_2 retention
• Reduced cricosternal distance, hyper-resonance and loss of cardiac dullness all indicate hyperinflation of the lungs, consistent with COPD
• Expiratory wheeze indicates airways obstruction
These findings would fit with the clinical diagnosis of acute exacerbation of COPD.

Do the examination findings exclude any of the other possible diagnoses?
• Lack of crepitations and bronchial breathing makes pneumonia less likely
• There are no positive features of lung cancer (clubbing, lymphadenopathy)
• There are no specific features of heart failure, although pulmonary oedema can cause wheeze by compressing small airways

Mr Harrison appears to have a respiratory infection. Is it important to make an exact diagnosis?
There are a number of key differences between infective exacerbations of COPD and pneumonia (Table 4), which lead to differences in treatment for patients with these conditions. Therefore, it is important to get the diagnosis right.

What investigations would you recommend to clinch the diagnosis and why?
• A chest X-ray. In clinical practice, pneumonia is usually diagnosed if there is consolidation on the chest X-ray and is less likely if the chest X-ray is clear. This test will also help to rule out lung cancer and heart failure
• An electrocardiogram (ECG) to look for ischaemic or right heart disease associated with COPD
• Full blood count to look for associated haemoglobin abnormalities and changes in white cell count indicative of infection
• Plasma biochemistry to allow detection of electrolyte abnormalities and underlying disease
• C-reactive protein (CRP) as an indicator of acute inflammation and infection
• Blood cultures to look for infection as he is pyrexial
• Sputum should be sent for culture and sensitivity testing as he has green sputum
• Arterial blood gases, particularly to look for type II respiratory failure and a metabolic acidosis

• Brain natriuretic peptide (BNP) may be useful if heart failure is suspected. A low value makes heart failure unlikely, although elevated concentrations could indicate ischaemic heart disease, right heart failure secondary to COPD or critical illness in general

His chest X-ray showed hyperinflation but his lung fields were clear.

Blood tests were normal apart from:

		Normal range
CRP	30 mg/L	(<4 mg/L)
White cells	$16 \times 10^9/L$	($4–11 \times 10^9/L$)
Neutrophils	$14 \times 10^9/L$	($3.5–7.5 \times 10^9/L$)
Arterial blood gases on 28% oxygen:		
pH	7.39	(7.35–7.45)
PaO_2	9.1 kPa	(10–13.1 kPa)
$PaCO_2$	5.2 kPa	(4.9–6.1 kPa)
HCO_3^-	24 mmol/L	(22–28 mmol/L)

How do you interpret his results?
• *Chest X-ray.* Mr Harrison's film shows hyperinflated lungs consistent with COPD. His lung fields are clear, therefore he does not have any evidence of pneumonia, cancer or cardiac failure
• *CRP.* Mr Harrison has a mild elevation of his CRP, which is much less than that seen in pneumonia. This is consistent with infection but could indicate other inflammation (Box 52). The elevated white cell count would also fit with infection (Box 53)
• *Arterial blood gases.* Oxygen therapy has resulted in satisfactory oxygenation ($PaO_2 >8$ kPa) without elevation of $PaCO_2$

Box 52 Causes of elevated C-reactive protein

CRP is an acute phase protein, which means its plasma concentrations increase by at least 25% during inflammatory conditions such as infection or autoimmune disease.

Values >100 mg/L
• Bacterial infection (80–85% cases)

Values >10 mg/L
Clinically significant inflammation, e.g. caused by:
• Infection
• Inflammatory conditions, such as rheumatoid arthritis

Box 53 Common causes of neutrophilia

- Acute infection
- Chronic inflammation, particularly during exacerbation
- Physiological stress (adrenaline)
- Drugs (glucocorticoids, β-agonists)
- Marrow stimulation or invasion

Box 54 Some causes of acute COPD exacerbations

- Infection
  - viral
  - bacterial
- Air pollution
- Smoking
- Allergens

What do you think is the most likely diagnosis now?

The clinical features and test results all point to an acute exacerbation of COPD. There is no evidence for any of the other diagnosis from the differential list.

What caused his COPD exacerbation?

Some causes of COPD exacerbations are shown in Box 54. Sputum purulence has been shown to be associated with infection, so a bacterial or viral cause should be suspected in Mr Harrison's case.

How should his exacerbation be managed?

He requires hospital admission as:
- He is not currently able to cope at home
- He requires acute oxygen therapy to maintain his oxygen saturations >90%

His exacerbation should be treated with:
- *Nebulized short-acting bronchodilators.* These relieve breathlessness by bronchodilatation
- *Oral corticosteroids.* These have an anti-inflammatory action. They modestly reduce the duration of exacerbation symptoms and reduce hospital stay by 1–2 days

Should he be given antibiotics?

Antibiotics are useful in exacerbations triggered by bacterial infections. A bacterial trigger is most likely in patients who have purulent (green/yellow) sputum, although viral infections can also cause purulent sputum. Mr Harrison has purulent sputum and so should receive antibiotics in addition to his nebulized bronchodilators and steroids.

Which antibiotic would you choose?

The bacteria most likely to cause a COPD exacerbation are:
- *Haemophilus influenzae*
- *Moraxella catarrhalis*
- *Streptococcus pneumoniae*

The antibiotic chosen by 'best guess' principles therefore needs to have a broad spectrum of action as it must cover Gram-positive cocci as well as Gram-negative cocci and bacilli. From the antibiotic chart (Figs 22 & 23, pp. 39 and 40) suitable choices include an aminopenicillin (e.g. amoxicillin), a macrolide (e.g. erythromycin) or a tetracycline (e.g. doxycycline). However, the majority of *M. catarrhalis* and some *Haemophilus* strains produce β-lactamases, making them penicillin resistant. If aminopenicillins are used they should be combined with clavulinic acid (e.g. co-amoxiclav), which has a structure similar to the β-lactam ring in penicillin. When clavulinic acid and amoxicillin are given together, the β-lactamase is used up by cleaving the β-lactam ring of the clavulinic acid, preserving the amoxicillin to kill the bacteria.

Mr Harrison is commenced on 2.5mg nebulized salbutamol 4-hourly and 250µg ipratropium 6-hourly. He remains on 28% oxygen. He is prescribed 625mg co-amoxiclav 8-hourly and 30mg/day prednisolone by mouth. He receives his first dose of antibiotics immediately while the nurses are waiting for his prednisolone to arrive from pharmacy. Mr Harrison calls for help 45min later. He is feeling more breathless and wheezy and has developed a red rash. His blood pressure is 90/40mmHg.

Summarize Mr Harrison's new problems

- Worsening airflow obstruction
- New hypotension
- Rash

How can these be explained?

These would be consistent with anaphylaxis (Box 55), an allergic reaction which has most probably been caused by antibiotics.

> **Box 55 Mechanism of anaphylaxis (Fig. 27, p. 47)**
>
> - Initial allergen exposure causes formation of immunoglobulin E (IgE) antibodies which become fixed to mast cells and leucocytes
> - On further exposure, allergen interacts with cell-bound antibody, activating cells to release histamine and other active mediators
> - Histamine stimulates H_1 receptors, causing smooth muscle contraction (bronchoconstriction), vasodilatation (hypotension) and increased capillary permeability (tissue oedema [e.g. larynx], skin rash)

What should be done to treat Mr Harrison?

This is an emergency and requires urgent treatment. Give:

- Intramuscular adrenaline (0.5–1 mL 1 in 1000)
- Intravenous antihistamine (chlorphenamine 10 mg IV)
- Intravenous hydrocortisone (100 mg)

How do these drugs work?

- Adrenaline causes vasoconstriction and bronchodilatation, reversing the effects of histamine (Box 55)
- Chlorphenamine blocks H_1 receptors and reduces the effects of histamine
- Hydrocortisone reduces vascular permeability, oedema and hypotension and suppresses further antibody–antigen reactions. Its actions require at least 30 min to take effect

Mr Harrison received adrenaline, chlorphenamine and hydrocortisone, intravenous 0.9% sodium chloride to elevate his blood pressure and a further salbutamol nebulizer. His breathlessness had settled 30 min later and his blood pressure was 116/84 mmHg. On questioning he admitted he had had a rash with antibiotics before. This had not been noted in his admission clerking.

> **KEY POINT**
>
> *Always* make a point of asking each patient about drug allergies *yourself* before writing a prescription. Only rely on records or relatives if the patient is unconscious.

How will you treat his COPD exacerbation now?

He must not receive any further drugs from the penicillin class. Of patients who are allergic to penicillins, 10% are also allergic to cephalosporins because of structural similarities between drugs. Cephalosporins can be used with caution if there is no alternative. However, in Mr Harrison's case better choices would be a macrolide, tetracycline or trimethoprim.

What advice should Mr Harrison receive about future treatment?

He should be advised that he is allergic to penicillin and should not receive this in the future. Ideally, this advice should be both verbal and in writing as a warning card, letter or worn as an alert bracelet. He should tell any health care professional he sees in the future about this allergy.

Additionally, his penicillin allergy should be recorded prominently in the hospital notes, on his drug chart during inpatient stay and his GP should be informed.

Over the next few days Mr Harrison was treated with 500 mg erythromycin q.d.s., nebulizers and steroids. He gradually improved and was able to mobilize around the bed and walk to the bathroom. His medication was changed to inhalers and community respiratory nurse input and home help were arranged to support him on discharge. Before going home he asks whether there is anything that can be done to make sure he does not end up in hospital with the same condition again.

How would you answer Mr Harrison's question?

Measures that could reduce future hospitalization for COPD exacerbations include:

- *Vaccination.* Patients with COPD should be vaccinated against *Streptococcus pneumoniae* and influenza (Box 56) because respiratory infection with these organisms may be life-threatening in patients with chronic respiratory disease. Mr Harrison should be advised to contact his GP for pneumonia vaccination when he has recovered from his acute illness and flu vaccination in the autumn
- *Outpatient review of COPD.* This should be performed after discharge to confirm the diagnosis, optimize therapy, promote smoking cessation and arrange pulmonary rehabilitation

---

Box 56 Pharmacology of respiratory vaccines

Pneumococcal vaccine

The pneumococcal vaccine used for patients with respiratory disease contains purified polysaccharide from 23 capsular types of pneumococci, which stimulates production of antibodies.

Use

Patients with chronic respiratory disease should receive a single dose and do not need a booster as:

- Repeat vaccination is associated with adverse reactions
- Pneumococcus is antigenically stable, therefore antibodies will be long-lasting

Contraindications

It should not be given to patients with acute illness or who have had a previous allergic reaction to a similar vaccine.

Influenza vaccine

Influenza viruses A and B constantly change their antigenic structure, hence new vaccines against new viral strains must be developed each year to generate appropriate immunity.

Uses

Patients with chronic respiratory disease should be vaccinated yearly in October/November so that they have developed immunity in time for the 'flu season' which reaches a peak in January.

Contraindications

Chicken eggs are used in vaccine production; hence patients allergic to eggs should not receive the flu jab. Other contraindications are the same as for pneumococcal vaccination.

- *Inhaled steroids.* High doses of inhaled steroids appear to reduce exacerbation rates in patients who have more severe COPD and have two or more exacerbations per year. Mr Harrison would be suitable for such treatment
- *Early treatment of exacerbation symptoms.* Mr Harrison could have antibiotics and steroids at home with written instructions on how to recognize an early exacerbation and when to start treatment. Prompt exacerbation treatment can speed recovery and prevent admission. Respiratory nurse support at home can also help reduce re-admission

Outcome. Mr Harrison was discharged home after 5 days to complete antibiotic and steroid treatment at home. He was visited 2 weeks later by the respiratory nurse, who found him to be less breathless. Over the next 4 weeks he increased his walking distance until he was able to buy his own paper. He then attended outpatients for review of his COPD.

CASE REVIEW

Mr Harrison is a life-long smoker who presents with acute shortness of breath and a cough newly productive of dark green sputum. A clinical diagnosis of an acute exacerbation of COPD is made. Investigations support this diagnosis and do not show any evidence of pneumonia. Mr Harrison is admitted to hospital for oxygen therapy, nebulized bronchodilators, corticosteroids and antibiotics, but develops an anaphylactic reaction to co-amoxiclav. This is treated with adrenaline, hydrocortisone and antihistamines. His antibiotic treatment is changed to erythromycin and he makes an uneventful recovery. On discharge, advice to prevent re-admission includes pneumococcal and influenza vaccination, smoking cessation, optimization of COPD treatment and early treatment of exacerbations.

KEY POINTS

- An acute exacerbation of COPD is defined as 'sustained worsening of symptoms from the stable state that is more than usual day-to-day variations, acute in onset and may require a change in treatment'
- Exacerbations are usually caused by viral or bacterial infection, but can be non-infective
- New purulent (green or yellow) sputum indicates an infective cause
- COPD patients may develop:
  - infective exacerbations of COPD, where infection is in the airways
  - pneumonia, where infection is in the alveoli
- Infective exacerbations of COPD should be differentiated from pneumonia by chest X-ray as causes, treatment and prognosis are different.
- Management of COPD exacerbations includes:
  - respiratory support
  - nebulized bronchodilators
  - systemic corticosteroids
  - antibiotics in patients with purulent sputum
- Future exacerbations requiring hospitalization can be reduced by:

- influenza and pneumococcal vaccination
- smoking cessation and optimization of COPD treatment
- inhaled corticosteroids
- early treatment of exacerbations at home
- respiratory nurse support
- **Anaphylaxis** is a type I hypersensitivity reaction to an allergen that can be life-threatening because of:
  - laryngeal oedema
  - bronchoconstriction
  - vasodilatation and hypotension
- Clinicians should always check for a history of drug allergy before prescribing any drug, particularly antibiotics, to patients to reduce the risk of drug-induced anaphylaxis
- Anaphylaxis should be treated immediately with intramuscular adrenaline, intravenous antihistamine and hydrocortisone
- Once the patient has recovered they should be given verbal and written information about their allergy and warned to avoid the causative allergen in the future

A 73-year-old woman, Mrs Briggs, is brought into accident and emergency. Her daughter is with her and explains that Mrs Briggs, who lives alone, has been increasingly confused over the past few days.

The following observations were performed on arrival:
- *Pulse 108 beats/min*
- *Blood pressure 120/84 mmHg*
- *Respiratory rate 12 breaths/min*
- *Oxygen saturations 78% on air*

What should you do first?

In an emergency always start with the ABC. Mrs Briggs' observations indicate that she is breathing and her circulation is intact. However, you should look at the patient for yourself as information may be inaccurate or her clinical condition may have changed.

How do you interpret her admission observations?

She is tachycardic, but is maintaining reasonable blood pressure. Although she has a 'normal' respiratory rate (normal range 12–18 breaths/min), she is markedly hypoxic.

What are the priorities for her management?

In an emergency situation it is vital that you take measures to save life and minimize potential disability even before you make a full assessment (Box 24, p. 36). Mrs Briggs is clearly in danger from her hypoxia, which can cause cell injury and death (Box 4, p. 8). Immediate measures for Mrs Briggs should therefore include:
- Oxygen therapy
- Insertion of an intravenous line
- Continuous monitoring:
  - oxygen saturation
  - cardiac rhythm
  - pulse
  - blood pressure
  - respiratory rate

She then needs more detailed assessment to identify and treat the underlying cause of her hypoxia.

On inspection Mrs Briggs' lips and tongue look blue, her hands feel warm and she has a bounding pulse. When her arms and wrists are extended there is a rhythmic flapping of her hands.

Mrs Briggs' arterial blood gases on air are:

		Normal range
pH	*7.24*	*(7.35–7.45)*
PaO$_2$	*5.6 kPa*	*(10–13.1 kPa)*
PaCO$_2$	*8.8 kPa*	*(4.9–6.1 kPa)*
Bicarbonate	*28 mmol/L*	*(22–28 mmol/L)*

How do you interpret her arterial blood gases?

- PaO$_2$ is low, indicating a problem with alveolar ventilation and/or capillary perfusion affecting gas exchange. Because PaO$_2$ is below 8 kPa, Mrs Briggs is in respiratory failure
- PaCO$_2$ is elevated, indicating hypoventilation. Mrs Briggs is in type II respiratory failure (Fig. 7, p. 7)
- pH is low (acidosis). When PaCO$_2$ is elevated [1], this drives the Henderson–Hasselbach equation to the left [2], increasing hydrogen concentration [3] and causing an acidosis. As the respiratory problem is the primary abnormality, this is called a respiratory acidosis

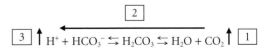

- HCO$_3^-$ is normal. In type II respiratory failure, normal bicarbonate concentrations indicate an acute problem. In patients with chronic CO$_2$ retention, there is renal retention of bicarbonate with correction of acidosis (compensation) and a rise in bicarbonate levels.

Can her examination findings be explained by her abnormal blood gases?

• The blue colour of her lips and tongue is central cyanosis caused by hypoxia
• The bounding pulse and flapping tremor can be accounted for by neurological and circulatory effects of hypercapnia (Box 5, p. 8)
• Her confusion could be caused by both hypoxia (Box 4, p. 8) and hypercapnia (Box 5)

Give a differential diagnosis for type II respiratory failure

Type II respiratory failure is caused by alveolar hypoventilation that is severe enough to impair both oxygenation of the blood and CO_2 excretion. The most common cause of type II respiratory failure is severe COPD. However, any severe lung, neurological, muscular or chest wall disease that impairs breathing can cause type II respiratory failure (Fig. 7).

What else would you look for when examining Mrs Briggs to establish the cause of type II respiratory failure?

The main differential is between severe lung disease and neurological, muscular or chest wall disease:
• *Severe lung disease.* You should perform a respiratory examination to look for signs of COPD (e.g. expiratory wheeze, lung hyperinflation) or other severe lung disease
• *Neurological, muscular or chest wall disease.* Reduction in consciousness suppressing respiration can be assessed by the Glasgow Coma Scale. A neurological examination should be carried out to assess spinal cord and motor nerve function. Visual inspection of the chest will reveal severe deformities (e.g. kyphosis), obesity or rib fractures

Mrs Briggs is slumped on the trolley but is able to cooperate with simple commands during examination. Her Glasgow Coma Score is 14. Neurological examination is otherwise unremarkable.

On chest examination she is thin with intercostal indrawing, a tracheal tug and reduced cricosternal distance. She has no obvious chest wall deformity. She has loss of cardiac dullness and downward displacement of her liver. She has quiet breath sounds with expiratory wheeze.

How do you interpret her examination findings?

• On respiratory examination she has classic signs of severe COPD with lung hyperinflation and airflow obstruction

• Her Glasgow Coma Score of 14 indicates a mild reduction in consciousness. Lack of other neurological or chest wall abnormalities indicates that this is most likely a consequence rather than a cause of her type II respiratory failure

The most likely cause of her type II respiratory failure is therefore severe COPD, probably worsened by an exacerbation.

Mrs Briggs is given 60% oxygen by the admitting team while other investigations are ordered. When they return her Glasgow Coma Score is 10. Repeat arterial blood gases are:

		Normal range
pH	7.18	(7.35–7.45)
PaO_2	6.8 kPa	(10–13.1 kPa)
$PaCO_2$	10.2 kPa	(4.9–6.1 kPa)
Bicarbonate	28 mmol/L	(22–28 mmol/L)

What has happened?

Mrs Briggs' Glasgow Coma Score has fallen from 14 to 10, indicating neurological deterioration. The most likely cause of this is worsening hypercapnia and acidosis.

Why does she have worsening hypercapnia and acidosis?

Ventilation is normally regulated through the chemosensitive area in the respiratory centre to maintain $PaCO_2$ within a tight range. Traditional teaching states that in patients with severe COPD, chronic CO_2 retention causes this chemosensitive area to become desensitized to changes in CO_2, which thus no longer controls breathing. These patients rely on the weaker stimulus of hypoxia for ventilatory drive. When they are given oxygen therapy that improves hypoxia they are no longer stimulated to breathe at an adequate rate and this hypoventilation worsens hypercapnia with toxic effects.

How could this have been prevented?

Oxygen therapy should be started cautiously in patients with a possible diagnosis of COPD who are at risk of CO_2 retention. One approach is to commence oxygen at 24–28% using a Venturi mask (Fig. 21, p. 37), then to adjust inhaled oxygen concentrations to correct hypoxia with careful monitoring of blood gases. The aim should be to maintain $PaO_2 > 8$ kPa or oxygen saturations >90%. If CO_2 retention develops or worsens with oxygen treatment, ventilatory support may be required. It is important to emphasize that even though oxygen treatment is difficult in these patients, correction of hypoxia is essential.

How should Mrs Briggs be treated now?

Mrs Briggs' most life-threatening problem is her hypoxia and this must be corrected. However, 60% oxygen therapy has worsened her condition by suppressing her hypoxic drive to breathe, increasing $PaCO_2$ and acidosis with toxic effects. Mrs Briggs now needs either non-invasive or invasive ventilation (Box 25, p. 37) to maintain her respiratory rate while she receives oxygen, allowing simultaneous correction of hypoxia, hypercapnia and respiratory acidosis.

Mrs Briggs is started on bi-level positive airway pressure (BiPAP) non-invasive ventilation (Fig. 38). The ward sister makes sure she is propped up comfortably at an angle of 30–45°, then puts on a face mask, which is connected by tubing to the ventilator. The ventilator is set to deliver 12 cm H_2O pressure during inspiration and 4 cm H_2O during expiration in spontaneous mode (Box 25). Supplemental oxygen is delivered through the face mask. The inspiratory pressure and inhaled oxygen concentrations are increased until her oxygen saturations are >90%. Her arterial gases are rechecked after 1 h to measure her $PaCO_2$ and pH. She also receives bronchodilators, antibiotics and steroid treatment for her COPD exacerbation.

What does non-invasive ventilation feel like?

It has been likened to trying to breathe while your head is out of the window of a moving car. Patients often find non-invasive ventilation uncomfortable and difficult to tolerate.

How does BiPAP work?

Positive inspiratory pressure (10–20 cm H_2O):
- Increases alveolar ventilation
- Reduces the work of inhalation, reducing oxygen demand

Positive expiratory pressure (4–8 cm H_2O):
- Prevents airway collapse during exhalation, which prolongs expiration, prevents hyperinflation and increases elimination of CO_2
- Reduces the amount of work required to start the next inhalation, reducing oxygen demand
- Opens up small airways, increasing the distribution of inspired air and improving ventilation

The advantages of BiPAP are that high inspiratory pressures (10–20 cm H_2O) can be generated to optimize beneficial effects, while expiratory pressures are kept relatively low to allow and support exhalation. Continuous positive airway pressure (CPAP) at pressures up to 12.5 cm H_2O in both inspiration and exhalation is used in patients without underlying lung disease with acute heart failure or obstructive sleep apnoea, who are capable of breathing out against these pressures.

Why non-invasive ventilation and not invasive ventilation?

- Non-invasive ventilation is an effective treatment for type II respiratory failure in patients with acute exacerbations of COPD, reducing length of hospital stay and death rate
- Patients receiving non-invasive ventilation are not intubated or receiving invasive monitoring, therefore they experience less complications, particularly hospital-acquired pneumonia and other infections, than patients receiving invasive ventilation
- If patients do not improve with non-invasive ventilation, invasive ventilation remains an option

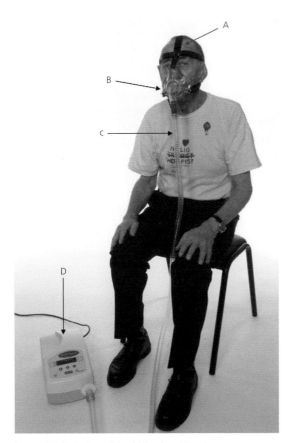

Figure 38 Patient receiving bi-level positive airway pressure (BiPAP). (A) Straps ensuring tight fit of mask; (B) tight fitting face mask; (C) tubing; (D) machine generating BiPAP.

Are there any patients who should not have non-invasive ventilation?

• COPD patients who do best with non-invasive ventilation are those who have moderately severe exacerbations. Patients with mild exacerbations recover without non-invasive ventilation and tolerate it poorly. Patients who are severely unwell with imminent respiratory arrest will need intubation and invasive ventilation

• Severely impaired consciousness is a contraindication to non-invasive ventilation. These patients cannot protect their airways or clear secretions and are at risk of aspiration

Are there any complications of non-invasive ventilation?

Non-invasive ventilation can cause:

• Aspiration in patients with reduced consciousness
• Pneumothorax
• Gastrointestinal distension and perforation

Non-invasive ventilation treatment fails in 10–20% patients with respiratory failure caused by COPD exacerbations.

What else can be done if non-invasive ventilation fails?

If non-invasive ventilation fails to correct respiratory failure, a decision must be made as to whether invasive ventilation on an intensive care unit should be started. This is a difficult decision as in this situation the patient may well not survive without invasive ventilation, but could potentially be in an even worse situation with invasive ventilation. Possible problems of escalating treatment to full intensive care could include loss of an opportunity for a dignified and comfortable death supported by family or a prolonged intensive care stay with difficulty weaning the patient from the ventilator and subsequent greatly impaired quality of life. In any

patient admitted with respiratory failure a decision should be made as soon as possible by a senior clinician as to what is the 'ceiling of therapy', i.e. the most invasive treatment the patient will receive. The main options are:

• Palliative care only
• Active medical treatment without ventilatory support
• Non-invasive ventilation
• Invasive ventilation and full intensive care

This decision is usually based on the patient's premorbid state, the patient's wishes, input from family and after discussion between admitting medical teams and the intensive care unit. The decision should be made early so that, if non-invasive ventilation fails, appropriate management can be implemented. However, it should also be reviewed regularly and could be altered if the patient's condition or wishes change.

Outcome. Mrs Briggs tolerates non-invasive ventilation and at 1 h her blood gases show improvement of her $PaCO_2$ to 7.4 kPa and pH to 7.30. She remains on non-invasive ventilation for 12 h and arterial gases show a sustained improvement in $PaCO_2$ and pH. Over the next 2 days she is weaned off BiPAP, initially by using it intermittently during the day then reducing to night only before stopping non-invasive ventilation completely. She continues bronchodilator, steroid and antibiotic therapy and mobilizes around the ward. Prior to discharge her arterial gases are rechecked and are:

		Normal range
pH	*7.39*	*(7.35–7.45)*
PaO_2	*8.4 kPa*	*(10–13.1 kPa)*
$PaCO_2$	*5.7 kPa*	*(4.9–6.1 kPa)*
Bicarbonate	*28 mmol/L*	*(22–28 mmol/L)*

She thus does not require long-term oxygen or home ventilatory support and is discharged home on medical therapy with respiratory nurse support.

CASE REVIEW

Mrs Briggs is brought to accident and emergency because she has become confused and difficult to rouse. On examination she is hypoxic with expiratory wheeze and right heart failure. Blood gases confirm that she is in type II respiratory failure with respiratory acidosis. The admitting team erroneously give her 60% oxygen which worsens her hypercapnia and acidosis by suppressing her hypoxic drive to breathe. She is started on non-invasive ventilation with

BiPAP. Inspiratory pressure and inhaled oxygen are increased until her oxygen saturations are >90%. She also receives bronchodilators, antibiotics and steroids for an exacerbation of COPD. BiPAP corrects her hypercapnia and acidosis and she is weaned off ventilation. After several days she is well enough to be discharged home on medical therapy with respiratory nurse support.

KEY POINTS

- Type II respiratory failure is defined as PaO_2 <8 kPa with hypercapnia
- Hypoxia causes cell damage and death
- Hypercapnia also has toxic effects, particularly on the brain and circulation
- Clinical features of hypercapnia include:
  - bounding pulse
  - flapping tremor
  - confusion
- Severe COPD and COPD exacerbations are the most common causes of type II respiratory failure. Other causes include neurological, muscular and chest wall disease
- In COPD patients with type II respiratory failure, respiratory drive is often altered:
  - chronic CO_2 retention reduces the sensitivity of the chemosensitive area in the brainstem and central control of breathing is lost
  - respiratory rate is maintained by hypoxic stimulation of peripheral chemoreceptors
  - injudicious correction of hypoxia with high concentrations of inhaled oxygen thus can suppress ventilation, worsening hypercapnia and causing acidosis
- Oxygen should be administered cautiously to COPD patients at risk of worsening CO_2 retention:
  - treatment should aim to improve PaO_2 to >8 kPa or oxygen saturations to >90%
  - patients should be started on oxygen at 24–28%
  - blood gases should be monitored to ensure that there is no increase in CO_2 or fall in pH before further increases in oxygen therapy
- COPD patients with CO_2 retention and respiratory acidosis usually require ventilatory support to correct hypoxia, hypercapnia and acid–base balance. Options are:
  - non-invasive ventilation (BiPAP)
  - invasive ventilation on an intensive care unit
- The underlying cause of type II respiratory failure should be treated and the patient weaned off ventilation as their underlying condition improves
- On admission a clear management plan should be decided for patients with respiratory failure to establish whether the 'ceiling of therapy' should be:
  - palliative care only
  - active medical treatment without ventilatory support
  - non-invasive ventilation
  - invasive ventilation and full intensive care
- Decisions regarding the 'ceiling of therapy' should be made by a senior clinician based on the patient's wishes and premorbid state and taking into account the opinions of the patient's family and clinicians from the intensive care unit

Case 9   A 78-year-old man with ankle swelling

Mr Shamin is a 78-year-old man referred to the clinic by the community respiratory nurse specialist for urgent medical review. Over the past 4 weeks he has noticed increasing ankle swelling and is now unable to put his shoes on. He was diagnosed with chronic obstructive pulmonary disease (COPD) 3 years previously. He has a 75 pack year smoking history and still smokes 5–6 cigarettes per day. He is breathless dressing or getting in and out of the bath and rarely leaves the house.

His medications are:

100 µg salbutamol inhaler, 2 puffs when required
18 µg tiotropium bromide inhaler, 1 puff daily
25 µg salmeterol, 2 puffs twice daily
500 µg fluticasone, 1 puff twice daily

What causes ankle swelling?

Ankle swelling (oedema) is usually caused by excess salt and water in the interstitium (Box 57). The ankles are the first place to swell in a mobile person as gravity causes interstitial fluid to accumulate at the lowest point. In a bed-bound patient oedema may present as sacral swelling.

How is the volume of interstitial fluid normally controlled?

There are four main forces controlling movement of fluid between blood and interstitium:
• Hydrostatic capillary pressure and interstitial osmotic pressure drive movement of fluid from capillaries to interstitium
• Osmotic pressure of plasma proteins and interstitial hydrostatic pressure drive movement of fluid into the capillaries

At the arterial end of the capillaries, the net effect of these pressures is to drive fluid out of capillaries into the interstitium. At the venous end of the capillaries, the net effect is to draw fluid back into the capillaries, where it is returned by veins to the right side of the heart. Excess water in the interstitium is cleared by the lymphatics.

How does oedema arise?

Disruption of any of the normal physiological processes controlling interstitial fluid volume can lead to oedema.

Increased capillary hydrostatic pressure

This is caused by downstream reduction in capillary drainage, e.g.
• Deep vein thrombosis
• Right heart failure
or an increase in sodium and water retention, e.g.
• Renal impairment

Reduced capillary oncotic pressure

This is caused by a reduction in plasma proteins, particularly albumin, e.g.
• Malnutrition
• Acute illness
• Liver failure
• Nephrotic syndrome

Increased leakiness of the capillary walls

This is caused by inflammation and allows leak of proteins and fluid into the intravascular space, e.g.
• Infection

Obstruction of lymphatics

This prevents clearance of fluid from the extravascular space and is caused by, e.g.
• Cancer
• Radiotherapy

What are the most likely causes of ankle swelling in a patient with COPD?

• Right heart failure secondary to lung disease
• Other heart disease caused by smoking
• Deep vein thrombosis resulting from immobility
• Hypoalbuminaemia brought about by malnutrition

Box 57 Body fluid compartments

Total body fluid volume is around 42 L. Fluid is compartmentalized as:
- Extracellular fluid (outside the cells, approximately one-third of body fluid)
  - circulating fluid (e.g. plasma, lymph)
  - interstitial fluid (among and between the cells, but not inside cells)
- Intracellular fluid (inside the cells, approximately two-thirds of body fluid)

Examination findings. Mr Shamin is short of breath getting onto the examination couch.

Body mass index 19 kg/m²

Cyanosed, oxygen saturations 87%

Pulse 104 beats/min regular, jugular venous pressure (JVP) +6 cm, blood pressure 112/68 mmHg

Bilateral pitting ankle oedema to his knees

Chest auscultation – poor air entry and expiratory wheeze bilaterally

Abdominal examination – liver palpable 2 cm below the right costal margin

How do you interpret these examination findings?
- His body mass index is reduced (normal range 20–25 kg/m²)
- He is hypoxic
- He has clinical evidence of right heart failure (raised JVP, ankle swelling)
- Chest examination is consistent with his diagnosis of COPD

How do you explain his palpable liver?
- The liver could be congested and enlarged because of right heart failure
- His liver could be a normal size but pushed down (displaced) by hyperinflated lungs

Can you tell between causes of a palpable liver on clinical examination?
The top of the liver should normally be percussed at the 5th intercostal space, midclavicular line on the right side of the chest. The bottom of the liver should not be palpable below the right costal margin.

- *Enlarged liver.* The top of the liver is percussed at the normal point but the liver is palpable in the abdomen
- *Displaced liver.* The top of the liver is percussed below the normal point and the liver is palpable 2–4 finger breadths below the costal margin

It is possible in a patient with COPD that the liver is both displaced and enlarged. This may be difficult to detect clinically and may require liver function tests and ultrasound to clarify the situation.

What is the differential diagnosis for Mr Shamin's clinical deterioration?
- Worsening COPD with hypoxia and right heart failure
  - exacerbation of COPD over past 4 weeks
  - progression of COPD with ongoing smoking
- Ischaemic heart disease
- Superimposed lung disease (e.g. cancer, pneumonia)
- Other disease including hepatic or renal impairment

What tests would you arrange immediately?
- Spirometry to reassess lung function
- Chest X-ray to look for pneumonia or lung cancer
- Electrocardiogram (ECG) to look for right heart strain
- Arterial blood gases to confirm hypoxia and determine whether there is CO_2 retention
- Blood tests:
  - C-reactive protein, white cell count to look for infection
  - haemoglobin and haematocrit to look for anaemia or polycythaemia
  - renal function, albumin and liver function to look for other causes of oedema

Mr Shamin's results are available 2 h later and show the following results.

Spirometry:
- *Today – FEV₁ 0.6 L (22% predicted), FVC 1.8 L (64% predicted), FEV₁/FVC % 33%*
- *1 year ago – FEV₁ 1.0 L (37% predicted), FVC 2.0 L (71% predicted), FEV₁/FVC % 50%*

Chest X-ray: hyperinflated lung fields, prominent pulmonary arteries

ECG: P pulmonale in lead II (Fig. 39)

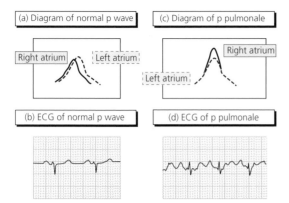

Figure 39 P pulmonale. The right atrium contains the sinoatrial node which initiates depolarization. If the atria are normal the right atrium therefore depolarizes slightly before the left atrium (a). A normal p wave (b) should be ≤2 small squares (2 mm) high. In patients with cor pulmonale there is right atrial dilatation and/or hypertrophy. Depolarization of the right atrium is delayed and occurs at the same time as the left atrium (c), making the p wave narrower and taller (>2 mm) (d).

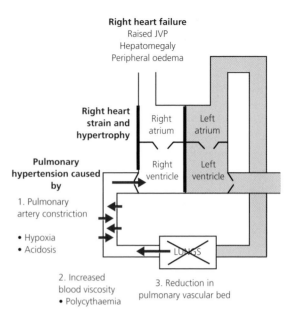

Figure 40 Cor pulmonale and right heart failure. Changes in the pulmonary circulation secondary to COPD cause pulmonary hypertension, leading to right heart strain and failure.

Arterial blood gases on air:		
		Normal range
pH	7.39	(7.35–7.45)
PaO_2	6.9 kPa	(10–13.1 kPa)
$PaCO_2$	5.7 kPa	(4.9–6.1 kPa)
Bicarbonate	28 mmol/L	(22–28 mmol/L)
Blood tests:		
Na	138 mmol/L	(135–145 mmol/L)
K	3.8 mmol/L	(3.5–5.0 mmol/L)
Urea	6 mmol/L	(2.5–8 mmol/L)
Creatinine	62 μmol/L	(60–110 μmol/L)
C-reactive protein	5 mg/L	(<8 mg/L)
Albumin	36 g/L	(34–48 g/L)
Gamma glutamyl transferase	73 U/L	(11–50 U/L)
Haemoglobin	18.6 g/dL	(13–18 g/dL)
Packed cell volume	0.6 L/L	(0.42–0.53 L/L)
White cells	$7.4 \times 10^9/L$	$(4–11 \times 10^9/L)$
Platelets	$290 \times 10^9/L$	$(150–400 \times 10^9/L)$
D-dimer	Negative	

How do you interpret these investigations?

• Spirometry shows severe airflow obstruction, which has deteriorated from a year ago. It is not possible to tell whether the deterioration is acute caused by an exacerbation or chronic as a result of disease progression

• The chest X-ray shows no evidence of other respiratory disease, such as lung cancer or pneumonia. However, he has prominent pulmonary arteries which could indicate pulmonary hypertension
• His ECG shows P pulmonale which indicates right heart hypertrophy and strain (Figs 39 & 40)
• Arterial blood gases show type I respiratory failure
• Blood tests show:
  ○ normal renal function and albumin
  ○ no evidence of infection
  ○ gamma glutamyl transferase is slightly raised, consistent with hepatic congestion or other non-specific pathology
  ○ haemoglobin and packed cell volume are elevated (polycythaemia)

Do these findings allow refinement of the differential diagnosis?

There is no evidence of respiratory disease other than COPD, or of primary cardiac disease, hypoalbuminaemia, hepatic or renal impairment.

The likely diagnosis is therefore:
• Deteriorating COPD complicated by right heart dysfunction and failure

How does COPD lead to right heart dysfunction and failure?

COPD causes changes in the pulmonary circulation, leading to increased blood pressure in the pulmonary arteries (pulmonary hypertension; Fig. 40). Mechanisms underlying this secondary pulmonary hypertension include:

• Loss of pulmonary arterioles and capillaries as part of the pathology of emphysema

• Pulmonary arterial vasoconstriction caused by hypoxia, secondary to COPD

• Increased viscosity of blood in the pulmonary circulation caused by polycythaemia, secondary to hypoxia

As the pressure in the pulmonary arteries rises, the right heart has to pump harder to force blood out of the right ventricle. The right ventricular muscle becomes thickened (hypertrophy) and problems extend to the right atrium, which can become dilated. Worsening hypoxia or secondary arrhythmias may cause 'decompensation' of right heart function, with systemic venous congestion, ankle oedema and hepatomegaly.

The clinical syndrome of right heart failure secondary to lung disease, associated with peripheral oedema is known as 'cor pulmonale'. Cor pulmonale is most commonly caused by COPD, but can also be caused by other chronic lung diseases that cause lung destruction and hypoxia (e.g. pulmonary fibrosis).

How could you assess his pulmonary arteries and right heart further?

• *Two-dimensional echocardiogram.* This studies cardiac structure and function and can detect right heart hypertrophy and strain

• *Doppler echocardiography.* This studies blood flow and can estimate pulmonary artery pressures from the velocity of blood regurgitating back through the tricuspid valve

• *Right heart catheterization.* A catheter inserted into the right heart and pulmonary artery via a large vein (internal jugular or femoral) can directly measure pressures in the right heart and pulmonary artery

Why does hypoxia cause polycythaemia?

Red blood cell production (erythropoiesis) is stimulated by erythropoietin, a hormone made by the kidney. Chronic hypoxia increases erythropoietin levels, over-stimulating the bone marrow and causing excessive red blood cell production. Polycythaemia increases blood viscosity, contributing to pulmonary hypertension and increasing the risk of systemic vascular events such as stroke.

Mr Shamin does have polycythaemia, as shown by his elevated haemoglobin and packed cell volume.

How would you treat Mr Shamin?

The first step is to write a problem list. Summarizing his problems will allow each one to be addressed.

Summarize Mr Shamin's medical problems

• COPD with worsening airflow obstruction
• Continues to smoke
• Hypoxia
• Right heart failure with symptomatic ankle swelling
• Polycythaemia
• Low body mass index

How should these problems be managed?
COPD with worsening airflow obstruction

This is the cause of all his other problems. Improvement in his COPD could improve oxygenation and reduce right heart failure. He is already on short- and long-acting bronchodilators and inhaled steroids. Reasonable options include:

• Check and optimize inhaler technique, advise use of volumatic

• Give short-acting bronchodilators as regular home nebulizers

• Treat him as if he is having an exacerbation with a short course of oral prednisolone

Ongoing smoking

He should receive strong advice and support to stop smoking because:

• Smoking will cause progression of his COPD

• If he needs home oxygen, smoking is dangerous as oxygen speeds burning and is a fire hazard. There are a number of reports in the literature of patients receiving severe burns from smoking while on oxygen. He must be advised of this before starting treatment

Hypoxia

Patients with COPD who have chronic hypoxia (PaO_2 <8 kPa) and develop signs of cor pulmonale have a 5-year survival of less than 50%. Oxygen treatment for at least

15 h/day can improve survival in this group of patients and in all COPD patients with PaO_2 <7.3 kPa:

• He should undergo treatment to improve COPD if possible, then should have his blood gases rechecked in at least 3 weeks to see if he is still hypoxic

• If his PaO_2 remains <8 kPa he should start on long-term oxygen therapy (Box 58)

Box 58 Long-term oxygen therapy

Indications

Long-term oxygen therapy (>15 h/day) improves survival in COPD patients who have persistent:

• PaO_2 <7.3 kPa; or
• PaO_2 <8 kPa with evidence of right heart failure or polycythaemia

It is not given to improve breathlessness.

Supply

Oxygen can be provided as:

• Cylinders
• Liquid oxygen
• Purified from room air by electrically driven concentrators

Concentrators are the cheapest and easiest way to provide oxygen where it is needed continuously. Patients may have back-up cylinders in case of power cuts.

Starting

Respiratory drive in patients with severe COPD may depend on hypoxia. Therefore, oxygen therapy should be tested with an oxygen trial to make sure CO_2 retention does not develop before the patient is started on oxygen at home. Arterial blood gases are tested before and 1 h after oxygen therapy at 1 L/min. The oxygen flow rate is adjusted upwards until a rate (usually 1–3 L/min) is identified that improves PaO_2 to >8 kPa without significant increase in $PaCO_2$.

What is it like?

Patients have to spend at least 15 h/day on oxygen. This can be made easier by:

• Sleeping with oxygen on
• Using nasal prongs to allow oxygen treatment while chatting and eating
• Having long oxygen tubing to allow them to wear oxygen while in bed, watching TV or doing household chores

Some patients find oxygen treatment very restrictive. Nasal oxygen tubing can rub their ears and oxygen treatment itself may dry their nasal membranes and cause nose bleeds.

Right heart failure

This often improves with treatment of hypoxia, either by optimizing COPD therapy or starting home oxygen treatment:

• Oedema can be controlled by diuretic treatment (e.g. 20–40 mg/day furosemide [frusemide]). However, watch out for the common side-effect of hypokalaemia which may precipitate cardiac arrhythmias.

Polycythaemia

Treatment of his polycythaemia may improve his cor pulmonale by reducing pulmonary artery pressure and pulmonary vascular resistance:

• *Venesection.* In the short term, removal of red blood cells to reduce his packed cell volume to <0.5 L/L could improve his cor pulmonale

• *Oxygen.* In the long term, improvement of oxygenation and reduction of exposure to carbon monoxide (smoking) could prevent recurrence of polycythaemia

Low body mass index

Patients with low body mass index (BMI) are more likely to die than heavier patients. He should receive dietary advice and supplements as necessary to encourage him to put on weight. Smoking cessation may also help.

How does the multidisciplinary team interact in management of COPD patients?

Primary and secondary care professionals (Box 27, p. 38) work together in the care of COPD patients and their roles may overlap. The patient should be at the centre of the team and should be as involved in the management as possible. For example, patients may have a self-management plan and be able to start antibiotics and steroids for an exacerbation themselves. Roles include the following.

Doctor

• Diagnoses disease, comorbidities and complications
• Provides education and information
• Prescribes therapy

Specialist respiratory nurse

• Supports and educates patients with new diagnoses
• Optimizes treatment, inhaler technique, nebulizer trials, oxygen assessment
• Manages exacerbations
• Provides home support

Physiotherapy

Provides:

- Pulmonary rehabilitation programmes
- Education and support
- Clearance of respiratory secretions

Dietitian

- Supports maintenance of normal BMI and good nutrition

Palliative care, including hospice

- Symptom control (e.g. management of chronic breathlessness)
- End of life issues

Social work

- Financial support, benefits, carer support

Occupational therapy

- Arrange support with activities of daily living, including shopping, washing and dressing

Outcome. Mr Shamin was started on nebulized bronchodilators and 30 mg/day prednisolone to improve his COPD. His ankle swelling was treated with co-amilofruse (furosemide combined with a potassium-sparing diuretic) and he underwent venesection. He was strongly advised to stop smoking and was prescribed nicotine patches to help him with this.

Three weeks later his ankle swelling was reduced but he remained hypoxic with PaO$_2$ of 6.9 kPa. After an oxygen trial he was started on oxygen treatment with flow rate 2 L/min for at least 15 h/day and had a concentrator installed at home. He was strongly advised not to smoke in the house because of the fire hazard.

Three months later he was much improved with no evidence of right heart failure. His packed cell volume was satisfactory at 0.48 L/L. He was managing oxygen therapy and receiving visits from the community respiratory nurse. He had reduced his cigarettes to 1–2 per day and smoked these outside, away from oxygen treatment. He was now felt to be fit enough to benefit from pulmonary rehabilitation and was referred to the programme.

PART 2: CASES

CASE REVIEW

Mr Shamin has severe COPD and now presents with a 4-week history of ankle swelling. Examination reveals right heart failure and hypoxia and a diagnosis of cor pulmonale is made. Mr Shamin is also found to have polycythaemia. He is initially treated with bronchodilators and steroids to optimize his COPD, diuretics to relieve his ankle swelling and venesection for his polycythaemia. He is commenced on long-term oxygen therapy for at least 15 h/day with the aim to improve prognosis from his COPD and reduce symptoms of right heart failure and recurrence of polycythaemia. Three months later he is fit enough to commence a pulmonary rehabilitation programme.

KEY POINTS

- COPD and other severe chronic lung diseases cause pulmonary hypertension by:
  - destruction of pulmonary arterioles and capillaries
  - hypoxia, causing pulmonary arterial vasoconstriction
  - increased blood viscosity in pulmonary circulation caused by hypoxia-induced polycythaemia
- Pulmonary hypertension leads to right heart hypertrophy, dilatation and failure
- Clinical features of right heart failure include:
  - raised JVP
  - hepatic enlargement brought about by congestion
  - peripheral oedema
  - pleural effusions
- Clinical trials have shown that long-term oxygen therapy >15 h/day improves survival of COPD patients with:
  - PaO$_2$ <7.3 kPa
  - PaO$_2$ <8 kPa with evidence of right heart failure or polycythaemia
- In clinical practice, long-term oxygen therapy improves symptoms of right heart failure and reduces incidence of polycythaemia
- Patients who require long-term oxygen therapy should be strongly advised to give up smoking as oxygen speeds burning and is a fire hazard. Home oxygen should only be given to patients who smoke if they are reliably able to keep smoking and oxygen apart
- Multidisciplinary teamwork by professionals including doctors, nurses, physiotherapists, dietitians, palliative care and social workers is essential to provide good care for patients with end-stage COPD

Case 10 A 72-year-old man with a hoarse voice

A 72-year-old man, Mr Cole, attends a routine appointment with his GP. As Mr Cole speaks his doctor notices that his voice is a hoarse whisper. Mr Cole explains that his voice has been like this for 3–4 weeks, but he had thought it was because of a cold. Mr Cole then produces a breathy cough.

What causes a hoarse voice?

Sound is made during speech by changes in air pressure in the larynx, which cause the vocal cords to snap together. A hoarse voice can be caused by the following.

Laryngeal or vocal cord lesions

• Laryngitis (e.g. viral infection, smoking, acid reflux)
• Voice overuse
• Inhaled steroids
• Vocal cord nodules
• Laryngeal carcinoma

Damage to nerves that supply the larynx

(Box 59)
• Lung cancer
• Thyroid surgery
• Thyroid cancer
• Dissection of the thoracic aorta

What is the most likely cause of Mr Cole's hoarse voice?

Mr Cole's voice is a hoarse whisper and he has a breathy cough. These signs indicate that his vocal cords are not coming together to make a proper sound. This is likely to be caused by recurrent laryngeal nerve palsy, preventing movement of one of the vocal cords. However, lesion of the cords themselves cannot be ruled out at this stage.

Laryngeal or lung cancer should be considered as the cause of hoarseness lasting more than 3 weeks in an adult. Mr Cole's hoarse voice has been present for 3–4 weeks so cancer is a possible diagnosis.

What other information does the GP need to assess Mr Cole fully?

The GP should establish in the history whether there is:
• Other information pointing to a vocal cord/laryngeal lesion:
  ○ voice overuse?
  ○ use of inhaled medication?
• Other information pointing towards a thoracic lesion:
  ○ respiratory symptoms?
  ○ vascular disease?
• History of exposure to risk factors causing laryngeal or lung cancer:
  ○ smoking history – this is the most important cause of laryngeal as well as lung cancer

The GP should also examine the thyroid gland, cervical lymph nodes and respiratory system.

Mr Cole has smoked 30 cigarettes per day since the age of 20 and still enjoys the habit. He has coughed up grey sputum in the morning on most days for several years and is short of breath walking uphill.

On examination his lungs are hyperinflated, but there are no other abnormal findings.

How many pack years has he smoked?

He has smoked 30 cigarettes per day for 52 years (i.e. approximately 78 pack years; Box 16, p. 19).

What do his other symptoms and signs indicate?

His chronic productive cough is chronic bronchitis, a component of chronic obstructive pulmonary disease (COPD) caused by smoking. He has MRC grade 2 shortness of breath (Box 12, p. 18) and hyperinflation, which are consistent with COPD. There are no other features of lung cancer.

PART 2: CASES

Box 59 Innervation of the larynx

- The 10th cranial nerve (vagus nerve) arises in the medulla of the brain
- Left and right recurrent laryngeal nerves are motor branches of the vagus nerve, which supply the vocal cords
- Anatomy:
  - left recurrent laryngeal nerve – this arises from the left vagus nerve as it passes in front of the thoracic aortic arch, then passes below and behind the arch
  - right recurrent laryngeal nerve – this arises from the right vagus nerve as it passes in front of the right subclavian artery, then loops round and behind the right subclavian artery
  - both nerves then ascend in grooves between the trachea and oesophagus on their respective sides behind the thyroid gland to reach the larynx
- Damage
  - the left recurrent laryngeal nerve is susceptible to damage from chest and aortic lesions, as it loops down into the chest
  - both recurrent laryngeal nerves are susceptible to damage from thyroid surgery or disease

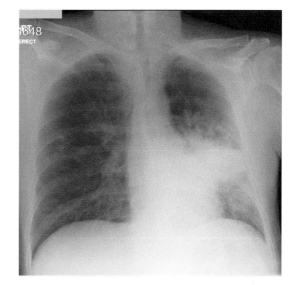

Figure 41 Mr Cole's chest X-ray.

How does this information help in Mr Cole's assessment?

His smoking history would be sufficient to cause laryngeal or lung cancer. Other negative findings are not sufficient to exclude a diagnosis of cancer and this needs further investigation.

What should his GP do now?

Department of Health guidelines state that anyone who has had a hoarse voice for more than 3 weeks should be referred urgently for chest X-ray and ENT examination, so Mr Cole should undergo this assessment.

!RED FLAG

Patients with a hoarse voice for >3 weeks should be referred urgently for chest X-ray and ENT examination to look for laryngeal or lung cancer.

Mr Cole's chest X-ray is carried out that day (Fig. 41). He receives an ENT appointment for the following week.

What does the chest X-ray show?

The X-ray shows a mass at the left hilum.

What could be causing this chest X-ray abnormality?

The most likely cause is primary lung cancer.
   Less likely causes include:
- Secondary tumour deposit in the lung (Box 60; Fig. 42)
- Tuberculosis
- Lymphoma
- Consolidation caused by pneumonia

Could the chest X-ray findings account for Mr Cole's hoarse voice?

The X-ray shows a hilar mass, which is probably lung cancer. This could be involving the recurrent laryngeal nerve, causing vocal cord paralysis and hoarseness. Mr Cole's hilar mass is on the left side. The left recurrent laryngeal nerve is more susceptible than the right to damage from chest lesions as it runs a longer course deeper into the chest (Box 59).

What are the priorities for Mr Cole's management now?

He needs a diagnostic work-up to:
- Determine the cause of his left hilar mass
- Determine treatment options for his left hilar lesion
- Establish whether the left hilar mass is sufficient to account for his hoarseness or whether alternative diagnoses should be sought
- His ENT appointment could be cancelled

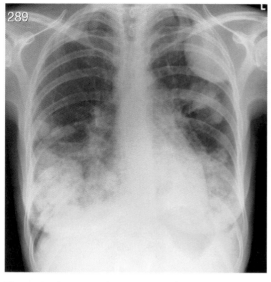

Figure 42 Chest X-ray showing cannon ball metastases in the lung from renal cell carcinoma.

Box 60 Secondary tumours in the lung

Haematogenous spread

Cancer cells enter tumour veins, are carried through the right side of the heart and are deposited in the lung parenchyma (Fig. 42). Tumours that metastasize in this way include:

- Renal
- Gastrointestinal tract
- Breast
- Cervix
- Ovary or testicle

Lymphatic spread

Tumour cells deposited in mediastinal nodes can spread along lymphatics into the lung. As the lymphatics become stuffed with tumour the patient becomes more and more short of breath (*lymphangitis carcinomatosis*). Cancers that spread in this way are usually adenocarcinomas and include:

- Stomach
- Colon
- Breast

  Lymphangitis carcinomatosis is also a recognized complication of primary lung cancer.

Mr Cole is seen urgently by a chest physician who arranges a bronchoscopy and a contrast-enhanced computed tomography (CT) scan of Mr Cole's chest and abdomen.

Why did the chest physician arrange a bronchoscopy?

The aim of the bronchoscopy is to attempt to visualize the lesion and take biopsies from it to obtain a tissue diagnosis which may guide treatment (see Part 1, Approach to the Patient, p. 33). As Mr Cole's lesion is central (at the lung hilum) it may be in a large airway where it will be accessible to biopsy. In patients with peripheral lesions arising from smaller airways inaccessible to the bronchoscope, cancer cells may be obtained by bronchial washings. Transbronchial needle aspiration can also be used to take samples from enlarged lymph nodes through the airway wall.

What information is needed before the bronchoscopy can be perfomed?

The main adverse events of bronchoscopy and biopsy are hypoxia and bleeding. Patients particularly at risk of complications include those with severely impaired lung function or bleeding disorders. These patients should be identified before the procedure and alternative tests arranged if the risks of procedure outweigh potential benefits. Prebronchoscopy assessment should include:

- Clinical assessment
- Oxygen saturations
- Platelet count
- Clotting function

What is the purpose of the CT scan?

In patients with possible lung cancer CT scanning can be used to:

- Characterize the lung lesion
- Stage the cancer, assessing local and metastatic spread of the tumour
- Direct bronchoscopy to the best area in the lung for sampling
- Identify enlarged lymph nodes for transbronchial needle aspiration
- Take a percutaneous CT guided biopsy from lesions inaccessible at bronchoscopy

At bronchoscopy, Mr Cole's left vocal cord was found to be fixed in a paramedian position and no laryngeal lesions were seen. A lesion with the appearances of lung cancer was seen in the left main bronchus (Fig. 43). The lesion was biopsied and brushings and washings were performed.

Bronchial biopsies revealed squamous cell carcinoma as the cause of his lung lesion.

His CT scan showed mediastinal lymphadenopathy and his tumour was staged at T2 N2 M0.

PART 2: CASES

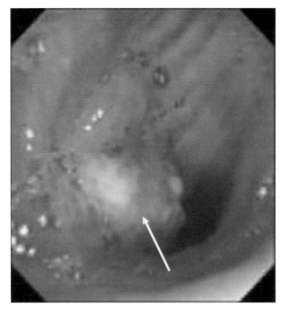

Figure 43 Lung cancer visualized by bronchoscopy. The picture shows the view down a bronchus seen through a bronchoscope. The arrow indicates a tumour protruding from the bronchial wall into the lumen.

How do you interpret the appearance of his vocal cord at bronchoscopy?

The fixed left vocal cord held in a paramedian position (half open, half closed) is a typical appearance of a cord affected by palsy of the supplying nerve. This, along with the absence of laryngeal abnormality, is strongly supportive of the diagnosis of recurrent laryngeal nerve palsy (Box 61).

What causes lung cancer?

Active cigarette smoking is the most important risk factor for the development of lung cancer. Overall, the risk of lung cancer is increased 13 times by active smoking. The risk of lung cancer increases with smoking load. A person who has a 40 pack year smoking history over 20 years has a 60–70 times greater risk of lung cancer than a non-smoker.

Other risk factors for lung cancer are given in Box 62.

What is squamous cell carcinoma of the lung?

Bronchi are normally lined by cuboidal epithelium. If the epithelium is subjected to repeated damage or

---

Box 61 Effects of direct local spread of lung cancer to adjacent structures

Chest wall
Local invasion causes:
- Pain
- Mass

Blood vessels
- Tumour compresses and obstructs the *superior vena cava*, reducing venous return from the head and upper limbs to the heart. This causes facial congestion, upper limb oedema and headaches

Nerves
Recurrent laryngeal nerve
- Involved by tumour in the hilum or mediastinum (left) or lung apices (left or right)
- Causes a hoarse voice and ineffective breathy cough

Sympathetic chain in neck
- Involved by tumour in the lung apex
- Causes constriction of the pupil of the eye on the affected side as a result of loss of sympathetic activation. The eye is also sunken (enophthalmos) and there is reduced sweating of the face on the affected side. This is called Horner's syndrome

Lower brachial plexus
- Tumours in the lung apex infiltrate the lower brachial plexus (Pancoast's tumour)
- This causes wasting of the small muscles of the hand and pain in the arm and hand

Oesophagus
- Mediastinal tumour can compress the oesophagus, causing difficulty in swallowing

---

Box 62 Risk factors for lung cancer other than active cigarette smoking

- Environmental smoke exposure (passive smoking)
- Marijuana and cocaine smoking
- Occupational carcinogens, including:
  - asbestos
  - arsenic
  - chromium
  - petroleum products and tar
- Environmental carcinogens
  - radon (gaseous decay product of uranium and radium that emits alpha particles, may accumulate in homes built above granite)

> **Box 63 Histological classification of lung cancer**
>
> The frequency of tumour types in the UK as a proportion of all lung cancer cases is given in brackets (information from Cancer Research UK statistics, November 2004).
>
> **Non-small cell lung cancer**
> - Squamous cell (35–45%)
>   - ∘ derived from bronchial epithelial cells
> - Adenocarcinoma (15%)
>   - ∘ derived from glandular tissue in the airway submucosa
> - Large cell carcinoma (10%)
> - Carcinoid (1%)
> - Bronchoalveolar cell carcinoma (rare)
>
> **Small cell lung cancer (~20%)**
> - Derived from endocrine cells in the lung

irritation (e.g. by cigarette smoking) it may change its form to squamous epithelium to withstand this (metaplasia). Early malignant changes (dysplasia) may arise during this process which may progress to cancer (neoplasia).

What other pathological types of lung cancer are there and how are they classified?

Lung cancer is generally classified by histological findings (Box 63), which allows planning and standardization of treatment. The main distinction is between non-small cell and small cell lung cancers as these respond differently to treatment:

- Non-small cell cancer:
  - ∘ responds poorly to chemotherapy
  - ∘ surgery can be curative for patients with localized disease
- Small cell lung cancer:
  - ∘ grows fast, therefore initially is responsive to chemotherapy
  - ∘ metastasizes early, therefore surgery has no role in the management of this condition

What does tumour staging mean and why is it done?

Tumour staging is an assessment of tumour spread and metastasis. It allows accurate prediction of response to therapy and prognosis and is used in combination with histological findings to decide on appropriate treatment for individual patients.

Mr Cole's tumour was staged at T2 N2 M0. What does this mean?

The TNM system is used for staging non-small cell lung cancer:

- 'T' is a measure of local invasion by the tumour and ranges from 0 (no evidence of primary tumour) to 4 (local spread of tumour to mediastinum or pleura)
- 'N' is a measure of spread of tumour to lymph nodes and ranges from 0 (no lymph node spread) to 3 (spread to more distant nodes)
- 'M' is a measure of distant tumour metastasis and ranges from 0 (no metastasis) to 1 (distant metastasis is present)

The more the tumour has spread or metastasized, the worse the prognosis and the lower the chance of curative treatment. In Mr Cole's case his T2 N2 M0 tumour is associated with a 23% 5-year survival rate.

How is non-small cell lung cancer treated?

Surgical resection of localized tumour gives the best chance of cure.

Suitability for surgery is determined by:
- Tumour resectability (lack of local spread or metastases)
- Physiological fitness of patient to survive major surgery

Surgical options include:
- Lobectomy or pneumonectomy
- Limited resection (segment or lung wedge containing tumour) if patients are physiologically compromised
- Mediastinal nodes are also removed for treatment and disease mapping

The decision to operate should be made by a thoracic surgeon with expertise in oncology as part of the multidisciplinary team. Unfortunately, 80% of patients with non-small cell lung cancer present with disease that is too advanced for surgery.

Radiotherapy can be used as:
- An adjunct to surgery in patients with potentially curable disease
- Radical therapy in patients with potentially curable disease who are considered inoperable
- Palliative therapy in patients with local or metastatic complications of their lung tumour

The clinical team considered that Mr Cole's tumour was probably too advanced for surgical treatment. However, to confirm this they arranged a positron emission tomography (PET) scan to examine his mediastinal lymph nodes. While waiting for the scan Mr Cole was admitted as an emergency complaining of pain in his lower back and difficulty passing urine.

How is a PET scan performed?
• A radiolabelled sugar (fluorodeoxyglucose [FDG]) is injected into the patient's veins
• There is a delay of around 1 h while FDG is taken up by the tissues
• The scan is performed to identify areas of high FDG uptake, then correlated with CT findings to relate anatomy to metabolic function
• Tumours grow and metabolize rapidly, therefore they take up more FDG than normal adult tissues
• Lymph node enlarged by tumour may be seen on the PET scan as areas of high isotope uptake, whereas lymph nodes enlarged for other reasons may not be detected by PET scanning

Why was Mr Cole asked to undergo a PET scan?
Mr Cole appears to have node involvement on his CT scan which stages his tumour at an advanced stage. PET scanning will help establish whether his lymphadeno-pathy is caused by cancer or other causes. If his PET scan is negative he could still be a candidate for surgical treatment.

What should you think of as the cause of Mr Cole's new symptoms?
You should immediately think of spinal cord compression in a patient with back pain and a change in bladder or bowel function. In Mr Cole's case the most important possible cause is spinal metastases from his lung cancer causing cord compression through effects of tumour bulk or by causing vertebral collapse.

What should the doctors do next?
Spinal cord compression is a clinical emergency and requires urgent diagnosis and treatment to prevent permanent neurological damage. Mr Cole should undergo a neurological examination, then X-ray and magnetic resonance imaging (MRI) of his spine to establish whether this has occurred.

!RED FLAG
Acute spinal cord compression is a medical emergency and requires rapid diagnosis and treatment before permanent neurological disability occurs.

It should be considered in patients with changes in control of bladder or bowel or neurological symptoms in their legs.

On examination Mr Cole had normal tone in his legs. Power was 5/5 in all muscle groups, coordination and sensation was normal and plantars were downgoing. He had a palpable bladder on abdominal examination. Rectal examination revealed normal anal tone, a smooth enlarged prostate and impacted faeces.

Does he have spinal cord compression?
Neurological examination is reassuring as there is no evidence of increased tone, weakness, upgoing plantars or sensory loss in his legs. Examination findings provide the alternative explanation of constipation and prostatic hypertrophy for his urinary retention. His back pain still requires investigation, although now not as an emergency.

What tests would be useful in investigating his back pain?
• Plain X-rays
• Bone scan
• CT or MRI of the spine
Serum calcium should be measured to exclude hyper-calcaemia, which can be caused by bone destruction by metastases or by secretion of parathyroid hormone related peptide or parathyroid hormone by the tumour.

Mr Cole's spinal X-rays and CT scan are shown in Fig. 44. His serum calcium is normal.

Have the X-rays identified a cause for his back pain?
He has a compression fracture of L2 which looks abnormal on CT scanning and contains metastasis (Box 64) from his primary lung cancer.

How should Mr Cole be treated?
As he has spinal metastases curative surgical resection of his lung tumour is not an option. His PET scan is cancelled.

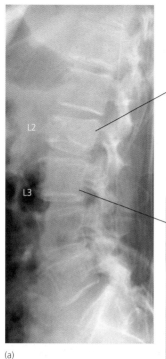

(a)

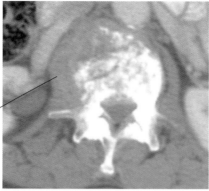

(b)

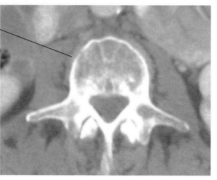

(c)

Figure 44 Plain X-rays and computed tomography (CT) scan of lumbar spine showing metastases. (a) Plain X-ray of lumbar spine showing compression fracture of L2. L3 is normal. (b) CT appearance of L2 showing abnormality in the vertebral body and fracture resulting from metastasis. (c) Normal CT appearances of L3 vertebral body for comparison.

> **Box 64 Metastatic complications of lung cancer**
>
> **Bone**
> • Causes pain, hypercalcaemia, pathological fractures, compression of adjacent neurological tissue
>
> **Liver**
> • Causes hepatomegaly, obstructive jaundice
>
> **Brain**
> • Causes headache, fits, confusion, raised intracranial pressure, focal neurological deficit (e.g. hemiplegia, hemianopia, depending on site of metastasis)
>
> **Adrenals**
> • May cause hypoadrenalism

He should receive palliative and supportive care including:
• Radiotherapy for painful metastases
• Analgesia
• Nutritional support
• Psychological and spiritual support
• Financial and practical help
• Legal and other advice

Is this the first time in Mr Cole's treatment that he has been considered as a person and not just 'a case of lung cancer'?

Patients with suspected lung cancer go through a rapid series of tests to establish the diagnosis, stage the tumour and decide on treatment. The reason for this haste is to offer as many people as possible treatment with some chance of cure or prolonged survival before their disease has progressed too far. Mr Cole went from discussing a routine problem with his GP to an urgent chest X-ray, respiratory referral, bronchoscopy, diagnosis and staging CT in around 2 weeks. A key part of Mr Cole's management is that he should be informed and contribute to the decision-making about his care. At each step of his investigation doctors and other professionals should discuss possible diagnoses, explain procedures and discuss benefits and risks of investigations and treatments with him. Mr Cole should be invited to involve a family member or other close person in his consultations if he wishes and be offered written information, support and symptom relief at all stages.

Outcome. Mr Cole received radiotherapy to his back with good pain relief. He was discharged home with outpatient support from his local hospice. Over the next 8 months he deteriorated with marked loss of weight and increasing

shortness of breath. He died at home of a respiratory infection supported by his wife and Macmillan nurses.

KEY POINT

Lung cancer is difficult to treat but relatively easy to prevent.

It is the responsibility of all doctors to advise people not to smoke.

CASE REVIEW

Mr Cole is noticed to have a hoarse voice on a routine visit to his GP. An urgent chest X-ray shows a left hilar mass and he is referred to secondary care for urgent investigation. At bronchoscopy, left vocal cord palsy and tumour in the left main bronchus are seen. Biopsy shows squamous cell car-cinoma. Staging CT shows metastasis to mediastinal lymph nodes. He subsequently develops back pain and an MRI demonstrates spinal metastases. He receives palliative radiotherapy to his back with good relief and dies at home with support from Macmillan nurses and his family.

KEY POINTS

- Patients with a hoarse voice for more than 3 weeks should be referred urgently for chest X-ray and ENT examination to look for lung or laryngeal cancer
- Causes of a mass seen on chest X-ray include:
  - primary lung cancer
  - secondary tumour deposit in the lung
  - tuberculosis
  - lymphoma
- Hilar masses are more likely to involve the recurrent laryngeal nerve on the left than on the right because of the different anatomy of the nerve on the two sides
- Further investigations of a mass seen on chest X-ray include CT scanning and bronchoscopy to characterize the lesion, obtain tissue for histology and stage possible cancers

- Lung cancer is predominantly caused by tobacco smoking
- Histological types of primary lung cancer are non-small cell (squamous cell, adenocarcinoma, large cell, carcinoid, bronchoalveolar cell) or small cell
- Tissue diagnosis of lung cancer is important as it guides treatment
- Treatment for non-small cell lung cancer includes:
  - curative resection for localized lung cancer
  - radiotherapy
  - chemotherapy, although the response is poor
- Complications of lung cancer include:
  - local spread
  - distant metastases (bone, liver, brain, adrenals)
  - paraneoplastic phenomena (see Case 11)

Case 11 A 56-year-old woman with an abnormal chest X-ray

Mrs Gibson, a 56-year-old woman, sees her GP complaining of cough and weight loss and is sent for a chest X-ray (Fig. 45). The radiologist reporting the film finds an abnormality and contacts the respiratory team who arrange to see her that week in a rapid access clinic.

What does her chest X-ray show?

The most notable abnormality is a large mass in the midzone of her left lung. There is some associated pleural fluid or reaction obscuring the left costophrenic angle.

What is the differential diagnosis for this chest X-ray abnormality?

This appearance is most likely caused by cancer which is either:

- Primary lung cancer; or
- Secondary metastasis

   Lung abcess, tuberculosis or pneumonia are less likely possibilities.

What is a rapid access clinic?

The UK National Cancer Plan has recommended a series of waiting time targets to prevent treatment delays in patients with lung cancer. These targets include a maximum of 14 days from GP referral to hospital appointment and 62 days from GP referral to first treatment. To facilitate this many hospitals have set up specific clinics to ensure patients with possible lung cancer have rapid access to services.

Mrs Gibson attends the clinic with her husband. She is extremely concerned about her abnormal chest X-ray and immediately asks the doctor whether she has cancer.

How should the doctor respond?

There is no easy response to such a question, particularly at this stage. The doctor already knows that cancer is the most likely diagnosis; however, it has not yet been proven

and non-cancer diagnoses are possible. He has just met Mrs Gibson and has had no opportunity to establish a doctor–patient relationship with her or predict how she may react. His response to her question may affect their future interaction and could facilitate or damage future communication.

   A reasonable approach could include some or all of the following:

- Asking Mrs Gibson what she has been told already and what her suspicions are
- Following this up by admitting that cancer is a possible diagnosis, but there are other differentials
- Explaining that the purpose of the clinic is to find out what is wrong with her, but this will require questions, examination and investigations
- Reassuring her that the assessment will be performed as quickly as possible and she will be informed of the results
- Establishing how much she would like to be told as information becomes available

Mrs Gibson tells her doctor that she knows she has a shadow on her chest X-ray. She has jumped to the conclusion that it is lung cancer as her father died of this condition. She agrees to further assessment, on the condition that she is fully informed of all results and involved in any decisions about her treatment.

What features in her history would point to a diagnosis of lung cancer?

Mrs Gibson presented to her GP with cough and weight loss. Further characterization of these and enquiry about associated symptoms are important to support the diagnosis.

   Most patients with lung cancer present with respiratory symptoms, generally coming on over weeks. It is helpful to establish:

- Whether Mrs Gibson's cough is recent or has changed at all. A long-standing cough over months or years indi-

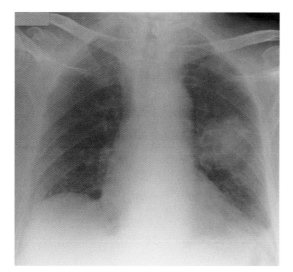

Figure 45 Chest X-ray.

PART 2: CASES

> **Box 65 Lymphatic drainage of the lung**
>
> Lymphatic drainage of the lung occurs via:
> - The superficial lymphatic plexus, which is deep to the visceral pleura and drains around the periphery of the lungs to bronchopulmonary nodes in the hila
> - The deep lymphatic plexus, which follows vessels and airways to the hila and also drains into the hilar (bronchopulmonary) nodes
>
> Efferent lymph channels carry lymph from the bronchopulmonary nodes to (sequentially):
> - Tracheobronchial nodes at the bifurcation of the trachea (carina)
> - Paratracheal nodes (alongside the trachea)
> - Mediastinal lymph trunks
>
> The right mediastinal lymph trunk joins right subclavian (from the right upper limb) and right jugular (from the right side of the head and neck) trunks and all three have a common opening into the origin of the right brachiocephalic vein via right supraclavicular lymph nodes.
>
> The left mediastinal lymph trunk, left subclavian (from the left upper limb) and jugular (left head and neck) trunks usually join the thoracic duct (from the lower limbs and abdomen), which drains via supraclavicular lymph nodes into great veins at the root of the neck.

cates another diagnosis (e.g. chronic obstructive pulmonary disease [COPD])
- Whether she has associated respiratory symptoms:
  - chest pain – chest wall involvement
  - haemoptysis – bleeding from the tumour
  - chest infection – tumours may partially obstruct airways, impeding mucociliary clearance and causing recurrent or intractable chest infection
  - shortness of breath – this may be caused by large airway obstruction or development of associated pleural effusion
  - malaise, weight loss and anorexia occur in almost all patients with lung cancer at some point in their illness Risk factors for lung cancer should also be established.

Mrs Gibson's cough started around 4 weeks ago and is non-productive. Over that time she has lost around 1 stone in weight. As a child both her parents smoked heavily and she started smoking aged 12. She currently smokes around 40 cigarettes per day.

On examination Mrs Gibson looked cachectic. She had a palpable lymph node in the left supraclavicular fossa. There were no abnormal findings on chest examination. Her liver was palpable at 3 cm below the costal margin.

How many pack years has Mrs Gibson smoked?

She has smoked 2 packets of cigarettes per day for most of 44 years (i.e. approximately 88 pack years; Box 16, p. 19).

How do you explain the enlarged lymph node in her left supraclavicular fossa?

Supraclavicular lymphadenopathy, especially in patients over 40 years, is most commonly caused by malignancy. The route of lymphatic drainage to the supraclavicular nodes is outlined in Box 65. An enlarged left supraclavicular lymph node is often caused by metastatic stomach cancer and is known as Virchow's node. However, in Mrs Gibson's case the combination of left supraclavicular lymphadenopathy and an abnormal chest X-ray is most likely to be because of a primary lung malignancy (Box 66).

Why might her liver be enlarged?

This could be explained by metastases from primary lung or abdominal/pelvic malignancy.

What investigations should be performed to make a diagnosis?

As cancer is likely to be the cause of Mrs Gibson's illness it is important to obtain tissue to make a histological diagnosis. This could be performed using a number of different approaches.

> **Box 66 Differential diagnosis of supraclavicular lymphadenopathy**
>
> **Malignancy** (most common, particularly in patients over 40)
> Right sided:
> • Lung
> • Mediastinum
> • Oesophagus
> • Lymphoma
>   Left sided:
> • Abdominal and pelvic malignancies (e.g. stomach, pancreas, ovaries, prostate)
> • Lung (left side of thorax)
> • Lymphoma
>
> **Other**
> • Tuberculosis

Fine needle aspiration of supraclavicular nodes

A fine needle is inserted into the node and negative pressure applied using a syringe to suck cells out of the node. The sample is smeared on a slide and examined cytologically. This is said to be no more painful than having blood taken by venepuncture, does not usually require anaesthetic and has few if any complications.

Liver ultrasound and biopsy

If radiology demonstrates that a mass is causing her hepatomegaly, percutaneous liver biopsy could be used to obtain tissue to make a diagnosis. Local anaesthetic is used to numb the overlying skin and ultrasound guides the biopsy needle into the abnormal part of the liver. The main complication is haemorrhage.

Fibreoptic bronchoscopy

If the tumour arises from a large airway this procedure will allow direct visualization of the tumour, which can be biopsied using forceps inserted along the bronchoscope. The main complication is haemorrhage. If the tumour is peripheral it will not be seen, but bronchial washings can be taken from the affected segment and examined cytologically for cancer cells.

CT guided biopsy

Peripheral lung tumours not accessible by bronchoscopy can be sampled by percutaneous transthoracic needle biopsy (i.e. a biopsy needle inserted through the chest wall into the tumour under CT guidance). Local anaes-

thetic is required and the procedure may be complicated by pneumothorax or haemorrhage.

Which of these investigations would be best for Mrs Gibson?

Fine needle aspiration of her palpable supraclavicular node is a very low risk procedure that has a good chance of making a positive diagnosis. The other techniques all carry risks of complications, with a real (although very low) risk of mortality. An initial approach would be to sample her supraclavicular node and arrange a contrast enhanced CT scan of her chest and abdomen to assess and stage her tumour and examine her liver. If the lymph node aspirate was unhelpful, further investigations could be planned based on the CT result. These investigations should be carried out as quickly as possible so as not to delay the diagnosis.

> *Mrs Gibson underwent fine needle aspiration of her left supraclavicular node. Cytological examination revealed small cell lung cancer. Her CT scan showed a large mass in her left hemithorax with mediastinal lymphadenopathy. Her liver was pushed down by hyperinflation of her lungs but not enlarged and no metastases were seen. Her adrenal glands looked normal.*

What is small cell lung cancer?

Small cell lung cancer arises from endocrine cells in the lung which are members of the APUD system (amine precursor uptake and decarboxylation). Small cell tumours comprise 20–30% of lung cancers and are rapidly growing and highly malignant. These tumours have usually metastasized, either overtly or occultly, at the time of presentation. As the tumour cells have an endocrine origin they often secrete hormones which have systemic effects.

Why did the radiologist comment on her adrenal glands?

Bronchogenic carcinoma often metastasizes to the adrenal glands, therefore examination of these is an important part of tumour staging.

> *Mrs Gibson's adrenal glands and liver look normal on CT scan so she has no overt evidence of distant tumour metastasis.*

What is the importance of staging a patient's lung cancer?

Tumour staging is helpful for planning treatment and can give an indication of prognosis.

> **Box 67 Staging of small cell lung cancer and prognostic indicators**
>
> **Staging**
> - *Limited disease.* Disease limited to the hemithorax of origin, mediastinum and supraclavicular nodes
> - *Extensive disease.* Widespread tumour beyond the extent of limited disease
>
> **Prognostic factors**
> - *Better prognosis.* Good performance status, female gender, limited disease
> - *Poor prognosis.* Poor performance status, liver or central nervous system (CNS) involvement

Mrs Gibson has limited disease (Box 67) which involves the left hemithorax, mediastinum and supraclavicular nodes but has not extended beyond these. As she is female and has good performance status she is in the best prognostic group.

What is the prognosis of small cell lung cancer?

This is an aggressive disease with a terrible prognosis. At presentation median survival is:
- *Limited disease.* 12 weeks
- *Extensive disease.* 4 weeks
  With best treatment:
- Survival is increased four- to fivefold.
- 10% of patients will remain disease-free for 2 years from start of therapy
- 5–10% of patients will survive for 5 years

  Investigation and start of treatment must therefore be as rapid as possible to give patients with small cell lung cancer the best chance of disease-free survival.

Mrs Gibson returns 1 week after her first appointment. Her husband has become concerned as she is irritable, nauseated and confused. He feels this is brought about by more than anxiety about her diagnosis.

What might account for Mrs Gibson's new confusion?

Possible causes include:
- Cerebral metastases from her small cell lung cancer
- Hormone excretion by the tumour causing hyponatraemia and confusion

- Secondary respiratory infection
- Hypoxia or hypercapnia secondary to lung disease
- Hypercalcaemia secondary to malignancy or bony metastases

What investigations would you order?
- CT brain scan
- Plasma biochemistry, calcium, full blood count and inflammatory markers
- Pulse oximetry, with arterial blood gases if abnormal

Mrs Gibson underwent these tests on the same day. Her results were as follows:
CT head. Normal
Blood tests:

		Normal range
Sodium	108 mmol/L	(135–145 mmol/L)
Potassium	4.2 mmol/L	(3.5–5.0 mmol/L)
Urea	5.6 mmol/L	(2.5–8 mmol/L)
Creatinine	94 µmol/L	(60–110 µmol/L)
Calcium	2.42 mmol/L	(2.2–2.6 mmol/L)
Liver function	Normal	
CRP	2 mg/L	(<8 mg/L)
Serum osmolarity	250 mosm/kg	(280–296 mosm/kg)
Urine osmolarity	600 mosm/kg	(350–1000 mosm/kg)
Full blood count	Normal	
Oxygen saturations	98%	

How do you interpret these results?
- She is hyponatraemic, which is sufficient to cause her symptoms
- There is no evidence of cerebral metastases or hypercalcaemia
- Inflammatory markers and oxygen saturations are normal

Why is she hyponatraemic?
- Her serum osmolarity is very low, indicating excess water in the blood
- In this situation, feedback to the posterior pituitary should turn off secretion of antidiuretic hormone (ADH), allowing water to be excreted in the urine. This should be seen as a low urine osmolarity
- Mrs Gibson has normal urine osmolarity, which indicates that she has failed to switch off ADH appropriately
- It is likely that Mrs Gibson has inappropriate ADH secretion from her small cell lung cancer that is not susceptible to normal regulation

---

> **Box 68 Paraneoplastic phenomena associated with lung cancer**
>
> **Cachexia**
> - Weight loss and wasting
>
> **Musculoskeletal and skin**
> - Finger clubbing
> - Hypertrophic pulmonary osteoarthropathy with pain, tenderness and swelling over affected bones
> - Acanthosis nigricans (localized hyperpigmentation)
>
> **Endocrine**
> - Inappropriate ADH secretion
> - Ectopic adrenocorticotrophic hormone secretion
> - Hypercalcaemia caused by secretion of parathyroid hormone-like substance
> - Gynaecomastia resulting from secretion of human chorionic gonadotrophin
>
> **Neurological**
> - Eaton–Lambert syndrome (antibodies to voltage-gated calcium channels causing proximal muscle weakness)
> - Peripheral neuropathies
> - Subacute cerebellar degeneration
> - Cortical degeneration
> - Polymyositis

This is a paraneoplastic complication of her lung tumour. Paraneoplastic syndromes are caused by factors produced by cancer cells that act at a distance from the primary cancer site or metastases. Other paraneoplastic phenomena associated with lung tumours are given in Box 68.

How should her hyponatraemia be treated?

Treatment of her small cell tumour to reduce cancer bulk may reduce ADH secretion and improve her hyponatraemia. She is not currently fit for this and needs restriction of water and fluid intake, monitoring and possibly demeclocycline, a drug that reduces renal sensitivity to ADH and allows water excretion.

In view of her confusion and urgent need to commence cancer treatment, Mrs Gibson is admitted to hospital to stabilize her condition. Over the next few days her serum sodium normalizes with water restriction and demeclocycline. As her confusion clears she is told the diagnosis. After a long discussion with the oncologists she and her husband decide that she should have chemotherapy

and radiotherapy as advised by the specialist. She prepares for treatment and also sees the palliative care team.

Why is she being given chemotherapy?

Small cell cancer is responsive to chemotherapy as it is rapidly growing. It also metastasizes early and so systemic treatment is required as local treatments such as surgery have little chance of curing or controlling her disease.

Why will she also receive radiotherapy?

In patients with limited stage small cell carcinoma, combination chemotherapy and radiotherapy of tumour have been shown to produce a modest improvement in prognosis in comparison to chemotherapy alone.

Does referral to the palliative care team at this stage indicate that there is no hope of cure?

The palliative care team can help with symptom control in patients with cancer, even during active treatment. A rapport built up at this stage may help later in the illness if it becomes necessary to withdraw active treatment. Patients with cancer and their families often need support with coming to terms with the diagnosis and dealing with end of life issues.

Mrs Gibson starts her first cycle of chemotherapy 2 weeks after her initial referral. She tolerates the treatment well apart from some diarrhoea and fatigue. The doctors monitor her blood count and during treatment she loses her hair.

Why does her chemotherapy cause diarrhoea and hair loss?

Chemotherapy kills cancer cells and normal cells that divide rapidly. In adults, most cells are non- or slowly dividing. Hair and intestinal cells do divide and so are most commonly affected, hence hair loss and diarrhoea. Blood cells are also rapidly dividing and a common side-effect of chemotherapy is bone marrow suppression which can increase susceptibility to infection. Her blood count is monitored to detect this.

Outcome. Mrs Gibson completes four cycles of chemotherapy and has thoracic radiation. However, 4 months later she is readmitted to hospital with worsening shortness of breath. She is found to have a large pleural effusion and liver metastases. At this point she refuses further chemotherapy and is transferred to the local hospice for palliative care. She dies comfortably 2 weeks later.

CASE REVIEW

Mrs Gibson presents to her GP with cough and weight loss. A chest X-ray shows a large mass in the midzone of her left lung and she is referred to the rapid access lung cancer clinic. Examination reveals an enlarged left supraclavicular lymph node and fine needle aspiration of this node gives a histological diagnosis of small cell lung cancer. On staging, she is found to have limited disease, but while awaiting chemotherapy she is admitted with confusion, caused by hyponatraemia secondary to inappropriate ADH secretion. Once her condition is stabilized, her cancer is treated with four cycles of chemotherapy and thoracic radiotherapy. Despite this she re-presents 4 months later with a pleural effusion and liver metastases. She is treated palliatively and dies comfortably in the local hospice.

KEY POINTS

- Small cell lung cancers are rapidly growing and highly malignant, hence have usually metastasized at time of presentation and carry a poor prognosis
- Small cell lung cancer arises from endocrine cells in the lung which are members of the APUD system. Therefore, they may secrete hormones that have a systemic effect, e.g.
  - antidiuretic hormone
  - adrenocorticotrophic hormone
  - parathyroid hormone-like hormone
- Small cell lung cancer is responsive to chemotherapy, although is unlikely to be cured

- The multidisciplinary team caring for patients with lung cancer includes:
  - doctors
  - nurses – hospital palliative care nurses and community Macmillan nurses
  - dietitians
  - occupational therapists
  - physiotherapists
  - social workers
  - religious leaders
  - counsellors

Case 12 # A 68-year-old man with shortness of breath and chest pain

Mr Stainson is a 68-year-old man who attends the chest clinic with the following referral letter from his GP.
Dear Doctor,
Thank you for seeing Mr Stainson who presented to the surgery last week complaining of shortness of breath and some dull left-sided chest pain. An urgent chest X-ray has been reported as showing pleural plaques suggestive of asbestos exposure and a left-sided pleural effusion. I would be grateful for your further assessment.

What is asbestos?

Asbestos is naturally occurring and is made up of silicates of iron and magnesium. It is obtained from the earth by mining and there are three main types:
- Chrysotile – white asbestos
- Crocidolite – blue asbestos
- Amosite – brown asbestos

Asbestos has heat-resistant and insulating properties, hence was used extensively as an insulating material until it was banned in 1989 (UK). It is still used elsewhere in the world.

How does exposure to asbestos occur?

- Direct asbestos exposure occurs in people working with asbestos (Box 69).
- Indirect exposure occurs in:
  - families of asbestos workers (e.g. through fibres brought into the home on work clothes)
  - people who live in an environment close to or contaminated by asbestos dust

In the UK, asbestos imports and hence exposure reached a peak in the 1970s.

How could you determine whether Mr Stainson has been exposed to asbestos?

A detailed occupational history should be taken to establish the possibility of asbestos exposure. This is important both medically, to assist with diagnosis, and legally because if Mr Stainson has asbestos-related lung disease

he might be eligible for compensation. At the first consultation the doctor should make a list of Mr Stainson's employers and the start and end dates of his employment with each one.

Mr Stainson's employment history is as follows:
1954–1957   Errand boy, local shop
1957–1975   Dockworker
1975–1985   Heavy goods vehicle driver, number of different companies
1985–present Black cab driver, self-employed
As a dockworker he remembers unloading sacks of raw asbestos, which often split and spilled dust. No one wore masks at that time to protect themselves as they did not know it was dangerous.

How does asbestos affect the lungs?

Asbestos exists in the form of fibres, which are at least three times longer than they are wide. Asbestos is a health risk when free fibres are present in the atmosphere as dust that can be inhaled. As they are breathed in, the long thin fibres become orientated longitudinally with the airways and so are able to descend right down into the small bronchioles. Here they are engulfed by macrophages and coated with ferritin granules, resulting in the formation of asbestos bodies. Pulmonary exposure to asbestos can cause several different pulmonary diseases (Box 70), which occur many years after the exposure.

Could any of these conditions account for Mr Stainson's presentation?

Mr Stainson has evidence of asbestos exposure (pleural plaques, Fig. 46) and a pleural effusion. His effusion could be caused by asbestos-related pulmonary disease:
- Mesothelioma
- Lung cancer
- Benign pleural disease

Box 69 Some occupations associated with asbestos exposure

Production and transport of asbestos fibres
- Mining
- Milling
- Transport and unloading (e.g. dockworkers)

Manufacture of insulation products
- Roofing
- Flooring
- Textiles
- Cements

Work with insulation products
- Building/demolition
- Shipping/aircraft/motor vehicles – manufacturers and mechanics
- Firefighters – asbestos dust may be released from fires in insulated buildings
- Other (e.g. people working with sheet metal, electrics, boilers, railways)

Box 70 Pulmonary conditions caused by asbestos exposure

Pleural plaques
- These are patches of pleural thickening, which become calcified over time
- They indicate asbestos exposure, but are benign
- They do not generally cause symptoms, although extensive benign pleural thickening encasing the lung can cause shortness of breath

Asbestosis
- Inflammation and fibrosis of the lung parenchyma occurs
- May be mild with minor symptoms or severe enough to cause death from respiratory failure
- Occurs 20–30 years after exposure

Lung cancer
- Asbestos exposure increases the risk of small cell and non-small cell lung cancer by several times in both smokers and non-smokers

Pleural mesothelioma
- This is a malignant tumour arising from the pleura
- Mean time from exposure to occurrence is 41 years
- Mean survival from diagnosis is 8–14 months

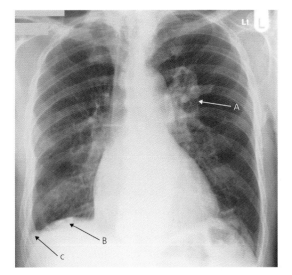

Figure 46 Chest X-ray from a different patient with pleural plaques. (A) The outline of a large calcified pleural plaque can be seen adjacent to the aortic arch. Its left border is indicated by the tip of the arrow. (B) On the top of the right hemidiaphragm there is a white line of calcification. This is a sign of pleural plaque. (C) The right costophrenic angle is blunted by pleural thickening.

However, it could also be caused by disease unrelated to asbestos exposure (e.g. infection or heart failure), with the pleural plaques being an incidental finding.

An unusual feature of Mr Stainson's pleural effusion is that it is associated with chest pain, whereas most effusions are painless. Dull diffuse chest pain is a common feature of mesothelioma and this diagnosis should be considered as a cause of his symptoms.

> **!RED FLAG**
>
> A diagnosis of mesothelioma should be considered in patients with pleural fluid or thickening who complain of chest pain.

How would you investigate his pleural effusion?

Pleural aspirate, pleural biopsy and further imaging including thoracic computerized tomography (CT) scanning could all be useful in diagnosing the cause of his pleural effusion. However, the diagnostic approach in Mr Swainson's case should be designed around the possibility that he has a mesothelioma. This condition requires

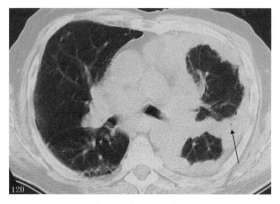

Figure 47 CT scan showing irregular pleural thickening around the left lung (arrow).

special care as any pleural intervention (e.g. aspirate, biopsy) can seed mesothelioma cells through the chest wall, spreading the tumour. The number of invasive pleural procedures should thus be minimized in patients investigated for mesothelioma and if the diagnosis is subsequently proven, patients should have radiotherapy to biopsy tracks to prevent tumour spread.

> *Mr Swainson's chest physician explained to him that there were a number of possible causes for his condition, but that disease caused by asbestos exposure was one possibility. Mr Swainson agreed to undergo CT scanning to assist with further diagnosis. At CT scanning irregular pleural thickening around the left lung was seen (Fig. 47) and was reported as showing some invasion of the chest wall. Pleural fluid was aspirated and a biopsy was performed of the irregular area under CT guidance.*
>
> *Pleural fluid:*
> | | |
> |---|---|
> | pH | 7.4 |
> | Protein | 40 g/L |
> | Glucose | 4 mmol/L |
> | Cytology | Negative |

How do you interpret his results?

• On CT scanning irregular pleural thickening with chest wall invasion indicates a malignant process. The differential diagnosis is:
  ○ local invasion by mesothelioma
  ○ pleural and chest wall spread from a primary lung tumour
  ○ invasive infection such as tuberculosis
• Pleural fluid shows:
  ○ an exudate (protein >30 g/L) – this would be consistent with malignant pleural disease or tuberculosis

  ○ the glucose, pH and cytology are unremarkable – which does not help us to distinguish between possible causes. Negative cytology does not exclude malignant disease

Why was the biopsy performed under CT guidance?

Mesothelioma tends to affect patches of the pleura and therefore biopsy without radiological guidance may miss the disease and may need to be repeated. CT guidance increases the chance of making a positive diagnosis and should reduce the number of pleural interventions required.

> *Mr Stainson's pleural biopsy showed malignant mesothelioma. He attends clinic with his wife to find out the results of his investigations. The respiratory consultant breaks the news to him that he has a malignant pleural tumour. He is stunned by the news, but after a few moments he asks how long he has to live and whether there is any treatment that could offer him chance of a cure.*

How should the consultant answer Mr Stainson's questions?

• Patients with mesothelioma usually survive about a year (8–14 months), although it can be longer or shorter
• There are no treatments available that have been proven in randomized controlled trials to cure mesothelioma
• There is some evidence that triple therapy (radical surgery to remove pleura and lung, chemotherapy and radiotherapy) can improve survival for patients with less malignant cell types. However, radical surgery carries a high mortality
• There are clinical trials currently ongoing that are looking for better treatments for mesothelioma. Mr Stainson could be considered for these if he wishes (www.mesothelioma.uk.com)
• Otherwise, the best treatment available is symptom control

> *Mr Stainson and his wife go away to discuss their situation and return to clinic 1 week later. They have decided to opt for symptom control to maximize the quality of Mr Stainson's remaining months, but Mr Stainson would like to be referred to a specialist centre to participate in a clinical trial.*

How could Mr Stainson's symptoms be controlled?

Pleural effusion

Treatment should aim to drain the effusion and prevent recurrence using one of the following:

- Video-assisted thoracoscopy (VATS procedure)
- Open surgery
- Closed chest drain

Recurrent effusions are prevented by sticking the visceral and parietal pleura together (pleurodesis):

- Medically – talc is put into the pleural space
- Surgically – part of the visceral pleura is scraped off

Both methods cause inflammation and adhesion of the pleural layers.

Radiotherapy

- Radiotherapy to the mesothelioma may reduce chest pain
- Radiotherapy to tracks made by invasive procedures will prevent growth of the tumour along the tracks

---

Box 71 WHO analgesic ladder

Patients in pain should receive regular analgesia with additional drugs available for breakthrough pain.

Step 1
Regular simple analgesia (e.g. paracetamol)

If pain persists

Step 2
Add mild opioid analgesia (e.g. codeine)

If pain persists

Step 3
Use stronger opiate (e.g. morphine)

If pain persists

Increase dose of opiate until pain relieved
Adjuvant drugs such as non-steroidal anti-inflammatory drugs, steroids or drugs used for nerve pain can be added to any step.

Other measures

- Pain control – the World Health Organization (WHO) analgesic ladder (Box 71) should be used when prescribing drugs to achieve pain control
- Support:
  - Mr Stainson would benefit from referral to palliative care services for physical, psychological and emotional support
  - he could also be put in contact with asbestos support groups (www.mesothelioma.uk.com) to help him deal with practical issues and come to terms with his condition

Is Mr Stainson entitled to financial compensation?

Yes – he should be advised to pursue one or both of the following.

Government benefit

Patients are eligible if:

- They have a diagnosis of mesothelioma, lung cancer or asbestosis
- They have a history of occupational exposure to asbestos
- They were not self-employed when exposed

Patients have to complete application forms successfully to obtain these.

Common law compensation

Patients may get compensation from the employer or their insurance company. This is trickier to obtain as:

- The action must be started within 3 years of knowledge of the diagnosis
- Claiming requires the assistance of an expert solicitor
- The claimant must prove that:
  - injuries were caused by asbestos exposure
  - the employer was negligent or did not comply with health and safety requirements

---

Outcome. Mr Stainson was referred to a mesothelioma specialist, but unfortunately was not considered to be suitable for any current clinical trials. He underwent VATS pleurodesis and radiotherapy for pain control. He remained comfortable for 6 months, but presented again with worsening breathlessness. At this time he was found to have extensive mesothelial tumour encasing the lung, pericardium and superior vena cava. His symptoms were palliated with opiates and he died at home 2 weeks later.

CASE REVIEW

Mr Stainson presents with shortness of breath and dull right-sided chest pain. Chest X-ray shows pleural plaques and a left-sided pleural effusion. His history reveals extensive asbestos exposure starting 40 years ago. He undergoes thoracic CT scanning with aspiration of pleural fluid and biopsy and a diagnosis of malignant mesothelioma is made. Mr Stainson is treated symptomatically with VATS pleurodesis and radiotherapy, but dies 6 months later from progressive disease.

KEY POINTS

- Asbestos exposure occurs in a wide range of occupational and domestic environments
- Pulmonary disease caused by asbestos usually presents decades after exposure and includes:
  - pleural plaques
  - asbestosis (interstitial fibrosis)
  - lung cancer
  - pleural mesothelioma
- A diagnosis of mesothelioma should be considered in patients with pleural fluid or thickening who complain of chest pain
- The diagnosis of mesothelioma is made by histological examination of a sample of affected pleura obtained under CT guidance or by VATS
- Mesothelioma has a poor prognosis (8–14 months survival) and treatment is usually symptomatic including:
  - drainage of pleural fluid and pleurodesis
  - radiotherapy
  - pain control
  - palliative support
- Patients with asbestos-related illness may be entitled to financial compensation from government or employer

Case 13   A 16-year-old boy with right-sided chest pain

Marcus Sakura is a 16-year-old boy who presents to accident and emergency complaining of right-sided chest pain. On questioning he tells the casualty officer that the pain is sharp in nature and came on suddenly. He now feels slightly short of breath and the pain is worse if he tries to breathe deeply. He has no cough and has previously been completely well.

What type of pain is this?

This sounds like pleuritic chest pain, which is a sharp localized chest pain, worse on deep inspiration or coughing.

Why does pleuritic chest pain occur?

Inflammation of the pleura (Fig. 2, p. 3) causes pain, felt via the parietal pain fibres. The pain is thus localized over the affected part of the pleura and exacerbated by movement of the pleura when the patient takes a deep breath or coughs.

What conditions cause pleural inflammation?

Pleural inflammation may be caused by disease of the pleura or by conditions affecting the peripheral lung immediately underlying, and hence involving, the pleura (Box 72).

His observations are as follows:

Temperature	*36.8°C*
Pulse	*88 beats/min, regular*
Blood pressure	*125/70 mmHg*
Respiratory rate	*16 breaths/min*
Oxygen saturations	*96% breathing room air*
Chest examination:	
Trachea	*Midline*
Expansion	*Right < left*
Percussion	*Increased resonance on right side*
Auscultation	*Reduced air entry into right lung*
Vocal resonance	*Reduced on the right side*

How do you interpret these findings?

Respiratory rate, oxygenation, pulse and blood pressure are normal. There is no evidence of respiratory failure or cardiovascular compromise. He therefore does not require resuscitation before further assessment.

In his chest:

• Examination findings are asymmetrical (different on the right and left sides), indicating a disease affecting one, rather than both lungs (Table 2, p. 28)

• Reduced expansion on the right side and reduced air entry into the right lung indicates that the right lung is inflating less than the left and is the abnormal lung

• When the normal left lung is percussed the action causes air in the underlying lung to resonate to an extent limited by its containment within lung tissue. This percussion note is described as resonant. When the abnormal right side of the chest is percussed the note is hyper-resonant, indicating the presence of free air not contained by lung tissue (i.e. air in the pleural space [pneumothorax])

• Vocal resonance is sound transmitted from the larynx via the lung tissue to the chest wall where it is heard as a vibration. Vocal resonance is reduced when air or fluid is present in the pleural space and buffers the transmitted sounds

What is the most likely diagnosis?

In summary, Marcus has a poorly expanding right lung with evidence of air in the pleural space. This is most likely to be a pneumothorax.

What basic investigations would you perform immediately?

• Chest X-ray to confirm the presence of pneumothorax and assess its size

• Full blood count and C-reactive protein (CRP) to look for evidence of infection or inflammation

Marcus's chest X-ray is shown in Fig. 48. Full blood count and CRP were normal.

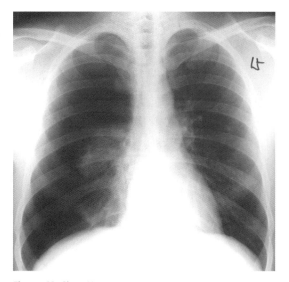

Figure 48 Chest X-ray.

Box 72 Causes of pleuritic chest pain

Pleural disease
- Pneumothorax
- Pleural malignancy (e.g. mesothelioma)
- Pleural inflammation in connective tissue disease, e.g.
  - rheumatoid arthritis
  - systemic lupus erythematosis
- Pleural infection
  - viral (e.g. Coxsackie B)
  - bacterial (empyema)

Conditions affecting the peripheral lung
- Pulmonary embolus
- Pneumonia

What does his chest X-ray show?

If you look carefully you can see that the vascular markings of the normal left lung extend all the way from the mediastinum to the chest wall. On the right side, however, there is a small ball of collapsed lung around the hilum with a clear edge, which is separated from the chest wall by a large black rim of air. This is illustrated more clearly in Fig. 49. The X-ray confirms that Marcus has had a pneumothorax.

What is normally in the pleural space?

There is normally a thin layer of fluid between the visceral and parietal pleura. The surface tension of this fluid

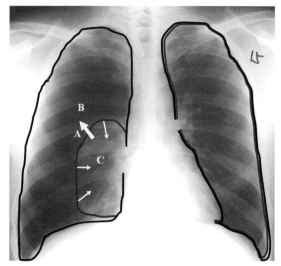

Figure 49 Pathogenesis of pneumothorax. The darker line indicates the position of the parietal pleura lining the chest wall. The lighter line indicates the position of the visceral pleura covering the surface of the lung. On the left side, the two pleural layers are stuck together by the negative intrapleural pressure generated by continual reabsorption of the intervening fluid which keeps the lung expanded. On the right side, there is a hole in the visceral pleura (A), allowing air to leak into the pleural space (B). As intrapleural pressure now equals atmospheric pressure there is nothing to oppose elastic recoil of the lung, which has caused the lung to collapse into a small ball of tissue at the hilum (C).

couples the pleural layers together and creates a negative pressure between them. In a normal chest there is nothing else between the pleural layers, thus the pleural space is a 'potential', rather than an actual space.

What is the function of the negative intrapleural pressure?

The negative intrapleural pressure keeps the lungs expanded and opposes their tendancy to collapse as a result of elastic recoil.

How does air get into the pleural space?

Pneumothoraces are caused when a hole in either visceral or parietal pleura occurs that allows air into the pleural space. Causes of pneumothorax are given in Box 73.

What happens to the lung when air enters the pleural space?

- When a hole in the pleura occurs, air enters the pleural space and the intrapleural pressure becomes less negative

Box 73 Causes of pneumothorax

Traumatic pneumothorax
Entry of air into pleural space is through a wound in chest wall and parietal pleura (wound may also penetrate visceral pleura), e.g.
- Rib fractures
- Stab wound

Spontaneous pneumothorax
Entry of air into pleural space is through a hole in lung and visceral pleura, which often occurs because of rupture of a pleural bleb or bulla (small bubbles of lung with thin covering of pleura).
- Primary:
  - occurs in people without underlying lung disease. This is more common in tall thin young men
- Secondary to underlying lung disease, e.g.
  - chronic obstructive pulmonary disease (COPD)
  - more rarely, asthma, bronchogenic carcinoma, lung abscess

Iatrogenic
- Central line insertion
- Transbronchial biopsy

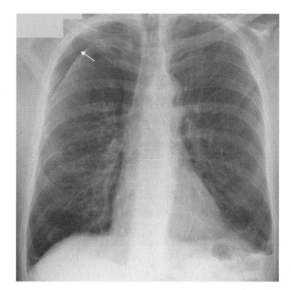

Figure 50 Partial (small) pneumothorax. The arrow indicates the edge of the right lung. There is a small rim of air seen in the pleural space at the right apex in a patient with underlying lung disease.

Box 74 Treatment options for pneumothorax

Air can be removed from the pleural space and the lung allowed to re-expand by:
- Spontaneous reabsorption without intervention
- Simple aspiration (thoracocentesis)
- Chest drain (thoracostomy)
- Surgical intervention, e.g.
  - open chest surgery (thoracotomy) and removal of pleura (pleurectomy)
  - video-assisted thoracoscopy and pleurodesis

- As the intrapleural pressure becomes less negative it is less able to oppose the elastic recoil of the lung. The lung therefore starts to collapse
- The degree of lung collapse depends on the amount of air entering the intrapleural space, which in turn depends on the size of the hole and whether the hole closes spontaneously:
  - if the hole closes as the lung collapses, the intrapleural pressure will remain somewhat negative, preventing the lung from collapsing completely (Fig. 50)
  - if the hole is large or remains open until intrapleural pressure equals atmospheric pressure, the lung will collapse completely into a small ball around the hilum (Figs 48 & 49). This has occurred in Marcus's case.

What is the most likely cause of Marcus's pneumothorax?

He was previously well without underlying lung disease and does not give a history of trauma. This is therefore likely to be a spontaneous primary pneumothorax.

How should his pneumothorax be treated?

The aim of treatment is to remove the air from the pleural cavity to allow his lung to re-expand (Box 74). If this is not carried out he may develop infection in and chronic damage to his collapsed lung, with severe consequences for his health.

Marcus is admitted to hospital and started on high flow oxygen at 10 L/min. His doctor advises him that his pneumothorax should be aspirated to allow his lung to expand.

Why was he started on high flow oxygen?

Air in his pleural cavity is made up of approximately 79% nitrogen and 21% oxygen. Inhalation of high flow oxygen is thought to reduce the partial pressure of nitrogen in the pulmonary capillaries, increasing the gradient for reabsorption of gases from pleura to blood. Whatever the mechanism, while Marcus is breathing high flow oxygen he will be reabsorbing his pneumothorax four times more quickly than if he was breathing air.

Why has the doctor told him his pneumothorax should be aspirated?

The British Thoracic Society (BTS) has issued guidelines which are very helpful in deciding how to treat patients with spontaneous pneumothorax (http://www.brit-thoracic. org.uk/c2/uploads/PleuralDiseaseSpontaneous.pdf). The doctor has decided that Marcus has a large pneumothorax (Box 75) with complete collapse of the lung. This pneumothorax will take many weeks to resolve spontaneously and so intervention to remove the air from the pleural space is indicated to aid recovery and prevent complications. The BTS guidelines state that where intervention is required aspiration should always be tried first.

How do you aspirate a pneumothorax?

You need a large syringe (50 mL), a three-way tap and a venflon. The venflon is inserted through the chest wall into the pleural space under local anaesthetic using aseptic technique. The site of venflon insertion is the safe triangle area of the chest, so called as it is an area where a needle can usually be inserted without hitting blood vessels, breast or muscle (Fig. 51). Once in place the venflon needle is removed, leaving the plastic cannula which is connected to the syringe via the three-way tap. When the tap is turned in one direction it allows air to be sucked out of the pleural space into the syringe. The tap is then turned so it is closed to the patient, but open to the atmosphere. This allows air to be expelled into the atmosphere without taking the syringe off the venflon or allowing air to leak from the atmosphere back into the pleural space.

> ### Box 75 British Thoracic Society classification of pneumothoraces by size
>
> **Small**
> - <2 cm visible rim of air on chest X-ray between lung margin and chest wall (Fig. 50)
> - Occupy <50% of the volume of the hemithorax (half chest)
> - Resolve spontaneously in around 3 weeks (1.25–1.8% hemithorax volume reabsorbed per day)
> - Hole causing pneumothorax has often closed spontaneously
> - Insertion of a sharp needle into the pleural space may not be advisable as lung is close to chest wall
> - Usually treated by observation
>
> **Large**
> - ≥2 cm visible rim of air on chest X-ray between lung margin and chest wall
> - Occupy ≥50% of the volume of the hemithorax
> - Takes many weeks to resolve spontaneously (1.25–1.8% hemithorax volume reabsorbed per day)
> - Hole causing pneumothorax may still be open
> - Usually treated by aspiration initially
> - Chest drain or other intervention required if aspiration unsuccessful

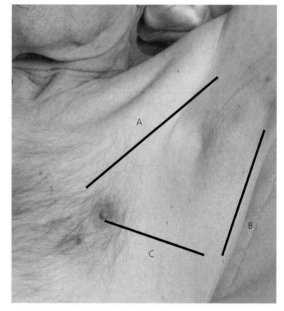

Figure 51 The safe triangle. The safe triangle is an area of the chest wall away from the usual course of the internal mammary artery and avoiding breast and muscle. The walls of the triangle are (A) the posterior border of pectoralis major, (B) the anterior wall of latissimus dorsi, (C) a line drawn at the horizontal level of the nipple. The tip (apex) of the triangle is in the axilla.

As the doctor prepares a trolley with equipment to aspirate the pneumothorax he is called back to the patient who has suddenly deteriorated. Marcus is distressed with rapid laboured breathing.

Marcus's observations are now as follows:

Temperature	36.8°C
Pulse	120 beats/min
Blood pressure	105/55 mmHg
Respiratory rate	30 breaths/min
Oxygen saturations 78% on high flow oxygen	
His trachea is deviated to the left	

What has happened?

It is very likely that he has developed a tension pneumothorax.

• The hole in his lung is acting as a one-way valve, opening on inspiration and allowing air into the pleural space but closing on expiration and trapping air in the pleural space. Thus, the volume of intrapleural air is expanding with every breath and the right-sided intrapleural pressure has increased above atmospheric pressure

• The expanding right-sided pneumothorax has reached the point of 'tension' as it is now causing respiratory and haemodynamic compromise:

  ○ the right pneumothorax is pushing Marcus's mediastinum to the left (detected as tracheal deviation)

  ○ this compresses major vessels in the mediastinum, reducing venous return and cardiac output, resulting in a fall in blood pressure with compensatory tachycardia

  ○ reduced ventilation (right lung collapse and compression of the left lung) and impaired pulmonary perfusion (mediastinal compression) cause hypoxia with compensatory tachypnoea

What do you need to do?

This is a medical emergency and cardiorespiratory arrest and death will occur unless the trapped air is removed.

A long cannula should be inserted immediately into the pleural space via the second intercostal space, midclavicular line to decompress the pneumothorax. The cannula should be left in place until a formal intercostal chest drain has been inserted.

Is it safe to do this without a chest X-ray first?

The diagnosis of tension pneumothorax is primarily a clinical diagnosis, based on either detection of or suspicion of a pneumothorax combined with cardiorespiratory compromise. There is often no time for a chest X-ray. Immediate needle decompression on clinical suspicion is thus considered best practice and recommended in the BTS guidelines. It should be remembered that needle decompression can have some complications including pneumothorax or bleeding.

The doctor inserts a cannula into Marcus's chest via the second intercostal space, midclavicular line. There is a hiss of air and Marcus rapidly improves. Over the next 15 min his observations return to normal. An intercostal chest drain is inserted and is attached to an underwater seal, which bubbles for 24h, then stops bubbling.

How is the intercostal drain inserted?

• The patient should give informed consent for the procedure

• The procedure can be painful, therefore premedication with opiates or benzodiazepines should be offered, taking care with the dosage as respiratory depression is a side-effect of these agents. Local anaesthetic is also used

• Aseptic technique is used to avoid causing infection

• The drain should be inserted between two ribs within the safe triangle (Fig. 51). Remember that the intercostal nerves and vessels run on the underside of the ribs so that needles and drains should be inserted over the top of a rib

• An incision is made in the skin, a dilator or forceps are used to make a track through the intercostal tissue, the pleura is perforated and a drain is fed into the pleural space

• The drain is held in place by sutures and transparent dressings as appropriate

• The free end of the drain is connected to an underwater seal (Fig. 52)

What is the purpose of the underwater seal?

Once the chest drain is inserted it is attached to a long tube and the open end is sited under water. When the patient breathes out, intrathoracic pressure increases above atmospheric pressure, forcing air out down the tube and bubbling out through the water. When the patient breathes in, intrathoracic pressure decreases, but water in the drain prevents air from re-entering the chest. As long as the underwater seal is below the site of entry of the drain into the chest, water is unable to rise up the drain sufficiently to enter the pleural space.

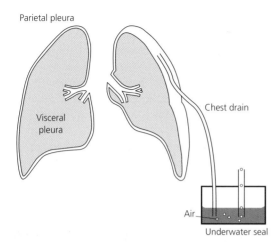

Parietal pleura

Visceral
pleura

Chest drain

Air

Underwater seal

Figure 52 Diagram of a chest drain with underwater seal. The chest drain is inserted into the pleural space. The other end is placed under 3–4 cm water. This allows air to leave the pleural space and the lung to re-expand. The water prevents air from re-entering the pleural space and does not pass along the tube into the chest unless the seal is raised above the level of entry of the drain into the chest.

KEY POINT

The underwater seal of a chest drain should always be kept below the site of entry of the drain into the chest to prevent water entering the pleural space.

What does bubbling of the drain for the first 24 h indicate?

When the drain is inserted the air in the pneumothorax is expelled, causing bubbles to come out of the end of the drain under the water. This should stop when the lung is re-expanded. Persistent bubbling indicates that the hole causing the pneumothorax has not sealed and air is still leaking from the lung into the pleural space.

How does the pleural hole seal?

Pleural inflammation leading to repair or scarring is probably responsible for the hole sealing.

Why might the drain have stopped bubbling after 24 h?

Possible reasons include:
1 The hole has sealed, air is no longer leaking into the pleural space and all residual air has been removed

2 The drain has dislodged and is no longer in the intrapleural space
3 The drain has become blocked

How can you find out which is the case?

If the drain is swinging (the water level rises in the drain with inspiration when intrathoracic pressure is reduced and falls with expiration when intrathoracic pressure increases) this indicates that it is in the right place and not blocked. Therefore, the first option is more likely.

A drain that is neither bubbling nor swinging is likely to be blocked or displaced.

These observations are best confirmed by a chest X-ray.

On observation of Marcus's drain a small amount of water from the drain bottle is seen to be 'swinging' up and down in the tube with respiration, indicating patency of the drain. His repeat chest X-ray shows that his lung has completely re-expanded and the drain is in the same position as before.

What should be done now?

His chest drain can be removed. If his lung remains re-expanded on repeat chest X-ray he can go home with follow-up in the chest clinic.

Prior to leaving the hospital Marcus tells you he is due to travel abroad with his father on a diving trip and wants to know the likelihood of recurrence of the pneumothorax.

What do you tell him?

• He should not fly until at least 1 week after resolution of his pneumothorax (current BTS guidelines)
• He can never dive without prior preventative surgery
• The chance of a recurrent pneumothorax on the same side is up to 50%
• He should not smoke cigarettes as this will increase his chance of pneumothorax recurrence
• He should seek medical help if his symptoms recur so that a recurrent pneumothorax can be dealt with promptly

Why are flying and diving dangerous in patients who have had a pneumothorax?

• Boyle's law states that the volume of a gas is inversely proportional to the pressure to which it is exposed

- Atmospheric pressure falls during flying and increases during deep sea diving
- Patients who have had one pneumothorax have a high risk of recurrence, probably because of other blebs and bullae on the surface of their lungs
- Changes in atmospheric pressure from flying or diving could cause expansion and rupture of these lesions and recurrence of the pneumothorax:
  ○ if a pneumothorax occurs when diving at depth this is particularly dangerous as it will expand and become a tension pneumothorax as the diver ascends
  ○ if a patient with a pneumothorax flies before it is fully recovered it can expand at high altitude, resulting in a tension pneumothorax

Outcome. Marcus returned to outpatients 6 weeks later with his father. His lung remained re-expanded and he had had no further problems. He had cancelled his diving holiday but remained concerned about the possibility of recurrent pneumothorax. Three months later he suffered a recurrence on the same side and was referred to the cardiothoracic surgeons who performed video-assisted thoracoscopy (VATS) and surgical pleurodesis on the right side.

CASE REVIEW

Marcus Sakura presented to hospital with pleuritic chest pain, which was found to be caused by a large right spontaneous pneumothorax. As the medical team prepared to treat him by aspirating the pleural air he deteriorated and required urgent treatment for a tension pneumothorax by blind insertion of a cannula. A chest drain was inserted and his lung re-expanded. On discharge he was advised not to fly or dive. Three months later his pneumothorax recurred and he underwent VATS pleurodesis to prevent further recurrence.

KEY POINTS

- Pneumothoraces most commonly occur spontaneously in tall thin young men (primary) or patients with underlying lung disease (secondary)
- Entry of air into the pleural space through a pleural hole makes the intrapleural pressure less negative and the lung collapses partially or completely because of elastic recoil
- If the lung remains collapsed it can become infected and scarred, therefore treatment is to remove pleural air, allowing lung re-expansion
- Small pneumothoraces (<2 cm visible rim of air on chest X-ray) can be allowed to resolve spontaneously in patients with primary, mildly symptomatic pneumothorax and asymptomatic secondary pneumothorax, and will do so more quickly if the patient breathes high flow oxygen
- Large pneumothoraces (>2 cm visible rim of air on chest X-ray) should be aspirated first. If they recur the patient requires a chest drain

- A tension pneumothorax is caused by a hole in the lung that allows air into but not out of the pleural space. It compresses the mediastinum causing cardiovascular and respiratory collapse
- A tension pneumothorax is an emergency and should be treated urgently by insertion of a cannula into the pleural space via the second intercostal space, midclavicular line without waiting for a chest X-ray
- On discharge, patients with spontaneous pneumothorax should be advised:
  ○ they have up to 50% chance of recurrence
  ○ they should not fly until at least 1 week after resolution of pneumothorax
  ○ they should never go deep sea diving

Case 14 A 62-year-old woman with breathlessness

Mrs Barbara Smith is a 62-year-old woman who is referred to the chest clinic by her GP with a 6-week history of increasing shortness of breath, which is now problematic at rest. Her history is otherwise unremarkable. Respiratory examination shows:

Trachea – midline

Expansion – slightly reduced on the left

Percussion – normal on right, stony dull on left side to midzone

Auscultation – decreased air entry on the left side

Vocal resonance – decreased on the left side to the midzone

How do you interpret her examination findings?

• Her abnormal chest examination findings are asymmetrical, indicating lung consolidation, collapse, pleural effusion or pneumothorax (Table 2, p. 28)

• The left side is abnormal with reduced air entry and expansion. The *dull* percussion note narrows the diagnosis to:
  ○ an abnormality in the lung – consolidation
  ○ an abnormality around the lung – pleural effusion

• The *stony* dull nature of the percussion note indicates that she has a pleural effusion:
  ○ *effusion* – fluid is around the lung in the pleural space and muffles the percussion note completely
  ○ *consolidation* – air in the alveoli and small airways is replaced by inflammatory exudates. The percussion note is partly muffled by this, but less completely than by a pleural effusion

• The other examination findings are consistent with the presence of a pleural effusion:
  ○ the effusion is occupying part of her left hemithorax, reducing air entry into the left lung which is detected as reduced expansion and air entry
  ○ vocal resonance is assessed by listening to sounds transmitted from the larynx through the peripheral lung and chest wall. Mrs Smith has reduced vocal resonance over the left lung because pleural fluid around

the lung is absorbing and preventing transmission of the sound

In summary, her clinical findings indicate that she has a pleural effusion.

Could a pleural effusion account for her presenting symptoms?

Yes. Dyspnoea is the most common symptom of a pleural effusion and usually indicates a large effusion (>500 mL). Pleuritic chest pain may also be a presenting complaint but becomes less intense as the effusion increases in size.

What test would you carry out initially to confirm your clinical suspicions?

The most useful initial investigation would be a chest X-ray.

Mrs Smith's chest X-ray is shown in Fig. 53. As she is so symptomatic she is admitted to hospital for rapid investigation and treatment.

What does her chest X-ray show?

Her left lung is obscured by a white shadowing. The upper border of the shadowing is clearly delineated, concave and highest laterally (meniscus). This is a classic appearance of a pleural effusion.

How do pleural effusions develop?

There is normally a thin layer of fluid between the visceral and parietal pleural layers (Fig. 2, p. 3) which holds the layers together by surface tension and allows them to slide smoothly over each other. Mechanisms keeping pleural fluid at the correct volume for normal function include:

• Normal pleural structure, acting as a barrier to uncontrolled fluid and solute movement

• Balanced hydrostatic and oncotic pressures, preventing excess movement of water into the pleural space

• Removal of excess pleural fluid by lymphatics

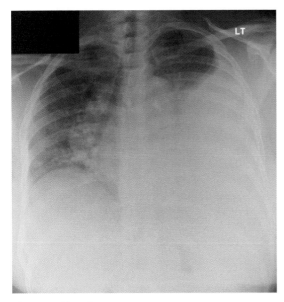

Figure 53 Chest X-ray.

A pleural effusion can be caused by any pathology that disrupts these normal processes (Box 76).

How would you investigate her pleural effusion?

A wide range of diseases cause pleural effusion. Investigation therefore needs to be planned carefully to make the diagnosis as quickly as possible, while minimizing invasive procedures.

The first step is to find out whether her pleural effusion is a transudate or an exudate. The reason for this is that these different effusion types have very different causes (Box 76) and treatments. As she has a unilateral pleural effusion she requires aspiration and analysis of the fluid to distinguish effusion types. Bilateral effusions are likely to be transudates and do not need aspirating unless they have atypical features or do not respond to treatment of the underlying disease.

How is pleural aspiration performed?

The site of the effusion is identified by percussion and the aspiration is performed at the bedside. If the effusion is small, ultrasound may be used to mark the effusion for bedside aspiration or the radiologist may aspirate fluid under ultrasound guidance. Aseptic technique is used and local anaesthetic is infiltrated if considered necessary. A fine bore (21 G) needle is inserted into the infusion and 50 mL pleural fluid is aspirated into a large syringe.

Box 76 Causes of pleural effusion

Pleural disease

Inflamed or diseased pleura allows fluid and solutes to leak from the blood and interstitium into the pleural space. These effusions usually have high protein content (>30 g/L) and are called *exudates*. Causes include:
- Infection:
  - pneumonia
  - tuberculosis
- Cancer:
  - pleural – mesothelioma
  - spread or metastasis from other cancers (e.g. bronchus, breast, gastrointestinal)
- Inflammation:
  - pulmonary embolus with pleural involvement
  - connective tissue disease (e.g. rheumatoid arthritis, systemic lupus erythematosus)
  - post-myocardial infarction syndrome
  - sarcoidosis
  - pancreatitis

Altered balance between hydrostatic and oncotic pressures

These effusions usually have low protein content (<30 g/L) and are called *transudates*.
- If intravascular hydrostatic pressure increases, water is forced out into the pleural space. Causes include:
  - cardiac failure
  - constrictive pericarditis
- If oncotic pressure (pull of water by proteins) in the blood decreases, water leaks out into the pleural space. Causes include:
  - nephrotic syndrome
  - liver failure
- Other transudates:
  - Meigs' syndrome associated with ovarian tumours
  - hypothyroidism

Failure of lymphatic drainage
- Trauma
- Malignancy

The appearance of the aspirated fluid should be noted (Table 5).

I *Mrs Smith's pleural aspirate revealed blood-stained fluid.*

What is the significance of the appearance of her pleural fluid?

Her pleural aspirate is blood-stained, which could be a result of slight trauma during the procedure.

Table 5 Appearance of pleural fluid.

Appearance	Possible pathology
Pale yellow (straw-coloured)	Non-specific
Pus	Empyema • infected pleural effusion
White (milky)	Chylothorax • lymph in the pleural space
Brown	Long-standing bloody effusion
	Ruptured amoebic liver abscess
Yellow/green	Rheumatoid pleurisy
Colour of enteral tube feed/central venous catheter infusate	Feeding tube/central venous catheter migration

Other causes of a blood-stained pleural effusion include:
• Malignancy
• Pulmonary infarction resulting from pulmonary embolus
• Trauma (haemothorax)
• Post-cardiac injury syndrome

What should be done with her pleural fluid?

The fluid should be divided and sent to three different laboratories to request the following tests.

Biochemistry

Send 10–20 mL in a sterile pot requesting analysis of:
• Protein
• Lactate dehydrogenase (LDH)
• Glucose
• Amylase – if oesophageal rupture or pancreatitis suspected

A small sample of fluid should be collected in a heparinized tube and analysed in a blood gas analyser for:
• pH

Microbiology

Send 10–20 mL in sterile pot for:
• Gram stain of pleural sediment for bacteria
• Alcohol and acid-fast bacilli (AAFB) stain if tuberculosis (TB) suspected

• TB culture
Also send 10–20 mL in blood culture bottles for:
• Culture and sensitivity for aerobic and anaerobic bacteria

Cytology

Send 20 mL of pleural fluid in sterile pot. Get this to the laboratory as soon as possible as it is best analysed fresh for:
• Differential cell count
• Malignant cells

The initial results of analysis of Mrs Smith's pleural fluid were:	
Biochemistry:	
Protein	*42 g/L*
LDH	*540 U/L*
pH	*7.45 (normal 7.60)*
Glucose	*2.9 mmol (normal >3.3 mmol)*
Microbiology:	
Gram stain	*Scanty lymphocytes seen, no bacteria*
AAFB	*Negative*
Cytology	*Awaited*

Is Mrs Smith's effusion an exudate or a transudate?

Mrs Smith's pleural fluid protein concentration is high (>30 g/L) so this is an exudate. Protein concentrations are high in exudative effusions because protein leaks from the blood into the pleural space across diseased pleura.

How does the serum protein concentration affect the pleural protein concentration?

If the serum protein concentration is low there is less protein to exude into the pleural space; an exudate may have a protein concentration of 25–35 g/L. It can thus be confused with a transudate and additional tests are required for pleural effusions with borderline protein concentrations to tell if they are transudates or exudates (Box 77).

Do Mrs Smith's other pleural fluid results give further useful information?
Lactic dehydrogenase

Normal serum LDH concentrations are around 240–460 U/L. Mrs Smith's pleural fluid LDH is 540 U/L which is more than two-thirds of normal serum upper limits, confirming her effusion is an exudate (Box 77).

Box 77 Use of Light's criteria to distinguish between an exudate and a transudate

If the protein level is borderline (25–35 g/L), Light's criteria should be applied. The effusion is an exudate if one or more of the following criteria are met:

- Pleural fluid protein/serum protein >0.5
- Pleural fluid LDH/Serum LDH >0.6
- Pleural fluid LDH >two-thirds upper limits of normal serum LDH

Very high levels of LDH (>1000 IU/L) may be found in:

- Empyema
- Rheumatoid pleurisy
- Malignancy (sometimes)

pH and glucose

If inflammatory or malignant cells are present in the effusion they use glucose and cause accumulation of hydrogen ions. Hence, effusions resulting from infection (empyema, TB), inflammation (rheumatoid arthritis) and malignancy tend to have low pH and glucose.

Mrs Smith's pleural fluid is slightly acidic and has a reduced glucose concentration, indicating an inflammatory or malignant cause for her effusion.

Microbiology

There are no neutrophils or bacteria seen on Gram stain, making empyema unlikely. TB microscopy is negative.

!RED FLAG

- If pleural glucose concentrations and pH are falling and LDH concentrations are rising, this is strongly indicative of pleural infection
- If the patient has pleural infection, a pleural fluid pH of <7.2 indicates the need for a chest drain

---

What is your differential diagnosis?

In summary, Mrs Smith has a blood-stained exudate with no evidence of infection but low pH and glucose concentration. The most likely diagnosis is a malignant pleural effusion, although other causes of an exudate are still possible.

What should the next steps in her investigation be?

She now requires a contrast-enhanced CT scan of her chest to look for underlying pleural or lung lesions and further sampling or analysis of pleural fluid or tissue to diagnose the cause of her pleural effusion.

What methods of pleural sampling can be used?

Percutaneous pleural biopsy

- *Blind biopsy*, using an Abram's needle inserted through the chest wall:
  - most useful for tuberculosis, makes diagnosis in 75% cases if sent for histology (granulomas) and TB culture
  - about 50% of cases of malignant pleural effusion are diagnosed on cytology of the pleural aspirate. Biopsy slightly increases the chance of a positive diagnosis of malignant pleural effusion
- *CT guided biopsy*. Required for focal pleural disease (e.g. mesothelioma)

Thoracoscopy

- If other techniques have failed to make a diagnosis, direct inspection of the pleura with a thoracoscope and biopsy of abnormal areas may be diagnostic.

Mrs Smith undergoes a contrast-enhanced CT scan of her thorax. Her scan shows normal lung fields, but there is a suspicion of an opacity in the left breast which was not detected on clinical examination. A mammogram confirms a left breast spiculated lesion, which is suspicious for a carcinoma of the breast. Mrs Smith's pleural fluid cytology results were reported as showing the presence of malignant breast cells. The pleural aspirate therefore made the diagnosis and she did not require pleural biopsy.

Mrs Smith was referred to the oncologists who staged her disease as stage IV metastatic breast carcinoma. She was advised that palliative chemotherapy and/or hormonal treatment could prolong her survival, although treatment would not be curative. Before discharge Mrs Smith was reviewed by the respiratory team for a decision regarding definitive management of her pleural effusion.

How should her large pleural effusion be treated?

Mrs Smith is very symptomatic from her large pleural effusion. She requires insertion of a chest drain to remove the fluid and relieve her symptoms. However, as the underlying cause of her pleural effusion has not been treated, the effusion is likely to recur once the chest drain is removed.

How can recurrent pleural effusion be prevented?
Medical pleurodesis
This is done by:
• Draining the pleural effusion to dryness
• Instillation of a sclerosing agent such as talc or doxy-cycline into the pleural space
• This causes aseptic inflammation with dense adhesions which stick the parietal and visceral pleura together, obliterating the pleural space and preventing reaccumulation of fluid
• This technique can be performed via a percutaneous chest drain or at thoracoscopy

Surgical pleurodesis (pleurectomy)
This involves surgical removal of pleura at thoracoscopy or open surgery, with subsequent scarring and loss of the pleural space.

Outcome. Mrs Smith has a chest drain inserted and obtains considerable relief from drainage of 2 L fluid. Once her effusion has drained completely, talc is inserted into her pleural space via the drain. She experiences some discomfort after the procedure, relieved by paracetamol. The chest drain is removed and she is discharged from hospital. She remains under the care of the oncologists and has no re-accumulation of her pleural fluid during her palliative chemotherapy.

CASE REVIEW

Mrs Smith presented with a 6-week history of breathlessness and was found to have a large pleural effusion on examination. A pleural aspirate showed that her effusion was an exudate and a diagnosis of malignant pleural effusion was made by cytological identification of malignant breast cells in the fluid. Her pleural effusion was drained to relieve her symptoms and, as her disease was incurable, medical pleurodesis was performed to prevent re-accumulation of pleural fluid and recurrence of her symptoms.

KEY POINTS

• A stony dull percussion note at the lung bases on examination indicates a pleural effusion
• On chest X-ray an effusion appears as white shadowing at the lung base. The upper border of the shadow is concave and highest laterally (meniscus)
• Pleural effusions may be exudates resulting from pleural disease or transudates caused by cardiac disease or hypoproteinaemia
• The first step in managing an effusion is to find out whether it is an exudate or transudate. This is done by aspirating pleural fluid and measuring the protein content (exudate >30 g/L protein, transudate <30 g/L)

• Aspirated pleural fluid should also be sent for further biochemical, microbiological and cytological analysis
• If a firm diagnosis is not made by pleural aspirate the next steps are:
  ○ CT scan of the thorax to look for pleural or lung lesions
  ○ sampling of pleural tissue
• Once the diagnosis is made treatment should aim to:
  ○ relieve symptoms by draining the effusion
  ○ prevent re-accumulation of fluid by treating underlying cause or by pleurodesis

Case 15 — A 24-year-old woman with pleuritic chest pain

A 24-year-old woman, Marie Lefevre, presents herself to the accident and emergency department complaining of sharp left-sided chest pain. She tells the triage nurse that it hurts to take a deep breath or cough.

What type of pain is this?
This is pleuritic chest pain (see Case 13).

Give a differential diagnosis for her presentation
• Pneumonia
• Pulmonary embolus
• Pneumothorax
• Pleural inflammation resulting from viral infection or connective tissue disease

Which of these conditions are most likely to occur in her because she is a young woman?
• Women are more likely than men to get pulmonary emboli as the oral contraceptive pill, pregnancy and hormone replacement therapy are all risk factors for this condition. Women are also more likely to develop connective tissue disease, whereas men are more at risk of pneumothorax
• Mesothelioma is a pleural malignancy that develops 20–40 years after asbestos exposure. At 24 years old she is extremely unlikely to have this disease

What features in the history may help to distinguish between these diagnoses?
• A cough productive of purulent sputum or blood may indicate underlying lung disease (i.e. pneumonia or pulmonary embolus)
• Fever, malaise and myalgia are suggestive of infection. Rigors (uncontrollable shaking) can occur in bacterial pneumonia
• Joint pains or skin rash could indicate connective tissue disease

• Calf pain could be caused by deep vein thrombosis as a source of pulmonary embolus
• Pulmonary emboli and pneumothoraces may be recurrent, so a previous history of disease is helpful
• You should ask about risk factors for the different conditions. Patients on immunosuppressive drugs or with a history of being immunocompromised (e.g. blood disorders, HIV) are at risk of pneumonia. Patients with underlying lung disease or who are tall and thin are at risk of pneumothorax. Risk factors for pulmonary embolus are given in Box 78

Miss Lefevre stated that the pain had been present for 24h. In addition, she had coughed up a small amount of bright red blood and found it painful to cough. She did not feel feverish; however, she had noticed some right calf discomfort which she had attributed to a 'pulled muscle'. Three days ago she had travelled to London from the South of France by coach.

On further questioning, she has smoked 20 cigarettes per day since the age of 21, she does not take the oral contraceptive pill but there is no potential for her to be pregnant. Her mother had a deep vein thrombosis during pregnancy 25 years previously.

What is the most likely diagnosis and why?
Deep vein thrombosis complicated by pulmonary embolus.

The clinical features of pleuritic pain and haemoptysis without fever are most likely to be caused by a pulmonary embolus. Right calf discomfort could indicate a deep vein thrombosis as a source of the embolus. She has several risk factors for thromboembolic disease including immobility (long distance coach travel), cigarette smoking and a positive family history (Box 78).

Box 78 Risk factors for deep vein thrombosis

Factors that cause venous stasis
- General immobility, e.g.
  - long distance travel
  - illness
- Compression of pelvic veins:
  - uterine fibroids
  - pelvic malignancy
  - pregnancy
- Obesity
- Cardiac failure

Imbalance of clotting factors
- Congenital:
  - thrombophilia (e.g. factor V Leiden, protein C or S deficiency)
- Acquired
  - malignancy
  - oestrogen (e.g. oral contraceptive, pregnancy, hormone replacement therapy)
  - infection
  - nephrotic syndrome
  - polycythaemia
  - smoking

Factors causing endothelial damage
- Recent surgery or trauma
- Pelvic disease (e.g. malignancy)
- Varicose veins
- Smoking

Table 6 Wells criteria for assessing clinical likelihood of pulmonary embolus (PE).

Clinical feature	Points	Miss Lefevre
Clinical symptoms of DVT	3	3
Other diagnoses less likely than PE	3	3
Heart rate greater than 100 beats/min	1.5	1.5
Immobilization or surgery within past 4 weeks	1.5	1.5
Previous DVT or PE	1.5	0
Haemoptysis	1	1
Malignancy	1	0
Total points		**10**

Wells criteria risk score interpretation (probability of PE):
>6 points: high risk (78.4%)

2–6 points: moderate risk (27.8%)

<2 points: low risk (3.4%)

DVT, deep vein thrombosis.

On examination the following observations were made:

Temperature	*36.4°C*
Pulse	*105 beats/min*
Blood pressure	*115/70 mmHg*
Oxygen saturations	*93% on air*
Respiratory rate	*20 breaths/min*

On chest auscultation she had a left-sided pleural rub

Calf diameters measured 10 cm below the tibia: right 36 cm, left 33 cm. The right calf was tender on palpation

Do these examination findings support your provisional diagnosis?

- She has a tachycardia with normal blood pressure, an increased respiratory rate and hypoxia. These features are consistent with, but not specific for a pulmonary embolus
- A pleural rub is a grating noise that occurs on breathing in and out and is caused by inflamed pleural surfaces rubbing over each other. It is localized to the affected area. Not all patients with pleural inflammation have an audible rub, but its presence is helpful in supporting this diagnosis. A pleural rub can be distinguished from a pericardial rub, which sounds similar, by asking the patient to hold their breath briefly. A pleural rub will stop, whereas a pericardial rub will continue
- The diameter of her right calf is greater than that of the left, indicating that it is swollen. This would fit with a diagnosis of deep vein thrombosis as venous occlusion causes oedema of the calf muscle. Calf tenderness is caused by muscle swelling and by inflammation of the thrombosed vein

Is there a formal method of assessing how likely it is that she has had a pulmonary embolus?

The Wells criteria can be used to estimate the likelihood of pulmonary embolus from information obtained at clinical assessment. Miss Lefevre's score is shown in Table 6.

Miss Lefevre's score is 10, therefore it is very likely that she has had a pulmonary embolus.

What is the purpose of clinical risk assessment?

In Miss Lefevre's case it is very likely that she has had a pulmonary embolus, so she should have the appropriate investigations and treatment. However, these tests and therapies themselves have potential risks for the patient. The clinical risk score is therefore useful in helping clinicians decide on a course of action for individual patients. For example, in patients with a low score an alternative diagnosis may be sought.

What basic investigations would you perform at the initial assessment?

The patient should have a chest X-ray and electrocardiogram (ECG) to exclude other diagnoses such as pneumonia, pneumothorax and myocardial disease. Arterial gases will be helpful to assess the need for oxygen and supportive treatment as well as in supporting the diagnosis.

Investigation results:

Chest X-ray – unremarkable

ECG – sinus tachycardia

Arterial blood gases on air:

		Normal range
pH	7.52	(7.35–7.45)
PO$_2$	9.2 kPa	(10–13.1 kPa)
PCO$_2$	3.9 kPa	(4.9–6.1 kPa)
HCO$_3^-$	22 mmol/L	(22–28 mmol/L)

How do you interpret her results?

The chest X-ray and ECG show no features consistent with alternative diagnoses.

Arterial gases:
- Mild hypoxia – respiratory impairment
- Hypocapnia – hyperventilation secondary to hypoxia
- Alkalosis secondary to hypocapnia driving the Henderson–Hasselbach equation to the right

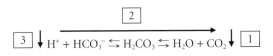

Further investigation also showed:
- D-dimer level 0.84 mg/L (normal range <0.3 mg/L)

What are D-dimers?

In the normal control of haemostasis, procoagulant, anticoagulant and fibrinolytic factors are balanced to prevent intravascular thrombosis. Plasmin stimulates breakdown of fibrin (Fig. 54) and cross-linked fibrin degradation products are called D-dimers. Where thrombosis is activated anywhere in the body, fibrinolysis is also activated and D-dimer levels become elevated.

Are elevated D-dimer levels in Miss Lefevre diagnostic of pulmonary embolus?

No. D-dimers are elevated in many clinical conditions (e.g. following trauma or surgery, as a result of myocardial infarction, renal impairment, pregnancy, stroke). Therefore, a positive D-dimer test is not informative and should not guide further investigation and treatment.

Why do a D-dimer test then?

If D-dimers are normal then *this* is a useful result as pulmonary embolus is unlikely. Negative (normal) D-dimers have >90% negative predictive value for pulmonary embolus (i.e. >90% of people with a negative D-dimer result do not have pulmonary embolus). However, the D-dimer test may give false negative results.

When should you do a D-dimer test in clinical practice?

Measuring D-dimer levels is controversial and if used indiscriminately can be more of a hindrance than a help in making the diagnosis and can lead to unnecessary investigation. A reasonable approach is to measure D-dimers *only* in patients with suspected pulmonary embolus who are assessed as being at low or moderate clinical risk of pulmonary embolus using Wells criteria (Table 6). In these patients a negative result can exclude a pulmonary embolus and prevent unnecessary investigation and treatment, whereas a positive result is supportive of the need for definitive tests for pulmonary embolus. If a patient is judged as being at high risk of pulmonary embolus, D-dimer measurement is unnecessary. If pulmonary embolus is not suspected clinically, D-dimers should not be measured.

> ### KEY POINTS
>
> - Elevated D-dimers are not useful in making a positive diagnosis of pulmonary embolus
> - However, normal (negative) D-dimers correctly exclude >90% of pulmonary emboli
> - D-dimer results should be taken in clinical context and not used alone

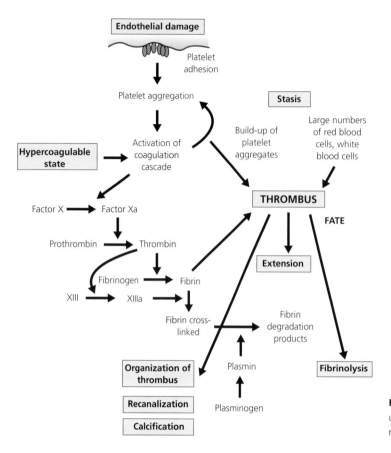

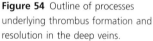

Figure 54 Outline of processes underlying thrombus formation and resolution in the deep veins.

How do you assess Miss Lefevre now?

She has a high clinical probability of pulmonary embolus and deep vein thrombosis and requires urgent treatment, followed by investigations to confirm the diagnosis.

How does deep vein thrombosis occur?

Deep leg veins are large veins that lie deep in the muscles of the leg and carry most of the deoxygenated, nutritionally depleted blood from the legs back up towards the heart. Movement of blood within these veins depends on compression by leg muscles and a system of valves that direct the blood out of the leg. Blood does not normally clot in the veins.

Thrombosis of blood in the deep veins can be precipitated by any of a triad of factors described by Virchow over 150 years ago (Box 78).

• *Venous stasis.* This promotes clotting as it allows more time for blood to clot, stops small clots from being washed away and increases blood viscosity

• *Imbalance of clotting factors.* In the blood, natural procoagulant, anticoagulant and fibrinolytic factors are bal-anced to prevent clots forming within the blood vessels. An imbalance of clotting factors (e.g. from hereditary abnormalities) can predispose to clots

• *Endothelial damage.* This triggers the coagulation cascade and forms a focus for clots

How does clot form in deep veins?

Clotting is initiated by one of Virchow's factors, which triggers the coagulation cascade and aggregation of platelets, fibrin and large numbers of red blood cells (Fig. 54). The process of thrombosis triggers fibrinolysis with breakdown of formed clot. During thrombosis and fibrinolysis the thrombus is fragile and may break away from the vein wall, becoming an embolus. Alternative fates for thrombi are complete removal by fibrinolysis, organization, recanalization or calcification.

Why do venous thrombi embolize to the lungs?

Free thrombus in the deep leg veins will embolize via the pelvic veins and inferior vena cava into the right side of

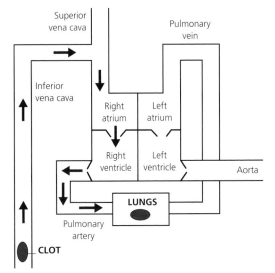

Figure 55 Circuit diagram of the heart and major vessels. Arrows indicate the route of embolism of the clot from the deep leg veins into the inferior vena cava, then through the right side of the heart and pulmonary artery to reach the lungs.

the heart, then into the pulmonary artery (Fig. 55). The embolus will come to rest at a point in the pulmonary arterial circulation where its diameter exceeds that of these vessels. Thus, a large embolus may impact in the main pulmonary arteries, whereas a small embolus may pass into smaller arteries supplying segments or subsegments of the lung.

Has Miss Lefevre had a large (massive) or small (non-massive) pulmonary embolus?

Miss Lefevre's symptoms are pleuritic chest pain and haemoptysis. These symptoms are caused by a small (correct term, non-massive) embolus that has impacted in a subsegmental or smaller artery, causing infarction of a small part of the lung (haemoptysis) and a patch of pleura (pleuritic pain). A large (correct term, massive) pulmonary embolus impacted in the main pulmonary arteries will block blood flow through the heart, causing shock and collapse. A massive pulmonary embolus does not immediately cause lung infarction because of dual blood supply to the lungs from the systemic circulation (bronchial arteries) and pulmonary arteries.

What treatment should she receive?
Supportive therapy
She should have oxygen to correct hypoxia and analgesia for her chest and calf pain.

Therapy for thromboembolic disease
She requires immediate anticoagulation with low molecular weight (LMW) heparin (Box 79; Fig. 56).

What effect will anticoagulation with low molecular weight heparin have?
Heparin will inhibit further extension of the deep vein thrombus. This will allow existing leg thrombus to become organized by natural processes, reducing the risk of further embolus.

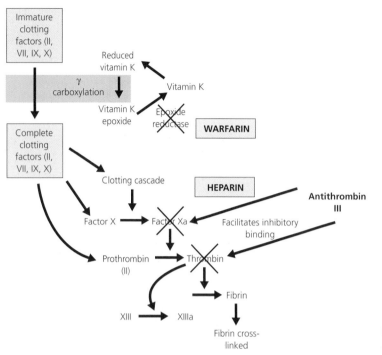

Figure 56 Mechanisms of action of anticoagulants.

What will happen to the pulmonary embolus?

The pulmonary embolus will be dealt with by natural processes, either being cleared by fibrinolysis or remaining in the affected artery and organized, recanalized or calcified (Fig. 54). The LMW heparin will have no effect on the pulmonary embolus.

Why is Miss Lefevre not being given treatment to 'dissolve' her pulmonary embolus?

Where the pulmonary embolus is non-massive, natural processes are the safest and most effective way to clear the clot, as treatment to dissolve the clot (thrombolysis) carries a risk of major bleeding as a side-effect. However, if she had a massive pulmonary embolus causing circulatory collapse then thrombolysis to dissolve the clot would have been indicated.

KEY POINT

In patients with non-massive pulmonary emboli without evidence of cardiac compromise, the aim of therapy is anticoagulation to prevent further, potentially fatal emboli and not to remove emboli that have already occurred.

What is low molecular weight heparin?

Heparins are mucopolysaccharides lining the inner surface of blood vessels. They were first discovered in liver (hence *hepar*in) and are extracted for clinical use from bovine lung and porcine intestinal mucosa. The extraction process causes degradation of the heparin into molecules with weights ranging 300–30,000 kDa. The low molecular weight components 1000–10,000 kDa are purified from the unfractionated preparation to obtain LMW heparin (Box 79).

Miss Lefevre was treated with 35% oxygen and 1 g paracetamol 6-hourly. As she weighed 65 kg, she was commenced on 13,000 units dalteparin subcutaneously once daily (200 units per kg). The following day she underwent ventilation–perfusion (V/Q) scanning to confirm the diagnosis of pulmonary embolus. The scan showed multiple unmatched perfusion defects, giving high probability of pulmonary emboli. Example images from the scan are shown in Fig. 57.

How is ventilation–perfusion scanning performed?

This test is made up of two parts.
• *Lung perfusion.* Albumin labelled with the radioactive isotope $^{99}Tc^m$ is injected intravenously and distribution of label throughout the pulmonary arterial tree is assessed with an external gamma camera.

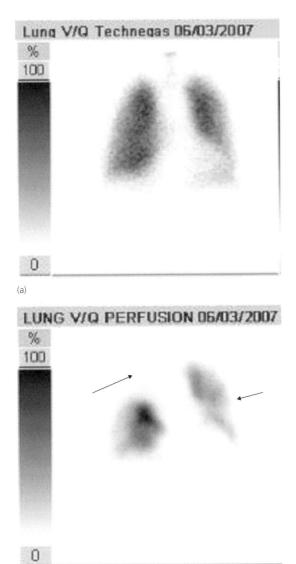

(a)

(b)

Figure 57 Ventilation–perfusion lung scan. (a) The ventilation scan shows the airspaces of the lung outlined clearly in black. (b) The perfusion scan shows areas without contrast (unperfused) in left and right lungs.

- *Lung ventilation.* The patient inhales nebulized $^{99}Tc^m$ diethylene triamine-pentacetic acid (DTPA) and distribution of label in the airways and alveoli is assessed with an external gamma camera.

If pulmonary emboli are present there will be areas of lung that are ventilated but not perfused (ventilation–perfusion mismatching; Fig. 57). The V/Q scan is interpreted by a radiologist who looks for areas of V/Q

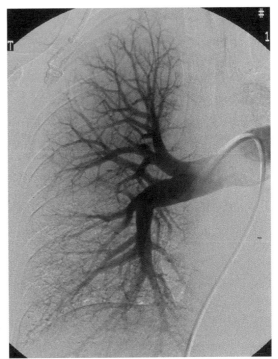

Figure 58 Pulmonary angiogram from a different patient.

mismatching and reports their findings as 'high', 'intermediate' or 'low probability' of pulmonary embolus.

Are there any other tests that can be used to diagnose pulmonary embolus?

- *Pulmonary angiogram.* In this test a catheter is inserted via the femoral or brachial vein into the right side of the heart, then through into the pulmonary arteries. Radiographic contrast is injected into the pulmonary arteries and the pulmonary arteries are visualized by repeated X-rays to look for clot (Fig. 58)
- *Computed tomography pulmonary angiogram (CTPA).* In this technique an X-ray beam moves around the chest as the patient lies on a table, taking multiple pictures which are collated in a series of 2D images on a monitor. To obtain a CTPA, images are taken after intravenous injection of contrast

What are the risks to the patient of these tests?

- *Radiation exposure.* CT involves the greatest radiation exposure (2–3 times the annual exposure to background radiation), which itself is associated with a 150–300 in 1,000,000 increased annual chance of death. Radiation exposure is less with V/Q scanning and least with angiography

• *Allergy.* Radiographic contrast (CT and non-CT angiography) contains iodine which may induce allergy and anaphylaxis if patients are sensitive to this

• *Dangers of intervention.* Pulmonary angiography requires insertion of a catheter through the right side of the heart into the pulmonary arteries. This has the risk of introducing infection and damaging myocardium, valves or vessels

How do you decide which test to use?

Hospitals usually have a policy to use either V/Q scanning or CTPA as first line and only exceptionally use pulmonary angiography. These tests are roughly comparable in their ability to diagnose pulmonary emboli and availability generally depends on resource allocation by individual hospitals. Specific uses are:

• *V/Q scan* – patients with iodine allergy

• *CTPA* – patients with structural lung disease that will affect the V/Q scan

How could you confirm the diagnosis of deep vein thrombosis?
Duplex ultrasound of the veins

This non-invasive rapid technique is a combination of:

• *Standard ultrasound.* Sound waves are reflected off the vessel walls, allowing visualization of the vascular structures

• *Doppler ultrasound.* Bursts of sound waves are reflected off moving red blood cells, allowing detection of blood flow

Clots may be visualized directly and as alteration in venous blood flow, although not all are detected.

Venogram

These are rarely performed these days but can be used if duplex ultrasound is not helpful. A foot vein is cannulated and radiographic dye is injected to show the leg veins. Clot appears as filling defects in the delineated veins. Complications include contrast allergy and phlebitis (inflamed veins).

Miss Lefevre had a positive duplex of her right leg, confirming a right calf deep vein thrombosis. LMW heparin was continued while she commenced oral anticoagulation with warfarin. By day 4 of her inpatient stay she was well and pain-free and her international normalized ratio (INR) was 1.6. She was discharged with follow-up in the anticoagulant and respiratory clinics, remaining on self-administered dalteparin until her INR was >2.0.

Why was her heparin (dalteparin) treatment changed to warfarin?

Standard practice is to anticoagulate patients for 3–6 months after a pulmonary embolus to minimize the risk of recurrence. Over a 3–6 month period tablets are preferable to (and cheaper than) daily injections. Also, heparin given for a prolonged period can cause osteoporosis.

Why was she not given warfarin instead of heparin in the first place?

After her pulmonary embolus she required immediate anticoagulation to prevent further clot. As warfarin inhibits synthesis of clotting factors (Fig. 56; Box 80) and

---

Box 80 Pharmacology of warfarin

Mechanism of action

In the final stages of synthesis of clotting factors II, VII, IX and X, the factors undergo gamma carboxylation, a process that oxidizes vitamin K. Vitamin K is recycled for further clotting factor synthesis by reduction catalysed by epoxide reductase. Warfarin inhibits clotting factor synthesis by inhibiting regeneration of reduced vitamin K.

Uses

• Prevention of recurrence of pulmonary emboli or deep vein thrombosis

• Prevention of intracardiac thrombosis in atrial fibrillation, mechanical heart valves

Pharmacokinetics

• Warfarin is metabolized by the liver, which terminates its action

• It has a narrow therapeutic range (i.e. the plasma concentration at which warfarin prevents clotting is close to the concentration at which major bleeding side-effects occur)

• Drug interactions are common in patients taking warfarin:

  ○ drugs that induce activity of liver enzymes increase warfarin metabolism and increase the risk of clotting (e.g. phenytoin, rifampicin and regular alcohol use)

  ○ drugs that inhibit activity of liver enzymes reduce warfarin metabolism and increase the risk of bleeding (e.g. erythromycin, ciprofloxacin, sodium valproate)

Side-effects

• Bleeding

• Skin necrosis

• Teratogenesis (fetal abnormalities when given to pregnant women)

existing clotting factors have to be used up, it can take 3–4 days after starting warfarin before anticoagulation is achieved. Heparin causes immediate anticoagulation as it promotes the natural anticoagulant effect of antithrombin III (Fig. 56), therefore it is used to bridge the gap while full warfarin anticoagulation is achieved.

What is the international normalized ratio?

Patients taking warfarin have blood sampled regularly for measurement of the prothrombin time, which is used to calculate the INR. During sampling, calcium is removed from the blood, then the sample is spun to remove blood cells. The resulting plasma is recalcified in the presence of a reagent with tissue factor activity which activates the clotting cascade. The time to production of a clot (prothrombin time) is measured, normally 11–15 s.

The INR is calculated by dividing the prothrombin time of the patient taking warfarin by the prothrombin time of a control subject. An INR of 1.6 indicates that Miss Lefevre's blood was clotting 1.6 times more slowly than a person not taking warfarin. In general, INR values of 2.0–4.0 are considered to indicate adequate anticoagulation, hence she was able to stop her heparin when her INR was >2.0.

KEY POINT

Before prescribing other drugs with warfarin, *always* check for potential interactions in Appendix 1 of the *British National Formulary* and adjust prescribing accordingly.

How long should she remain on warfarin for?

• Standard practice is for patients to take warfarin for 6 months following a deep vein thrombosis or pulmonary embolus to minimize the risk of recurrence
• Warfarin treatment should continue for longer than 6 months if the risk factor for clots (e.g. untreated uterine fibroids, persistent immobility, hereditary thrombophilia) is still present
• Warfarin treatment is often life-long in patients who have a recurrence of their deep vein thrombosis or pulmonary embolus
• Patients with deep vein thrombosis may stop warfarin earlier than 6 months if the risk factor has been removed

---

Box 81 Overview of hereditary thrombophilia

Patients with hereditary thrombophilia have an increased tendency to clot. The most common abnormalities are caused by deficiencies in the natural anticoagulant system.

Factor V Leiden is a genetic variant of factor V which is resistant to natural inactivation by activated protein C.

Proteins C, S and antithrombin inactivate clotting as part of the natural anticoagulant system. Genetic variants causing protein deficiencies result in anticoagulant defects and increased clotting tendencies.

Box 82 Prevention of deep vein thrombosis during prolonged travel

The aim is to maintain venous flow and minimize hypercoagulability.

Maintain venous flow
• Leg exercises, short walks, journey breaks if possible, avoid immobility
• Use travel compression stockings

Reduce hypercoagulability
• Keep hydrated
• Single dose prophylactic heparin with medical advice

Does she need further investigation?

• *Thrombophilia screen.* As Miss Lefevre is young and has a family history of thrombosis she may have an underlying genetic coagulation abnormality (Box 81) and should be tested for this after stopping warfarin as anticoagulation will affect the results
• *Pelvic ultrasound.* Miss Lefevre probably developed her thrombus because of immobility from a long coach journey. Patients without detectable risk factors (particularly women) should undergo pelvic ultrasound to look for predisposing masses or malignancy

Outcome. Miss Lefevre stopped her warfarin after 6 months and remained completely well. Her thrombophilia screen did not detect a heritable clotting abnormality. She was therefore given advice to help avoid recurrence of her thromboembolic disease (Box 82), encouraged to stop smoking and discharged from follow-up.

CASE REVIEW

Marie Lefevre presents with left-sided pleuritic chest pain and haemoptysis following a long distance coach journey. She has also noticed some right calf discomfort. A clinical diagnosis of deep vein thrombosis and pulmonary embolus is made and she is treated with LMW heparin. The following day these diagnoses are confirmed by a duplex ultrasound demonstrating right calf deep vein thrombosis and a V/Q scan showing high probability of a pulmonary embolus. She receives anticoagulation with warfarin for 6 months. Her thromboembolic disease is attributed to her long distance journey and cigarette smoking and a heritable clotting abnormality is excluded. She is advised to stop smoking and take precautions when immobile for long periods to reduce the risk of recurrence.

KEY POINTS

- Deep vein thrombosis can be precipitated by any of 'Virchow's triad' of factors:
  - venous stasis
  - imbalance of clotting factors
  - endothelial damage
- Thrombi in the deep veins can break free, becoming emboli that travel to the lungs – pulmonary emboli
- Pulmonary emboli impact in the pulmonary circulation at the point where the diameter of the embolus exceeds that of the vessels
- Smaller pulmonary emboli impact in peripheral pulmonary arteries where they may cause infarction of the supplied lung and overlying pleura with symptoms of pleuritic chest pain and haemoptysis
- Pulmonary emboli can be difficult to diagnose:
  - at presentation, clinical features are used to estimate the likelihood of pulmonary emboli (Wells criteria)
  - D-dimer measurement can be used to rule out pulmonary emboli in patients with low or moderate likelihood of emboli

  - definitive investigations including V/Q scanning and CTPA are often not available out of hours except in severe emergencies, so patients at moderate or high risk of emboli are usually treated until diagnosis can be confirmed
- Patients with suspected or proven deep vein thrombosis and/or pulmonary embolus are initially treated with subcutaneous LMW heparin to prevent further pulmonary embolus
- Existing thrombus or embolus is usually cleared or organized by intrinsic (natural) mechanisms
- Once the diagnosis has been confirmed, patients receive oral warfarin for 3–6 months to prevent recurrence
- Investigations including pelvic ultrasound scanning and hereditary thrombophilia testing should be performed to look for an underlying cause of thromboembolic disease
- Patients with recurrent thromboembolic disease should receive life-long anticoagulation

Case 16   An elderly woman who collapsed suddenly

An elderly woman is rushed into accident and emergency by ambulance having collapsed at home. Her husband, Mr Khan, told the ambulance crew she had been well previously with no relevant past medical history and that this had happened without warning.

On arrival at accident and emergency:

Her airway is patent and she is breathing spontaneously with respiratory rate 20 breaths/min

Oxygen saturations are 74% on 35% oxygen

Her pulse is 140 beats/min and blood pressure 60/36 mmHg

She has a Glasgow Coma Score of 11/15 and has an intravenous cannula in her right arm inserted by the ambulance crew

What is the first priority in her management?

Mrs Khan needs urgent resuscitation. Her life-threatening problems are hypoxia and hypotension, which cause tissue damage. Her brain is particularly at risk as it can only survive anoxia for 4–5 min before permanent damage occurs. Her reduced Glasgow Coma Score may indicate this is already occurring.

How should she be resuscitated initially?

Hypoxia

She should immediately receive higher concentrations of inhaled oxygen via a mask with a reservoir bag (15 L/min will deliver an oxygen concentration of 75–90%). Blood gas tests should be performed as soon as possible to look for CO_2 retention which may be contributing to her impaired consciousness. If high flow oxygen does not correct her hypoxia or is contraindicated by CO_2 retention she will require ventilatory support.

Hypotension

Initially, she should be given intravenous fluid to attempt to raise her blood pressure. A crystalloid such as isotonic saline or a colloid solution of macromolecules such as dextrans or gelatin, which stay in the circulation longer, should be used.

After an increase in oxygen therapy to 15 L/min via mask and reservoir bag and 1 L isotonic saline, Mrs Khan's observations were as follows:

Oxygen saturations 86%

Pulse 125 beats/min and blood pressure 90/60 mmHg

Glasgow Coma Score 14

How do you interpret these new observations?

There is some improvement after her initial resuscitation, which has created time to identify and treat the underlying cause of her collapse.

What mechanisms might explain her sudden collapse?

She has hypoxia, hypotension and confusion. Any of these could have been the primary abnormality that caused her clinical presentation:

- *Hypoxia.* This could have developed rapidly as a result of any of the conditions that cause respiratory arrest (Box 28, p. 42). If hypoxia is severe, cardiac and brain function are impaired, leading to hypotension and confusion
- *Hypotension.* Low blood pressure can be caused by hypovolaemia (e.g. haemorrhage), cardiac impairment (e.g. post myocardial infarction), infection (septic shock) or anaphylaxis. Reduced cerebral and pulmonary perfusion could cause secondary confusion and hypoxia
- *Confusion.* A primary brain problem, such as haemorrhage or stroke could impair consciousness. This could lead to hypoventilation and hypoxia

How would you approach her assessment?

The next step is to establish which of these mechanisms has caused her collapse and whether her primary disease is cardiovascular, respiratory or neurological. This requires rapid systematic assessment by clinical examination and initial investigation.

> *The examination findings were as follows.*
> *Cardiovascular system:*
> • *Jugular venous pressure (JVP) elevated to +10 cm*
> • *Right ventricular heave*
> *Respiratory system:*
> • *Normal breath sounds*
> *Nervous system:*
> • *No focal abnormalities, plantars flexor bilaterally*
> *Other:*
> • *Evidence of recent weight loss*

How do you interpret these examination findings?

• The major abnormality is in the cardiovascular system, with the lungs and nervous system seemingly intact
• An elevated JVP with right ventricular heave indicates that the right side of the heart is overloaded
• On the left side of the heart, output is reduced (low systemic blood pressure), but there is no evidence of pulmonary oedema, indicating poor left heart filling rather than left heart failure
• Overload of the right heart with reduced left heart filling and clear lung fields indicates that the abnormality is most likely to be in the pulmonary circulation

What is the differential diagnosis?

The most likely diagnosis is a massive pulmonary embolus (Fig. 59).
 Less likely diagnoses include:
• Infarction and failure of the right side of the heart
• Tricuspid valve disease
• Pericardial tamponade

Why are these other diagnoses less likely than massive pulmonary embolus?

• Right heart infarction is relatively unusual. Damage to the right ventricle would cause systemic venous congestion (raised JVP) and poor left heart filling (low blood pressure) but the right ventricle would pump more weakly, rather than more strongly (right ventricular heave)
• Rapid destruction of the tricuspid valve (e.g. resulting from infective endocarditis) could cause overwork of the right ventricle (heave) and reduce left heart filling (hypotension). However, this patient does not have a murmur

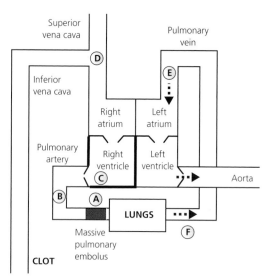

Figure 59 Circuit diagram illustrating the pathophysiology of massive pulmonary embolus. (A) The massive pulmonary embolus is shown impacted in the main pulmonary arteries. (B) This prevents blood entering the lungs, causing hypertension in the pulmonary arteries. (C) The right ventricle strains to push blood through the lungs and (D) blood backs up into the systemic veins, which become congested. (E) As blood cannot get through the lungs, filling of the left side of the heart is reduced. (F) This reduces left ventricular output, causing low blood pressure.

of tricuspid regurgitation and this condition is generally less common than pulmonary embolus
• Pericardial tamponade occurs when fluid in the pericardium compresses the heart, reducing contraction. This would cause a more global reduction in cardiac function and a right ventricular heave would be unlikely

> *The results of Mrs Khan's initial investigations are as follows:*
> *Chest X-ray. Clear lung fields*
> *ECG – see Fig. 60*
> *Arterial blood gases on 15 L/min oxygen via mask and reservoir bag:*

		Normal range
pH	7.36	(7.35–7.45)
PO_2	7.4 kPa	(10–13.1 kPa)
PCO_2	4.5 kPa	(4.9–6.1 kPa)
HCO_3^-	23 mmol/L	(22–28 mmol/L)
D-dimers	1.8 mg/L	(<0.3 mg/L)
Troponin T	0.6 ng/mL	(<0.01 ng/mL)

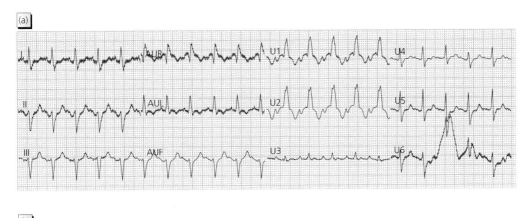

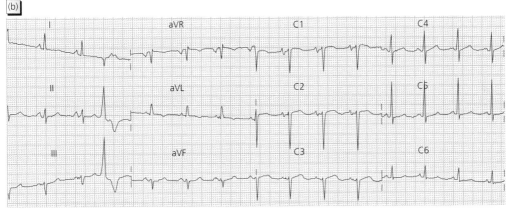

Figure 60 Electrocardiograms. ECG (a) was taken during the acute admission and is shown compared with ECG (b), found in Mrs Khan's old notes from a previous hospital visit. The notable differences are: 1. The heart rate is faster (~150 beats/min) in (a) than in (b) (~100 beats/min). 2. (a) shows new big R waves (first upward deflection) in leads V1 and V2, which are the leads that look at the right ventricle and new S waves in leads V5 and V6. As the QRS complexes are also wider (2.5–3 small squares) this is new right bundle branch block. These ECG abnormalities are features of right heart strain. 3. In ECG (a) there is a new S wave in lead I and Q wave in lead III. These abnormalities which can occur with an inverted T wave in lead III are the classic SIQIIITIII of acute pulmonary embolus. In practice this is not often seen.

Can these investigations be interpreted to make a firm diagnosis?

• The normal chest X-ray and abnormal ECG support the deduction that the abnormality is somewhere in the heart or circulation rather than in the lungs

• The ECG shows features of right heart strain (Fig. 60) consistent with the clinical findings of right ventricular heart strain and raised JVP

• Arterial gases show type I respiratory failure, which has been poorly corrected by high flow oxygen therapy. This is consistent with a massive pulmonary embolus because increasing oxygen concentrations in the alveoli will have little impact if there is insufficient perfusion of pulmonary capillaries for oxygen uptake into the blood.

However, any other disease causing severe ventilation–perfusion (V/Q) mismatch could account for these results

• Elevated D-dimers indicate breakdown of clot somewhere in the body, but are raised in a wide range of clinical conditions and are unhelpful in making a diagnosis. It could be argued in this situation that testing them is simply a waste of money

• Troponin T is specifically released from cardiac myocytes and so indicates myocardial damage. In this patient raised troponin T could indicate a primary cardiac event (e.g. right ventricular infarction). However, massive pulmonary embolus causes secondary cardiac ischaemia by reducing coronary perfusion with elevation of troponin T

Thus, the initial investigations give information that is supportive, but not specific for a diagnosis of massive pulmonary embolus so further investigations are required to make a firm diagnosis and guide therapy.

How long should it have taken to arrive at this point?

The results of clinical examination, chest X-ray, ECG and blood gases can all be available in about 20 min, sufficient to guide decision-making. Blood test results take longer, depending on the hospital laboratory. However, the clinicians should not wait for these to make a decision regarding further care.

What tests could be used to make a firm diagnosis of massive pulmonary embolus?
Echocardiogram
This can confirm the diagnosis by:
• Visualizing thrombus in the right heart or main pulmonary artery
• Demonstrating right ventricular strain
• Excluding cardiac diagnoses (infarction, valve disease)

Computed tomography pulmonary angiography
Computed tomography pulmonary angiography (CTPA) is most useful for direct visualization of the thrombus in the pulmonary arteries.

How do you decide which of these tests to use?
Both tests will give diagnostic information. The considerations are:
• Which test is available most quickly?
• Is the patient stable enough to undergo testing?

For example, it may be safer to bring a portable echocardiography machine to the patient if an operator is available, than move the patient to the CT scanning department away from resuscitation facilities. The most suitable test will therefore vary depending on local resources.

Mrs Khan was judged stable enough to undergo further investigation and, as echocardiography was not available, an urgent CTPA was arranged. The medical registrar accompanied her to the radiology department with the resuscitation trolley in case of rapid deterioration. However, Mrs Khan tolerated the scan, which is shown in Figs 61 and 62. A diagnosis of massive pulmonary embolus was confirmed and she was transferred to intensive care for consideration of urgent thrombolysis. A right pleural effusion was also seen on the scan, presumed secondary to her massive pulmonary embolus. As Mrs Khan remained drowsy and unwell the medical team spoke briefly to her husband to determine whether she had any contraindications to this treatment (Box 83).

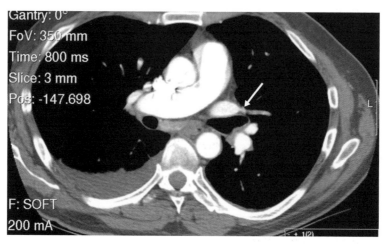

Figure 61 Computed tomography pulmonary angiogram (CTPA). This is a single slice taken from a CTPA at the level of the aortic arch. The patient is supine, so their front is at the top of the picture. Ribs and vertebrae appear white, soft tissue is grey and lung fields are black. The vessels show white as they contain radiographic contrast injected intravenously. The arrow indicates a point in the left pulmonary artery where it narrows suddenly and a grey area can be seen in the contrast (shown in more detail in Fig. 62). Clot is occluding the artery and preventing perfusion of the vessel beyond. There is also a right-sided pleural effusion which could be secondary to pulmonary emboli in this patient.

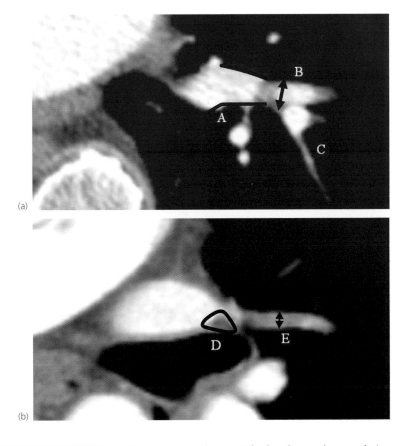

Figure 62 Comparison of pulmonary arteries imaged using computed tomography pulmonary angiogram (CTPA). (a) Normal. (b) Pulmonary embolus. In the normal artery there is (A) unoccluded vessel allowing contrast to (B) pass distally into (C) tributaries. In the abnormal artery (D) embolus can be seen as a grey protrusion into the white (contrast) arterial lumen (E). There is little run off from the occluded artery into the distal pulmonary circulation.

Box 83 Contraindications to thrombolysis

Absolute contraindications
- Previous history of intracranial haemorrhage
- Active intracranial neoplasm
- Recent (<2 months) intracranial surgery or trauma
- Current or recent (<6 months) internal bleeding

Relative contraindications
- Other coagulation disorder with increased bleeding risk
- Uncontrolled severe hypertension (blood pressure >200 mmHg systolic or >110 mmHg diastolic)
- Non-haemorrhagic stroke (<2 months)
- Surgery (≤10 days)
- Low platelet count (<100 × 10⁹/L)

How could thrombolysis help Mrs Khan?

Mrs Khan's massive pulmonary embolus is causing severe hypoxia and hypotension and she already has signs of end organ damage including confusion (brain) and raised troponin T (heart). In theory, removal of the pulmonary embolus by thrombolysis would correct her hypoxia and hypotension and prevent further damage by reperfusing the pulmonary arteries and increasing left heart filling.

How could this be achieved by thrombolysis?

Thrombolytic drugs are infused into an arm vein and circulate to the pulmonary artery. They activate plasminogen to plasmin, a naturally occurring thrombolytic molecule (Fig. 63), which dissolves thrombus and recanalizes the main pulmonary artery.

Do clinical trials show that thrombolysis is beneficial in massive pulmonary embolus?

Although it seems intuitive that removing pulmonary thrombus would be a good thing, clinical trials showed that thrombolysis compared to anticoagulation with heparin produced:
- No significant reduction in mortality
- Short-term improvement in right ventricular function
- Possible longer term lower pulmonary arterial pressures (one study)

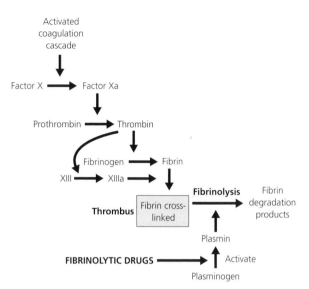

Figure 63 Mechanism of action of thrombolytic drugs. Fibrinolytic drugs activate plasminogen to plasmin. This degrades fibrin, hence breaks up thrombi.

However, clinical trials are difficult to perform and interpret in this group of patients because of small numbers and problems conducting trials in an emergency situation. Most clinicians therefore accept that thrombolysis can be life-saving in selected patients with major pulmonary embolus and would use it in this situation if the benefits appear to outweigh the risks of major haemorrhage (Box 83).

Which drugs are used for thrombolysis? (Box 84)
Some options include the following.

Streptokinase
This thrombolytic drug, derived from streptococci, has been available for clinical use for many years. As an 'old' drug it has several advantages:
• Its manufacture is no longer restricted by patent, so it is relatively cheap
• It has been widely studied in the clinical situation
However, as a bacterial product it is antigenic and can cause allergic reactions. It also has to be given as an infusion over 24 h, which may be too slow in this patient group.

Recombinant tissue plasminogen activator
This agent occurs naturally in tissues including endothelial cells. Pharmacological recombinant tissue plasminogen activator (rTPA) has also been widely studied in patients with pulmonary emboli. rTPA is more expensive than streptokinase, but can be given more quickly (≤2 h) and does not induce allergic reactions.

Box 84 Pharmacology of thrombolytic drugs

Mechanism of action
• Streptokinase binds to plasminogen, forming an active enzyme that activates plasmin. It is not well absorbed by fibrin thrombi, so acts generally in the circulation, which may increase risk of bleeding
• rTPA binds to fibrin, increasing its affinity for plasminogen and enhancing plasminogen activation. As rTPA binds to fibrin it is less likely to produce a general coagulation disturbance than streptokinase

Uses
Removal of thrombus in emergency situations including:
• Massive pulmonary embolus
• Myocardial infarction
• Acute stroke
• Arterial embolus

Pharmacokinetics
• Drugs given intravenously and have plasma half-life of 30 (rTPA) to 90 min (streptokinase)

Major side-effects
• Major bleeding, particularly intracranial (~1%)
• Allergy, hypotension (streptokinase)

Tenecteplase
This is a newer agent which can be given rapidly as a bolus. It is not yet licensed for use in patients with pulmonary emboli, but is currently being tested in clinical trials.

Is thrombolysis dangerous?

The major side-effect of thrombolytic drugs is bleeding, particularly from the gastrointestinal tract, into the retroperitoneal space and into the brain. Up to 3% of patients with massive pulmonary embolus who receive thrombolysis have a brain haemorrhage.

Patients with massive pulmonary embolus may be more at risk of bleeding from thrombolysis than patients with myocardial infarction because other disease, including malignancy and recent surgery, may underlie the development of their thromboembolism.

Before thrombolysis is given, the risk of bleeding should be assessed using a checklist of contraindications (Box 83). Thrombolysis should not be given to patients who have any of the absolute contraindications. The risks and benefits of thrombolysis for patients with relative contraindications need to be weighed up by the treating clinician.

Are there any alternatives to thrombolysis?

Thrombus can also be removed from the pulmonary artery using:
• *Catheter embolectomy.* The thrombus is physically broken up by a catheter inserted directly into the pulmonary artery, with fragments either retrieved by suction or allowed to pass into the distal pulmonary arteries where they do less damage
• *Surgical embolectomy.* The patient is put on to cardiopulmonary bypass and the thrombus is removed directly at operation

These options may be considered in patients with massive pulmonary embolus when thrombolysis either fails or is contraindicated.

> *Mr Khan told the clinical team that Mrs Khan did not have any contraindications for thrombolysis. However, Mr Khan was concerned that thrombolysis was dangerous and stated that he would rather she did not receive it.*

What are the ethical issues surrounding consent to treatment?

As a basic principle, patients have a right to autonomy (i.e. the right to make their own choices as to how their lives will be lived).

Health professionals must therefore:
• Respect their patients' autonomy
• Provide sufficient information to support patients in making an autonomous decision

---

> **Box 85 Re C test**
>
> The 'Re C' test refers to a legal case (regarding patient 'C').
>
>   Can the individual:
> • Understand and retain information
> • Believe it and
> • Weigh it up to arrive at a choice
>   If they are unable to do any one of these, they are considered to lack capacity or be incompetent to make autonomous choices.

> **Box 86 Useful websites for further reading about ethics of informed consent**
>
> General Medical Council. Seeking patients' consent: the ethical considerations. http://www.gmc-uk.org/guidance/current/library/consent.asp
>   UK Clinical Ethics Network. http://www.ethox.org.uk/Ethics/econsent.htm

• Obtain informed consent before performing any diagnostic or therapeutic intervention

Patients should be assumed to be able to make an autonomous choice (i.e. give or withhold consent). However, some patients, including those who are unconscious, confused or mentally ill, may lack capacity to make an autonomous choice. This should be tested using the Re C test (Box 85).

If an individual in England lacks capacity, the law states that no one can consent to treatment on their behalf (this law is different in other countries). However, in this situation the health professional has the duty of beneficence (i.e. is morally required to do good and may take decisions about medical treatment in the patient's best interests). In an emergency situation, health professionals should do no more than 'what is immediately necessary to save life or avoid significant deterioration in the patient's health' (General Medical Council [GMC]; Box 86).

Who should decide what treatment Mrs Khan receives?

Mrs Khan lacks capacity to decide on her treatment as she is drowsy and unwell and unable to retain and weigh up information regarding her thrombolysis.

Under English law, Mr Khan does not have the right to decide on her treatment. The clinical team caring for her must therefore act in her best interests.

How are Mrs Khan's 'best interests' established?

These are defined in the UK by the GMC (Box 86). The following should be taken into account:
• What investigations and treatment are clinically indicated?
• Does she have any previously stated preferences?
  ○ advance directive?
  ○ third party report (e.g. from husband)
  ○ indicated by cultural or other beliefs
• Which option least restricts her future choices?

The clinical team discussed the situation further with Mr Khan. He stated that Mrs Khan had no formal advance directive, but had always said she would like to keep going with her life as long as possible. She had agreed to treatments including surgery in the past, even when told she might not recover. The outcome of this discussion was that Mr Khan and the clinical team agreed that Mrs Khan would probably want treatment and in her case the chance of clinical benefit was felt to be greater than the risk of bleeding. A decision was made to go ahead and Mrs Khan received thrombolysis with rTPA, followed by anticoagulation with unfractionated heparin to prevent further thromboembolus as per treatment guidelines.

Observations before thrombolysis:
Oxygen saturations 84% on 15 L oxygen
Pulse 132 beats/min
Blood pressure 82/56 mmHg
Observations 2 hours after thrombolysis:
Oxygen saturations 96% on 15 L oxygen
Pulse 106 beats/min
Blood pressure 132/74 mmHg
Mrs Khan experienced bleeding from her gums, but no other complications.

Was the thrombolysis effective?

Increasing oxygenation and blood pressure and improvement in her tachycardia indicate that the pulmonary artery thrombus is no longer obstructing pulmonary arterial blood flow and left heart filling.

Why did she receive unfractionated, rather than low molecular weight heparin?

Unfractionated heparin comprises molecules of molecular weight 300–30,000 kDa and has different properties from low molecular weight heparin (LMW), which is purified to contain only molecules 1000–10,000 kDa:

• *Half-life.* Unfractionated heparin binds to a wide range of proteins and is thus rapidly deactivated and cleared from the plasma. It has a short plasma half-life of 30–60 min and thus anticoagulation wears off more quickly than for LMW heparin which is renally excreted, has a plasma half life of ~4 h and a longer effect duration
• *Reversibility.* The anticoagulant effect of unfractionated heparin can be reversed by protamine, which binds the heparin and neutralizes it. LMW heparin cannot be fully neutralized by heparin

Unstable patients with massive pulmonary embolus are therefore anticoagulated with unfractionated heparin as it can be stopped and reversed rapidly if the patient deteriorates.

In most other clinical situations LMW is preferred to unfractionated heparin because LMW heparin is easier to use, does not require monitoring with regular blood tests and can be self-administered by the patient at home.

Mrs Khan made a good recovery from her massive pulmonary embolus. On day 2 she was transferred out of intensive care to a medical ward. She mobilized and on day 3 was commenced on warfarin. An echocardiogram showed no residual right heart strain and an ultrasound of her pelvis was normal. No underlying cause for her embolus was identified. When her INR was 3.0 she was discharged home with follow-up appointments for the anticoagulation and respiratory clinics.

Are there any long-term complications of pulmonary emboli?

Pulmonary emboli can be fatal and are responsible for around 60 deaths per million people in the UK annually. Luckily, Mrs Khan survived. It is likely that her embolus has resolved either completely or with a small residual deficit. However, a small proportion of patients develop pulmonary hypertension, although the mechanisms underlying this are not fully understood.

Should Mrs Khan undergo any further tests?

Further tests can be helpful in deciding how long Mrs Khan remains on warfarin and checking for complications of pulmonary emboli. Useful tests include:
• *Lung function tests.* Reduced gas transfer may indicate a persistent perfusion defect preventing normal oxygenation of blood by the lungs
• *Echocardiogram.* This checks for residual right heart strain or pulmonary hypertension

- *Ventilation–perfusion scan.* This demonstrates persistent perfusion defects. It is useful to perform this when she is well to identify residual defects, which can then be distinguished from new defects if she presents with recurrent pulmonary embolus

If all of these tests are normal 6 months after her pulmonary embolus then it may be possible for her to stop warfarin if there are no residual risk factors for thrombus. If she has persistent pulmonary hypertension or gas transfer abnormalities then she may need further investigation and prolonged anticoagulation.

Mrs Khan will also be seen in the anticoagulation clinic for monitoring of her warfarin therapy by INR and thrombophilia testing (see Case 15).

Outcome. At 6 months Mrs Khan was well and was able to walk to the shops without breathlessness. She had a normal gas transfer and echocardiogram. However, as her massive pulmonary embolus remained unexplained, she elected on discussion with the haematologist to remain on warfarin to prevent recurrence.

CASE REVIEW

Mrs Khan collapsed at home and was hypoxic and hypotensive on arrival in accident and emergency. Examination and investigations showed right heart strain and a provisional diagnosis of massive pulmonary embolus was confirmed by an urgent CTPA. Mrs Khan was treated with rTPA to break down the clot (thrombolysis) followed by unfractionated heparin. Two hours later her oxygenation, pulse and blood pressure had improved considerably and Mrs Khan went on to make a good recovery. No underlying cause for her pulmonary embolus was identified. She was discharged home on warfarin and elected to remain on this treatment for life to prevent recurrence.

KEY POINTS

- 'Massive' pulmonary emboli impact in the main pulmonary arteries causing:
  - acute right heart strain as the right heart attempts to force blood past the clot
  - reduced left heart filling and output causing low systemic blood pressure and shock
- Where massive pulmonary embolus is suspected, urgent CTPA or echocardiogram should be performed to make a firm diagnosis
- Confirmed massive pulmonary embolus can be treated with thrombolysis to remove the clot. Clinical trials have shown that this produces short-term improvement in right ventricular function and possible longer term lower pulmonary arterial pressures
- Thrombolysis is associated with significant risk of major haemorrhage, including intracranial haemorrhage

- Patients should be screened carefully for risk of haemorrhagic complications before decisions about thrombolysis are made
- Thrombolysis should be followed by treatment with unfractionated heparin and patients should be started on warfarin when stable
- Patients who do not receive thrombolysis should still be anticoagulated, usually with LMW heparin
- Patients with massive pulmonary emboli should receive 6 months of anticoagulation
- The decision to continue or stop anticoagulation depends on many factors including:
  - underlying cause of thromboembolic disease (safer to stop if the cause has been removed)
  - presence or absence of pulmonary hypertension complicating the embolus (continue anticoagulation if present)

Case 17 A 45-year-old man with chest pain and breathlessness

Mr Sivakumaran is a 45-year-old man who presents to accident and emergency with worsening chest pain and shortness of breath over the past 24 h. The pain is in the left side of his chest and is particularly bad when he coughs or takes a deep breath. He is not usually short of breath, although he does not take much exercise, but is now breathless when climbing the stairs.

What type of pain is this?
Pleuritic chest pain (see Case 13).

What conditions are most likely to be the cause of his symptoms?
Three important common causes of pleuritic chest pain are:
• Pneumonia
• Pulmonary embolus
• Pneumothorax
For other causes see Box 72, p. 118.

What features will you ask for when taking a history to help you distinguish between these diagnoses?
Pneumonia
Patients may complain of fevers, shivers and aches or develop uncontrollable shaking (rigors). They may have a cough with or without purulent (yellow/green) sputum, which may contain blood (haemoptysis).

Pulmonary embolus
Patients may have a cough and haemoptysis, but do not produce purulent sputum. They may have pain or swelling in a calf (deep vein thrombosis) and give a history of immobility, trauma, pregnancy or oestrogen treatment (oral contraceptive, hormone replacement).

Pneumothorax
Pain is usually of sudden onset, cough is a less frequent feature and there is no sputum or haemoptysis. Patients are more often male (6:1 male:female) and may be young, tall and thin, older with underlying lung disease or a victim of trauma.

Mr Sivakumaran's cough has been present for the last 24 h and is now productive of a small amount of green sputum. He has no risk factors for pulmonary embolus but has smoked 10 cigarettes per day since he was 15. He has not taken any treatment for his condition.
His examination findings are:
Temperature 38.4°C
Pulse 102 beats/min
Blood pressure 110/80 mmHg
Respiratory rate 32 breaths/min
Oxygen saturations 90% on air
Chest:
Trachea – midline
Expansion – reduced on the left
Percussion note – dull left base
Auscultation – bronchial breathing and crepitations over left base

How do you interpret his examination findings?
His elevated temperature suggests infection and tachycardia is likely to be caused by fever. As a general rule, the pulse increases by 20 beats/min per degree rise in temperature.

Chest findings are consistent with airspace consolidation, brought about by pneumonia (Box 87). Alveoli in the infected lobe of the lung become filled with fluid and cells instead of air (Fig. 64) and the lobe becomes solid. In the affected lobe expansion is reduced, percussion note is dull and normal vesicular breath sounds are reduced. Harsher 'bronchial' breath sounds are transmitted to the chest wall from the large airways across the consolidated lung and crackles are caused when swollen lung tissue and fluid-filled alveoli are inflated on inhalation.

What is the most likely diagnosis?
Lobar pneumonia.

Box 87 Pathology of pneumonia

Pneumonia is alveolar inflammation caused by infection. It can affect alveoli uniformly from one or more lobes of the lung (lobar pneumonia) or spread from the terminal bronchioles to the alveoli in a more patchy distribution (bronchopneumonia).

Lobar pneumonia classically has four pathological phases, although these may be less distinct now antibiotics are widely used.

Phase 1. Congestion
1–2 days. Pulmonary capillaries vasodilate and serous fluid exudes out of the capillaries into the alveoli. The patient is feverish and develops shortness of breath and cough.

Phase 2. Red hepatization
2–4 days. This literally means that the lungs look like 'red liver'. The affected lobe of the lung is solid as the alveoli are full of red blood cells and fibrin strands instead of air. As there is no gas exchange in this lobe the patient becomes breathless and hypoxic. They may also cough up the red blood cells as blood-stained or rusty sputum.

Phase 3. Grey hepatization
4–8 days. The affected parts of the lungs remain solid but now look like 'grey liver'. The alveoli are full of neutrophils and dense fibrous strands. The patient coughs up purulent sputum and remains breathless.

Phase 4. Resolution
Beginning day 8–10. Monocytes clear the inflammatory debris and normal air-filled lung architecture is restored.

Pleuritic chest pain indicates involvement of the visceral and parietal pleura overlying the infected lung lobe (pleurisy). Fluid may exude through the inflamed pleura into the pleural space; hence pneumonia may be complicated by a pleural effusion.

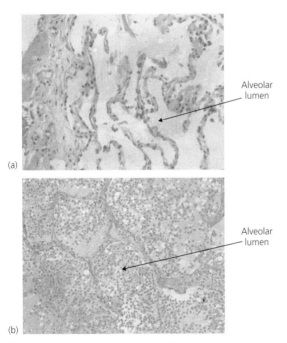

(a)

Alveolar lumen

(b)

Alveolar lumen

Figure 64 Pathology of pneumonia. (a) Normal air filled alveoli. (b) Alveoli in acute pneumonia filled with exudate and inflammatory cells.

What initial investigations will you request?
- Chest X-ray to confirm consolidation
- Renal function, electrolytes and glucose to assess illness severity
- Full blood count and C-reactive protein (CRP) to confirm infection
- Blood and sputum cultures to look for a causative organism
- Blood gases for further assessment of oxygenation and ventilation

His test results are as follows.
  Chest X-ray (Fig. 65):

		Normal range
Na	*140 mmol/L*	*(135–145 mmol/L)*
K	*3.9 mmol/L*	*(3.5–5.0 mmol/L)*
Urea	*11 mmol/L*	*(2.5–8 mmol/L)*
Creatinine	*89 μmol/L*	*(60–110 μmol/L)*
CRP	*230 mg/L*	*(<8 mg/L)*
Haemoglobin	*14 g/dL*	*(13–18 g/dL)*
White cells	*19.2 × 10^9/L*	*(4–11 × 10^9/L)*
Neutrophils	*14.8 × 10^9/L*	*(2.0–7.5 × 10^9/L)*
Platelets	*380 × 10^9/L*	*(150–400 × 10^9/L)*
pH	*7.50*	*(7.35–7.45)*
PaO$_2$	*7.8 kPa*	*(10–13.1 kPa)*
PaCO$_2$	*3.9 kPa*	*(4.9–6.1 kPa)*

What does his chest X-ray show?
The obvious abnormality is confluent, fairly homogeneous (uniform) white shadowing in the lower half of the left lung field. This is airspace shadowing which occurs in consolidation because the air in the alveoli has been replaced by inflammatory exudates (Fig. 64). The left

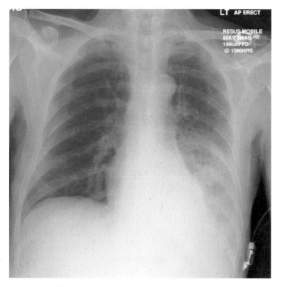

Figure 65 Chest X-ray.

hemidiaphragm is obscured by the shadowing, indicating that the pathology is in the left lower lobe of the lung (Fig. 66).

This confirms a diagnosis of left lower lobe pneumonia.

How do you know this is consolidation and not a pleural effusion?

A chest X-ray of a pleural effusion is shown for comparison in Fig. 67. The main differences are:

• The top of the effusion (Fig. 67) is a meniscus (curve) indicating a fluid level in the pleural space. The top of the consolidation (Fig. 65) is fluffy, indicating fluid (pus) in the alveoli

• Shadowing of the effusion is a dense white, completely obscuring the lung and costophrenic angle. Shadowing of the consolidation is a less dense light grey and the structure of the underlying lung can still be made out

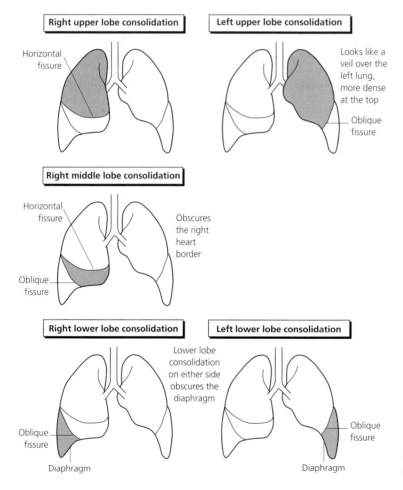

Figure 66 X-ray abnormalities in lobar pneumonia.

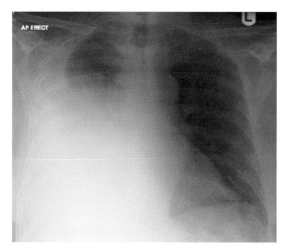

Figure 67 Chest X-ray showing pleural effusion.

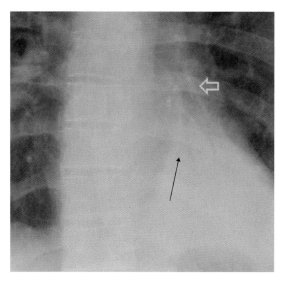

Figure 68 Chest X-ray showing air bronchograms (arrows).

• You may see air bronchograms in consolidation (Fig. 68). These occur because pus eliminates air from the alveoli, making them look grey–white, but not from the airways, which remain air-filled and black (see arrow in Fig. 68).

How severe is his pneumonia?

The severity of pneumonia is judged using the CURB-65 score (Box 88). This 5-point score is based on core adverse prognostic factors that have been shown to be associated with an increased risk of death from pneumonia. Mr Sivakumaran scores:

Box 88 CURB-65 Score

One point each for:

New **C**onfusion – mini mental test score <8

Urea >7 mmol/L

Respiratory rate ≥30 breaths/min

Blood pressure <90 mmHg systolic and/or ≤60 mmHg diastolic

Age ≥**65** years

The British Thoracic Society guidelines (http://www.brit-thoracic.org.uk/) state that:

• Patients with a CURB-65 score of 3 or more are at high risk of death and must be hospitalized and treated as having severe pneumonia

• Patients with a CURB-65 score of 2 are at increased risk of death and probably need at least a short hospital stay

• Patients with a CURB-65 score of 0 or 1 are at low risk of death and may be suitable for home treatment

Other worrying features in patients with pneumonia:

• Underlying disease

• Hypoxia – sats <92% or PaO_2 <8 kPa

• Bilateral or multilobe involvement

New confusion	0
Urea >7 mmol/L	1
Respiratory rate ≥30 breaths/min	1
Low blood pressure	0
Age ≥65 years	0

His CURB-65 score is 2. His hypoxia is also a concern. He has an increased risk of death and requires hospital admission.

What organisms cause pneumonia?

The most common cause of community-acquired pneumonia is *Streptococcus pneumoniae*. Pneumonia can also be caused by a variety of other bacteria and viruses (Fig. 69). The cause is never identified in at least 25% of patients.

What is 'atypical' pneumonia?

'Atypical' pneumonia is an old term used to describe pneumonias where symptoms were more systemic (headache, malaise, diarrhoea) than pulmonary (cough, sputum production, shortness of breath). 'Atypical' pneumonia was most often caused by pathogens such as *Mycoplasma*, *Chlamydia* and *Legionella* (Table 7), hence the term 'atypical' pathogens is applied to these organisms. Currently, it is recognized that symptoms do not reliably

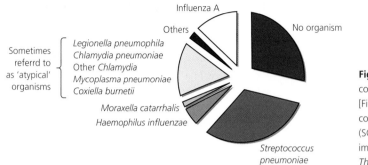

Figure 69 Microbiological causes of community acquired pneumonia in the UK. [Figure drawn from data in Lim *et al*. Study of community acquired pneumonia aetiology (SCAPA) in adults admitted to hospital: implications for management guidelines. *Thorax* 2001; **56**: 296–301.]

Table 7 Pneumonia caused by 'atypical' pathogens.

Pathogen	Clinical features associated with pathogen	Investigations other than serology
Legionella pneumophila	Pathogen lives in water (e.g. in hotel showers, cooling towers)	Urinary legionella antigen
	Most common in male smokers	
	Associated gastrointestinal and neurological symptoms	
	Causes severe pneumonia and multisystem involvement	
Mycoplasma pneumoniae	Outbreaks in young people living in institutions	Cold agglutinins (IgM antibodies that attach to red cells at low temperatures causing them to stick together)
	Prodromal headache and malaise	
	Hyponatraemia	
	Less severe pneumonia	
	Immunological extrapulmonary complications, e.g.	
	• Myocarditis/pericarditis	
	• Haemolytic anaemia/thrombocytopaenia	
	• Neurological abnormalities	
Chlamydia spp.	*C. pneumoniae* Milder illness, headache	
	C. psittaci Infection from affected birds, especially parrots May be a severe illness	
Coxiella burnetii (Q fever)	Zoonosis (infection spread by animals via dust, unpasteurized milk, etc.)	
	Acute flu-like illness	
	Chronic infection – systemic involvement of heart, eyes, testes and bone	

predict the infecting organisms and that bacteria in the atypical group commonly cause pneumonia (Fig. 69). However, the term 'atypical' has stuck as it is useful to think of these organisms in a separate group to *S. pneumoniae* as they require different investigation and treatment.

What microbiological tests can be carried out to identify the organism?
Blood and sputum cultures
These tests rely on the presence of living organisms in samples that can be grown, identified and tested for antibiotic sensitivity. Samples are most likely to give a useful result if:
- The patient has *not* had antibiotics before testing
- The patient has severe pneumonia
- Proper samples are taken – sputum should be purulent (yellow–green) and not clear (saliva)

Urinary antigen testing
Antigens from *S. pneumoniae* and *L. pneumophila* are excreted in the urine during active infection. Commercial kits are available which work in a manner similar to a pregnancy test. Urine is dropped on to a test booklet impregnated with antibodies and appearance of coloured lines indicates a positive test. These tests are useful as the results are rapidly available and they remain positive even after antibiotics, although antibiotic sensitivity testing is not possible. Their use is recommended in patients with severe pneumonia.

Serology
Atypical bacteria and viruses that cause pneumonia do not grow in laboratory culture. Infection is detected by testing for antibodies in blood from affected patients. Antibody titres are compared in acute and convalescent samples taken 7–10 days apart, with an increase in titres indicating infection. Results are usually available too late to influence treatment, but serology is useful for epidemiological surveillance and in patients in whom a diagnosis remains elusive.

Blood cultures are taken from Mr Sivakumaran. He is unable to produce any sputum so urine is sent for pneumococcal antigen testing. He is started on 35% oxygen by mask and his oxygen saturations rise to 94% (>92% is considered satisfactory). His raised urea indicates that he may be hypovolaemic and he is given 1 L intravenous normal saline over 6 h. Paracetamol 1 g is given for symptomatic relief of pain and pyrexia. He is started on antibiotic therapy.

How do you decide which antibiotic to give him?
The principles of antibiotic therapy are outlined in Part 1B. You should make a best guess as to the likely causative organism(s) and choose antibiotics effective against those organisms (Figs 22 & 23, p. 39 and 40). Other factors including local antibiotic resistance and patient allergies should be taken into account when making the final decision.

Box 89 Pharmacology of penicillins

Mechanism of action
Bacteria make cell walls by cross-linking peptidoglycans using a transpeptidase enzyme. Penicillins comprise a β-lactam ring which binds this transpeptidase, inhibiting cell wall production and killing the bacteria.

Uses in respiratory disease
Penicillins can be classified into four groups:
1 *Standard penicillin* (e.g. benzyl penicillin, phenoxymethyl penicillin) is used to treat streptococcal infection such as pneumonia and sore throat
2 *Antistaphylococcal penicillin* (e.g. flucloxacillin) is used to treat staphylococcal pneumonia (e.g. following influenza or acquired in hospital – unless methicillin or flucloxacillin-resistant)
3 *Aminopenicillins* (e.g. ampicillin, amoxicillin) are broad spectrum with activity against Gram-negative as well as Gram-positive organisms. Used to treat community-acquired respiratory tract infections (e.g. infective exacerbation of COPD, community-acquired pneumonia)
4 *Antipseudomonal penicillins* (e.g. piperacillin, azlocillin) are like aminopenicillins, but their spectrum of action is even broader. They are used to treat pseudomonal infection (e.g. in patients with cystic fibrosis or with hospital-acquired pneumonia)

Pharmacokinetics
- They are very water soluble; hence many of them have to be given intravenously as they are poorly absorbed
- They are rapidly excreted by the kidney, hence usually have to be given at least 3–4 times daily

Main side-effects
- Hypersensitivity
- Gastrointestinal upset
- *Clostridium difficile* diarrhoea (aminopenicillins)
- Rash in patients with Epstein–Barr virus infection (aminopenicillins)

The doctor assumes that Mr Sivakumaran's pneumonia is caused by S. pneumoniae or H. influenzae. Mr Sivakumaran is not allergic to antibiotics and has not previously received any for this infection so he is started on 500 mg amoxicillin t.d.s. (Box 89). The doctor fails to consider 'atypical' organisms as a cause for pneumonia and does not consult hospital guidelines before starting treatment.

Mr Sivakumaran remains very unwell 24 h later. His observations now are:

Temperature 38.1°C

Pulse 110 beats/min

Blood pressure 112/76 mmHg

Respiratory rate 28 breaths/min

Oxygen saturations 89% on air

His investigations today show:

		Normal range
Blood cultures	Negative so far	
Urinary pneumococcal antigen	Negative	
CRP	392 mg/L	(<8 mg/L)
White cells	21.1 × 10^9/L	(4–11 × 10^9/L)

How do you assess the situation?

The persistent temperature, tachycardia and rising white cell count and CRP suggest ongoing infection. Clinically, Mr Sivakumaran is not improving despite antibiotic therapy as he remains tachypnoeic and hypoxic.

How can you explain his failure to improve?

Antibiotic therapy may be failing because:

• The 'best guess' and antibiotic choice are wrong. Tests show no evidence of pneumococcal infection. Mr Sivakumaran could be infected with an organism insensitive to amoxicillin such as *L. pneumophila* or *M. pneumoniae*

• The 'best guess' was right but the organism is resistant to the antibiotic chosen:

  ○ penicillin resistance in *S. pneumoniae* is caused by changes in bacterial penicillin binding proteins which reduce the affinity of these proteins for penicillin

  ○ penicillin resistance in *H. influenzae* is caused by bacterial production of β-lactamase enzymes which break the β-lactam ring and inactivate the antibiotic

• The antibiotic is not 'strong' enough:

  ○ the dose is too low

  ○ he is not absorbing or receiving the treatment

• He may have developed an infected pleural effusion (empyema) secondary to pneumonia

What changes could you make to his treatment to overcome these problems?

• Adding erythromycin (Box 90) to amoxicillin will ensure organisms including *L. pneumophila* and *M. pneumoniae* as well as *S. pneumoniae* and *H. influenzae* are covered

• Increasing the dose of amoxicillin to 1 g t.d.s. will overcome penicillin resistance resulting from low affinity binding proteins in *S. pneumoniae*

• Adding clavulinic acid to amoxicillin (co-amoxiclav) can overcome resistance resulting from β-lactamase production. Clavulinic acid has a structure similar to the β-lactam ring in penicillin. When clavulinic acid and amoxicillin are given together the β-lactamase is used up by cleaving the β-lactam ring of the clavulinic acid, preserving the amoxicillin to kill the bacteria

• A chest X-ray should be performed to exclude pleural fluid

Box 90 Pharmacology of macrolide antibiotics (erythromycin, clarithromycin, azithromycin)

Mechanism of action

Drugs bind to the bacterial ribosome, inhibiting protein synthesis. They stop bacterial growth (bacteriostatic), allowing the host's immune system to clear the infection.

Uses

In respiratory medicine, macrolides are mainly used for treatment of community-acquired pneumonia caused by 'atypical' organisms or in people allergic to penicillin. Erythromycin is usually the first choice as it is 'off patent' and is much cheaper than the other drugs. Azithromycin or clarithromycin have better activity against *H. influenzae* and cause fewer gastrointestinal side-effects.

Pharmacokinetics

• Oral route is preferred. Can be given intravenously but erythromycin causes vein irritation

• Metabolized by and inhibit the cytochrome p450 system in the liver. Potential for drug interactions, particularly with warfarin (increased risk of bleeding) and theophylline (risk of toxicity including arrhythmias and convulsions)

Main side-effects

• Gastrointestinal upset

• Hypersensitivity

• Hepatitis

• Reversible hearing loss

KEY POINT

Community-acquired pneumonia severe enough to require hospital admission is usually treated with a combination of penicillin (e.g. amoxicillin) and macrolide (e.g. erythromycin) to cover *S. pneumoniae* and 'atypical' organisms that are the most common causes of this condition.

Erythromycin 500 mg orally q.d.s. was added to Mr Sivakumaran's treatment and amoxicillin increased to 1 g t.d.s. intravenously. A chest X-ray showed no pleural fluid. Over the next 48 h Mr Sivakumaran's temperature and tachycardia settled and he started to improve. On further testing Mr Sivakumaran's urine was positive for Legionella antigen. By day 6 Mr Sivakumaran was much better with oxygen saturations of 96% on air and was mobile on the ward. He was discharged home to complete 14 days of treatment and to be followed up as an outpatient 6 weeks later.

Why does he need outpatient follow-up?

Follow-up is booked to ensure that he has recovered from his pneumonia. At his appointment he will have a repeat chest X-ray to monitor resolution of his consolidation. Persistent consolidation could indicate an obstructing lesion in the airways (e.g. lung cancer) and may require further investigation. Follow-up will also provide the opportunity for further counselling regarding smoking cessation.

Outcome. At follow-up Mr Sivakumaran is better but not completely back to normal. His chest X-ray is now clear. He has not smoked since discharge and is using nicotine patches to support smoking cessation. He is advised that tiredness can persist for up to 3 months following pneumonia and is discharged.

CASE REVIEW

Mr Sivakumaran is admitted as an emergency with pleuritic chest pain and is found to have left lower lobe pneumonia. His CURB-65 score is 2 and he is judged to be at increased risk of death from his pneumonia. He is erroneously initially treated with 500 mg amoxicillin t.d.s. but becomes increasingly unwell over the next 24 h. Erythro-

mycin is added to his treatment to cover 'atypical' pathogens. A diagnosis of *Legionella* pneumonia is subsequently made by urinary antigen testing. With this treatment he makes a good recovery and his chest X-ray abnormality has resolved when he is reviewed 6 weeks later in the outpatient clinic.

KEY POINTS

- Community-acquired pneumonia is caused by bacterial or viral pathogens, most commonly *Streptococcus pneumoniae*
- 'Atypical' pathogens causing pneumonia (*Legionella pneumophila, Mycoplasma pneumoniae* and *Chlamydia* spp.) are 'atypical' because they:
  ○ cause more systemic symptoms than other bacteria
  ○ require serological testing rather than culture to confirm the diagnosis
  ○ do not respond to penicillins and require macrolide or tetracycline treatment
- *Legionella pneumophila* should particularly be considered as a cause in patients with severe pneumonia, although it can cause pneumonia of any severity
- Infections causing pneumonia trigger an inflammatory reaction, causing airspaces within affected alveoli to become replaced with inflammatory exudate
- Patients with pneumonia have symptoms of cough, haemoptysis, pleuritic chest pain, fever and shortness of breath

- Clinical signs of lobar pneumonia include dullness to percussion, crepitations and bronchial breathing over the affected area of lung
- The diagnosis of pneumonia requires demonstration of consolidation, usually on chest X-ray
- Severity of pneumonia is assessed by CURB-65 score and determines the site of treatment (home, hospital ward or intensive care)
- Community-acquired pneumonia severe enough to require hospital admission should be treated with a combination of penicillin and macrolide antibiotics to cover usual and 'atypical' pathogens
- Patients should return for an outpatient chest X-ray 6 weeks after discharge to ensure resolution of consolidation
- If pneumonia has not resolved at review, an underlying cause such as obstruction of an airway by lung cancer should be considered

Case 18 A 72-year-old man who becomes breathless during inpatient stay on a medical ward

Mr Virgil Simpson is a 72-year-old man from Jamaica, who was admitted 1 week ago with a dense right hemiplegia and expressive aphasia. A computed tomography (CT) brain scan demonstrated an infarction (stroke) caused by left middle cerebral artery thrombosis. He has been sleepy and unable to get out of bed since admission. Today the ward staff notice that he is breathless and call for a medical review.

His observations are:
Respiratory rate 28 breaths/min
Oxygen saturations 91% on air
Pulse 105 beats/min
Blood pressure 158/104 mmHg

Give a differential diagnosis for his breathlessness?

The most likely diagnoses are:
- Pneumonia
- Pulmonary embolus
- Cardiac disease

Why are these the most likely causes of his breathlessness?

Pneumonia

His stroke may have impaired his lung defences against infection by several mechanisms (Fig. 9, p. 10):
- He is sleepy and may not be protecting his airway with an adequate cough reflex
- His stroke may have impaired his swallowing, which, in combination with an inadequate cough reflex, could have resulted in aspiration of oral or refluxed gastric contents into his lungs
- He is unable to care for himself and maintain oral hygiene. Bacterial overgrowth in the mouth increases the likelihood that aspiration of oral secretions will result in lung infection
- He is immobile, which may be reducing his lung ventilation and clearance of lung secretions. Poorly cleared 'stagnant' secretions can block the airways causing mini lung collapses (atelectasis) and can become infected

- Patients with acute illness also have reduced activity of innate and acquired immune defences against infection

Pulmonary embolus

- He is immobile with reduced blood flow in his leg veins and this stasis could have caused deep vein thrombosis (DVT) and pulmonary embolus. Medical patients who are immobile should all receive prophylactic heparin and/or anti-embolus stockings to prevent this complication.

Cardiac disease

Cardiac disease may cause breathlessness because of pulmonary oedema, arrhythmias, ischaemia and infarction. In hospital patients, overenthusiastic intravenous fluid replacement should also be considered as a cause of pulmonary oedema.

What clinical signs would you look for to distinguish between your diagnoses?

As Mr Simpson has expressive aphasia and is unable to answer questions, the diagnosis depends on examination findings and investigation. Possible findings are as follows.

Pneumonia

- Pyrexia
- Purulent respiratory secretions
- Lung crepitations over the affected area
- Bronchial breathing
- Impaired gag reflex or unsafe swallow (Fig. 70)

Pulmonary embolus

Pulmonary emboli can be difficult to detect so you should have a 'high index of suspicion' whenever the diagnosis is even slightly possible. Look for:

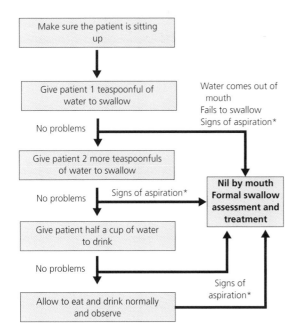

Figure 70 A simple clinical assessment of swallow. * Signs of aspiration include coughing, choking, breathlessness or a 'wet voice' after swallowing. This simple clinical assessment should be performed immediately in any patient where swallowing difficulties are suspected and can be carried out by any health professional with brief training. If in doubt hospitalized patients should be kept nil by mouth and given intravenous fluids until specialist assessment by a speech and language therapist can be arranged.

• Tachycardia, low blood pressure, right ventricular heave and raised jugular venous pressure (JVP) (large central embolus)
• Pleural rub (small peripheral embolus)
• Calf tenderness and swelling (DVT) – this may be clinically apparent as a source of emboli in some patients but absence of a DVT does not rule out pulmonary embolus

Cardiac disease

Check pulse rate and rhythm for arrhythmias and look for signs of left heart failure:
• Fine bibasal crepitations
and associated right heart failure:
• Raised JVP
• Hepatomegaly
• Peripheral oedema – do not forget to check for sacral oedema as this is the first affected site in bed-bound patients

Mr Simpson is difficult to examine as he is a large gentleman and requires two staff to sit him forward. His breathing sounds rattly and he has:
Temperature 38.6°C
Pulse 96 beats/min regular
JVP not elevated, looks dehydrated
Heart sounds normal
No oedema, calf swelling or tenderness
Breath sounds vesicular with widespread coarse crepitations, worse on the right
His swallow is felt to be unsafe when tested. A provisional diagnosis of aspiration pneumonia is made.

What would be your immediate management?

• Sit him up to optimize ventilation
• Oxygen to increase saturations >92%
• Nil by mouth to prevent further aspiration
• IV access and IV fluids to replace fluid losses and maintain hydration while he is nil by mouth
• Suction to help him clear respiratory secretions by nurses or physiotherapist

What investigations would you carry out?

• Culture of sputum obtained by suction
• Blood cultures
• Blood tests as below.

Plasma biochemistry:

		Normal range
Na	143 mmol/L	(135–145 mmol/L)
K	3.9 mmol/L	(3.5–5.0 mmol/L)
Urea	18 mmol/L	(2.5–8 mmol/L)
Creatinine	112 μmol/L	(60–110 μmol/L)
CRP	196 mg/L	(<8 mg/L)
Full blood count:		
Haemoglobin	15.2 g/dL	(13–18 g/dL)
White cells	21.4×10^9/L	$(4–11 \times 10^9$/L)
Neutrophils	18.2×10^9/L	$(2.0–7.5 \times 10^9$/L)
Platelets	274×10^9/L	$(150–400 \times 10^9$/L)
Arterial blood gases on air:		
pH	7.34	(7.35–7.45)
PaO_2	7.4 kPa	(10–13.1 kPa)
$PaCO_2$	6.9 kPa	(4.9–6.1 kPa)
HCO_3^-	26 mmol/L	(22–28 mmol/L)
Chest X-ray:		
See Fig. 71		
ECG:		
Sinus tachycardia		

PART 2: CASES

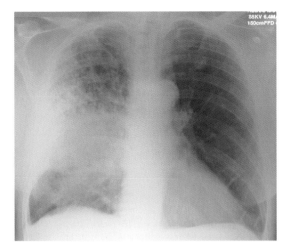

Figure 71 Chest X-ray.

How do you interpret these investigations?

• His raised white cell count (mostly neutrophils) and elevated C-reactive protein (CRP) support the clinical diagnosis of infection

• The raised urea and relatively normal creatinine could be accounted for by dehydration, although he may have some underlying renal impairment

• His blood gases show hypoxia on air. As the PaO_2 is <8 kPa this meets the definition for respiratory failure. His $PaCO_2$ is slightly elevated, indicating hypoventilation, which would fit with his immobility and stroke. This has caused a slight respiratory acidosis

• He has right midzone airspace shadowing consistent with consolidation and pneumonia

• His electrocardiogram (ECG) shows no evidence of a cardiac cause for his breathlessness

Is it significant that the pneumonia is in his right lung?

The right main bronchus is more vertical than the left main bronchus and so aspiration is more often into the right than the left lung.

Which organisms are most likely to be causing his aspiration pneumonia?

This is most commonly caused by:

• Anaerobes from the mouth (e.g. *Bacteroides*, *Fusobacterium* and *Peptococcus* spp.)

• Gram-negative bacteria (e.g. *Klebsiella* and *Pseudomonas* spp.)

However, Mr Simpson has been in hospital for 1 week and so his pneumonia could also have been caused by organisms that are commonly picked up in hospital, including:

• *Pseudomonas aeruginosa*

• *Staphylococcus aureus* (including methicillin-resistant strains)

Hospital-acquired pneumonia is also called 'nosocomial pneumonia'.

How does hospital-acquired pneumonia differ from community-acquired pneumonia?

In the community the most common pneumonia pathogens are *Streptococcus pneumoniae*, *Haemophilus influenzae* and 'atypical' pathogens (see Case 17). These are very different from the organisms causing hospital-acquired pneumonia (see above). This has important implications when choosing antibiotic treatment. Some reasons for these differences are given in Table 8.

What antibiotic treatment would you recommend for Mr Simpson?

A rational choice of antibiotic should be based on the most likely causative organism. In Mr Simpson's case the antibiotic regime must cover Gram-negative organisms including pseudomonas and anaerobes (see Figs 22 & 23, pp. 39 and 40). A possible choice would be a third generation cephalosporin such as cefotaxime (Box 91) with metronidazole to cover anaerobes (Box 92).

How should the antibiotics be given?

Seriously ill patients should be given antibiotics intravenously to ensure therapeutic plasma concentrations. Other considerations are:

• Mr Simpson is nil by mouth because of his swallowing problems, hence he cannot take oral medication

• Third generation cephalosporins can only be given parenterally as oral preparations are not absorbed

Mr Simpson was started on 1 g cefotaxime IV and 500 mg metronidazole IV t.d.s. He was made nil by mouth to prevent further aspiration and received intravenous rehydration. His oxygen saturations improved to 95% on 35% humidified oxygen and he had regular physiotherapy with suction to clear respiratory secretions. A nasogastric tube was inserted for enteral feeding and hydration.

Why was the oxygen humidified?

Oxygen is humidified by bubbling through sterile water. This appears to maintain hydration and ease clearance

Table 8 Some reasons for differences in pathogens causing hospital- and community-acquired pneumonias.

	Community-acquired pneumonia	Hospital-acquired pneumonia
Patient factors		
Pre-morbid state	Usually well before infection	Immunocompromised by acute illness or comorbidity
Exposure	Mostly in contact with well people	Close to other people with infection and illness
		Looked after by staff who may be colonized with pathogens and have poor hand hygiene
Organism factors		
Antibiotic resistance	Organisms live in community where antibiotic use is relatively low and resistance is uncommon	Organisms live in hospitals where antibiotic use is high and resistance is common
Persistence in environment	Pathogens fragile, need human host and are poorly persistent in environment	Pathogens persistent in hospital environment (e.g. *Staphylococcus aureus*, nasal and skin colonization, *Pseudomonas aeruginosa* in water). These organisms form biofilms (i.e. bacterial communities) which can survive when times are hard

---

Box 91 Pharmacology of cephalosporins

Mechanism of action

Cephalosporins come from a fungus called *Cephalosporium*. They are similar to penicillins as they have a β-lactam ring, impair bacterial cell wall synthesis and are bacteriocidal.

Uses

Cephalosporins are grouped together in generations according to their spectrum of action. In respiratory medicine they have the following main uses:
- *First generation* (e.g. cefaclor [oral]) – treatment of uncomplicated respiratory tract infections in the community
- *Second generation* (e.g. cefuroxime [oral or IV]) – treatment of community-acquired pneumonia

- *Third generation* (e.g. cefotaxime [IV]) for severe community-acquired and hospital-acquired pneumonias. Ceftazidime (IV) is particularly useful against *Pseudomonas*

Pharmacokinetics

Cephalosporins are renally excreted and dose reduction may be required in renal impairment.

Main side-effects
- Hypersensitivity. Note that 10% of patients who are allergic to penicillin will also be allergic to cephalosporins (and vice versa) because the two groups of antibiotics have structural similarities
- Diarrhoea and antibiotic-associated colitis

---

of respiratory secretions. Patients on oxygen therapy may also find oxygen treatment more comfortable if humidified as it causes less drying of the mucous membranes.

Mr Simpson initially appeared to improve. However, after 72 h he was unwell, pyrexial and had had two episodes of diarrhoea. His blood results were:

		Normal range
Na	143 mmol/L	(135–145 mmol/L)
K	3.2 mmol/L	(3.5–5.0 mmol/L)
Urea	9 mmol/L	(2.5–8 mmol/L)
Creatinine	118 μmol/L	(60–110 μmol/L)
CRP	255 mg/L	(<8 mg/L)
White cells	25.6 × 10⁹/L	(4–11 × 10⁹/L)
Neutrophils	22.0 × 10⁹/L	(2.0–7.5 × 10⁹/L)

> **Box 92 Pharmacology of metronidazole**
>
> **Mechanism of action**
> This drug is taken up by anaerobic organisms and activated by reduction of a nitro group. It binds to DNA, prevents nucleic acid formation and stops bacterial growth.
>
> **Uses**
> In respiratory medicine metronidazole is mainly used for the treatment of aspiration pneumonia or lung abscesses.
>
> **Pharmacokinetics**
> - Can be given orally, rectally or intravenously
> - Inhibits alcohol and aldehyde dehydrogenase in the liver. Patients should avoid taking alcohol with metronidazole as acetaldehyde will accumulate in the body, causing flushing, headache, tachycardia, nausea, vomiting and collapse. Patients do not need to avoid alcohol with other classes of antibiotics
>
> **Main side-effects**
> - Hypersensitivity
> - Gastrointestinal upset
> - Rarely, peripheral neuropathy and seizures

What do these blood results show?

Most notably his CRP and white cell count have risen rather than fallen in response to antibiotics. His serum potassium has also fallen, probably because of the diarrhoea.

How can you explain his failure to improve?

His pneumonia may not be resolving because:
- Best guess antibiotic therapy was wrong and the organism is untreated
- Underlying cause (e.g. aspiration, immunosuppression) persists

His symptoms may now be caused by his diarrhoea, which could be a result of:
- Colonic infection with toxin-producing *C. difficile* secondary to antibiotic treatment
- Initiation of hyperosmolar enteral feeding

How will you investigate him to distinguish between these possibilities?

- Send stool sample to microbiology to look for *C. difficile* toxin

- Repeat chest X-ray to look for worsening consolidation

> *Mr Simpson's oxygen saturations were 95% on 24% oxygen. His repeat chest X-ray showed some improvement in consolidation. His original sputum and blood cultures were negative. His stool sample was positive for C. difficile toxin.*

How do you interpret this new information?

His improving oxygenation and chest X-ray suggest that his pneumonia is responding to antibiotics. His cultures did not identify bacteria resistant to the antibiotics used. His stool sample indicates that his deterioration is caused by *C. difficile* diarrhoea.

How does *Clostridium difficile* diarrhoea occur?

Patients may become infected with a toxin-producing strain of *C. difficile* while in hospital. *Clostridium difficile* persists in the hospital environment in spore form and infection is spread by the faeco-oral route, facilitated by poor hand hygiene by staff, patients and visitors. *Clostridium difficile* is most likely to cause diarrhoea if an infected patient also receives a broad-spectrum antibiotic (cefotaxime in Mr Simpson's case) which kills normal bowel flora. This allows overgrowth of *C. difficile* and secretion of toxins A and B, which cause colonic mucosal injury and inflammation. Patients often have profuse debilitating diarrhoea that can impair recovery and increase mortality.

How should his diarrhoea be treated?

The antibiotic charts (Figs 22 & 23, pp. 39 and 40) indicate that metronidazole and vancomycin are effective against *C. difficile*. He is already on metronidazole so vancomycin would be the most sensible choice here. Vancomycin should be given down Mr Simpson's nasogastric tube to make sure it is in the gut, which is the site of infection. Treatment is for 10–14 days, although patients may still relapse after this time.

Why did he get *C. difficile* infection if he was already taking metronidazole?

- The strain of *C. difficile* he acquired may have been metronidazole-resistant
- Metronidazole given IV may not have reached sufficient concentrations in the gut lumen to prevent *C. difficile* overgrowth

Could anything have been done to prevent this *C. difficile* infection?

• Good hygiene and infection control to prevent the spread of hospital-acquired pathogens
• Limiting use of broad-spectrum antibiotics to prevent *C. difficile* overgrowth in the bowel
  ○ consider amoxicillin/macrolides/tetracyclines instead of broad-spectrum cephalosporins
  ○ use shortest course of treatment possible

KEY POINT

It is essential that *everyone* (staff, students, visitors and patients) on a hospital ward maintains excellent hand hygiene to prevent the spread of infection. Thorough handwashing is the most effective method of decontamination, although alcohol gels are also widely used. One approach is:
• Always wash hands *after* touching a patient
• Always apply alcohol gel *before* touching a patient

Outcome. Mr Simpson's treatment was changed to 625 mg co-amoxiclav t.d.s. and 125 mg vancomycin q.d.s. via nasogastric tube. Infection control measures were instituted to prevent spread of infection from Mr Simpson to other patients, including obligatory wearing of gloves and aprons by staff when caring for him. He received chest physiotherapy to help him clear chest secretions. Over the next week his diarrhoea settled and his pneumonia improved. His swallow was reviewed by the speech and language therapist and he was allowed to take a small amount of thickened fluids by mouth. Once he was free of infection and off antibiotics he was transferred to a rehabilitation ward.

CASE REVIEW

Mr Simpson became short of breath 1 week after suffering a stroke resulting from aspiration pneumonia, secondary to an unsafe swallow. His oral intake was stopped and he received intravenous antibiotics, fluid and chest physiotherapy. After initial improvement he deteriorated because of *C. difficile*-related diarrhoea. This was treated with oral vancomycin. As his pneumonia and diarrhoea resolved, oral intake was restarted under supervision of the speech and language therapist and he was transferred to a rehabilitation ward for further treatment of his stroke.

KEY POINTS

• Hospitalized patients often have compromised pulmonary defence, caused by
  ○ impaired cough reflex or swallow
  ○ reduced mucociliary clearance because of hypoventilation
  ○ impaired innate or acquired immunity
• Pneumonia secondary to aspiration is most commonly caused by
  ○ anaerobes from the mouth
  ○ Gram-negative bacteria
• Aspiration pneumonia should therefore be treated with antibiotics that cover:
  ○ anaerobes – metronidazole
  ○ Gram-negative organisms – amoxicillin, cephalosporin, macrolide

• Hospital-acquired (nosocomial) pneumonia may be caused by bacteria that persist in the hospital environment, particularly:
  ○ *Pseudomonas aeruginosa*
  ○ *Staphylococcus aureus* (including methicillin-resistant strains)
• *Clostridium difficile* diarrhoea is caused by:
  ○ bowel colonization with a toxin-producing strain of *C. difficile*
  ○ broad-spectrum antibiotics (particularly cephalosporins) which kill normal gut flora and allow *C. difficile* overgrowth
• The risk of *C. difficile* diarrhoea in hospital patients should be reduced by:
  ○ excellent hygiene to reduce transmission
  ○ minimizing use of cephalosporins and broad-spectrum antibiotics

Case 19 A 58-year-old woman with breathlessness following surgery

Mrs Elinor Aaronson is a 58-year-old woman who underwent an open cholecystectomy 48h ago and has now become short of breath.

What is the first thing you should do on arriving at her bedside?

You should perform an 'ABC' assessment. Does she have a patent airway, is she breathing and is her circulation intact?

Mrs Aaronson is fully responsive and has the following observations:
Pulse 110 beats/min
Blood pressure 115/65 mmHg
Respiratory rate 24 breaths/min
Oxygen saturations 93% on air

How do you interpret her observations?

She has an increased respiratory rate with mild hypoxia. She has a tachycardia but normal blood pressure and is not haemodynamically compromised. Her observations indicate that she is unwell but there is time to make a full assessment of her condition before commencing treatment.

What causes of breathlessness should you consider in her case?

The most notable feature of her case is that she has recently had upper abdominal surgery. It is therefore important to consider whether she might have developed a postoperative complication accounting for her breathlessness (Box 93).

What will you do next to narrow down the differential diagnosis?

You should take a focused history including symptoms, risk factors and past medical history to determine whether her breathlessness is respiratory or cardiac in origin, then explore possible diagnoses in more detail (Fig. 11, p. 18).

Mrs Aaronson has had difficulty breathing for the last 24h. Her shortness of breath occurs in all positions, is not worse on lying flat, but is associated with a troublesome cough. She is experiencing pain from her abdominal wound, particularly on taking a deep breath or coughing. She is not producing sputum and has not coughed up any blood. She has no chest pain, palpitations or ankle swelling.

In the past she has had chest infections requiring antibiotics from her GP about twice per year for the last 5 years and has a chronic productive cough in the winter. She has never been admitted to hospital and does not normally take any medication. She started smoking when she was 15 years of age and smoked 10 cigarettes per day until she gave up 3 years ago. She does not to her knowledge have high blood pressure or cholesterol and is not diabetic. In her family her father had emphysema and her son has asthma.

Is her shortness of breath more likely to be caused by cardiac or respiratory disease?

Her history points to a respiratory rather than a cardiac cause of her postoperative breathlessness because:
• Associated symptoms are respiratory (cough) and there are no other cardiac symptoms (no chest pain, palpitations or oedema)
• Lying flat does not exacerbate her breathlessness (this is most often a feature of pulmonary oedema)
• She is a smoker, which can cause both heart and lung disease, however:
  ○ she has no family history of cardiac disease and has no other cardiac risk factors
  ○ her past medical history indicates previous recurrent respiratory illness

Which respiratory causes should be considered?

Mrs Aaronson complains of abdominal pain that is preventing her from coughing and taking a deep breath. This predisposes her to (Box 94):

Box 93 Postoperative complications causing breathlessness

Respiratory complications
- Atelectasis
- Infection, including bronchitis and pneumonia
- Bronchospasm
- Ventilatory failure
- Exacerbation of underlying chronic lung disease

Cardiac/vascular complications
- Ischaemia/infarction
- Arrhythmia
- Pulmonary oedema (heart failure/fluid overload)
- Pulmonary embolus

Other
- Postoperative anaemia
- Fluid overload

Box 94 Mechanisms underlying development of respiratory postoperative complications

Factors affecting the respiratory system postoperatively include:
- Pain from the surgical wound inhibiting deep breathing and coughing
- Muscle dysfunction preventing effective ventilation caused by:
  - surgical damage
  - prolonged neuromuscular blockade
- Drugs that reduce the respiratory drive:
  - opiates
  - anaesthetic drugs

These factors reduce tidal volume and deep sighing breaths, limiting lung expansion. The cough is less effective and there is reduced mucociliary clearance. This causes:
- *Atelectasis* – obstruction of small airways with distal collapse (Figs 72 & 73) causing hypoxia.
- *Infection* – stagnation of respiratory secretions which become infected
- *Ventilatory failure* – weakness of respiratory muscles leading to inadequate ventilation

- Atelectasis
- Infection

She appears to have underlying lung disease, so could also have:
- Exacerbation of underlying chronic lung disease

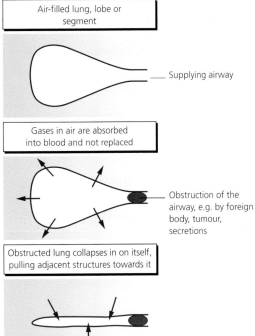

Air-filled lung, lobe or segment

Supplying airway

Gases in air are absorbed into blood and not replaced

Obstruction of the airway, e.g. by foreign body, tumour, secretions

Obstructed lung collapses in on itself, pulling adjacent structures towards it

Figure 72 Pathophysiology of pulmonary collapse and atelectasis.

At this stage, further information from examination and investigations is still required to exclude other diagnoses.

What underlying lung disease may she have?

Her chronic productive cough and regular need for antibiotics could be consistent with chronic bronchitis. Mrs Aaronson has smoked around 10 cigarettes per day for 40 years (i.e. ~20 pack years). It is likely that she has underlying chronic obstructive pulmonary disease (COPD).

On examination she has:
Temperature 37.9°C
Dry mouth and decreased skin turgor
Pale conjunctivae
  Respiratory system:
Decreased air entry throughout both lung fields
Inspiratory and expiratory crackles at both lung bases with
  some expiratory wheeze
  Abdominal examination:
Soft abdomen, but tender around the wound site which
  looks clean

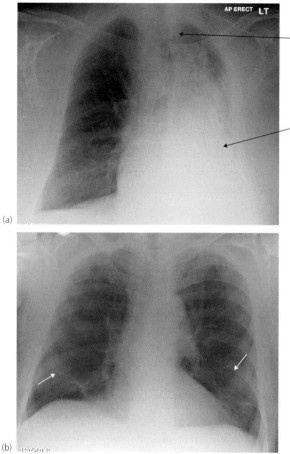

(a)

(b)

Figure 73 Chest X-rays illustrating lobar collapse and subsegmental collapse (atelectasis). (a) Lobar collapse. (b) Basal atelectasis. Arrows indicate linear shadows of pulmonary atelectasis – collapse of very small segments of lung.

Trachea and mediastinum pulled towards affected side

Collapsed lower lobe – opaque as does not contain air

Audible bowel sounds

Urinary catheter in situ and the bag contains 150 mL concentrated urine which she has passed over the last 4 h. Urinalysis shows blood +, nil else.

She is wearing anti-embolism stockings.

How do you interpret these examination findings?

Mrs Aaronson has mild pyrexia. This could indicate infection in her:

• *Chest.* She has poor air entry consistent with reduced lung expansion postoperatively. Crepitations could be caused by retained secretions which could have become infected (Box 94)

• *Abdomen.* This is soft and bowel sounds are heard. There is no evidence of postoperative peritonitis or wound infection

• *Biliary tree.* This could have become infected from surgery. There is no clinical evidence of biliary obstruction as she is not jaundiced

• *Urine.* Urinalysis shows no evidence of leucocytes or nitrates which are present in urine infection

Her dry mucus membranes, reduced skin turgor and concentrated urine indicate hypovolaemia. Bilateral inspiratory and expiratory crepitations on chest examination are most likely to indicate retained secretions and infection as there is no evidence of heart failure or fluid overload. Expiratory wheeze is consistent with bronchospasm.

What is the purpose of anti-embolism stockings?

Deep vein thrombosis and pulmonary emboli may occur postoperatively as a result of immobility, vascular trauma and hypercoagulability. Anti-embolism stockings and prophylactic low molecular weight heparin are used to prevent these complications. Thromboembolic complications usually occur at least 5 days postoperatively and are unlikely to be causing Mrs Aaronson's breathlessness 48 h after surgery, although early emboli have been described.

What is your differential diagnosis now?
• Atelectasis
• Pulmonary infection
• Underlying COPD

What investigations would you request and why?
• *Chest X-ray* – to visualize atelectasis or pneumonia
• *Full blood count and C-reactive protein (CRP)* – to look for infection and postoperative anaemia
• *Arterial blood gases* – to look for CO_2 retention resulting from underlying COPD or postoperative ventilatory failure
• *ECG* – to exclude cardiac ischaemia or arrhythmias
• *Troponin T or I* – to look for myocardial damage
• *Peak flow recording or spirometry* – to look for airflow obstruction
• *U and Es* – to look for renal impairment and electrolyte imbalance

Her investigation results were as follows:
Chest X-ray – poorly expanded lungs with atelectasis at both lung bases
ECG – sinus tachycardia, nil else
Troponin T – normal
Peak flow – not performed because of abdominal pain
Blood tests (Table 9)

Arterial blood gases on 4 L oxygen:

		Normal range
pH	7.49	(7.35–7.45)
PaO_2	10.4 kPa	(10–13.1 kPa)
$PaCO_2$	4.4 kPa	(4.9–6.1 kPa)
HCO_3^-	22 mmol/L	(22–28 mmol/L)

How do you interpret these results?
• Chest X-ray – bi-basal atelectasis has occurred postoperatively, impairing gas exchange and predisposing her to infection
• Normal cardiac investigations support the clinical suspicion that her breathlessness is respiratory in origin
• Airflow obstruction could not be assessed because of pain
• Her rising neutrophil count and CRP are consistent with developing infection
• Her haemoglobin has fallen postoperatively and she is anaemic
• Her rising plasma urea and sodium concentrations confirm dehydration
• Mrs Aaronson's $PaCO_2$ is low, indicating hyperventilation in response to hypoxia rather than ventilatory failure or CO_2 retention. She is maintaining normal PaO_2 with supplemental oxygen
• None of these investigations rule out a pulmonary embolus. However, her rising inflammatory markers and early presentation make infection more likely. She should remain on prophylactic heparin and the diagnosis should be reviewed regularly

How do her test results modify your differential diagnosis?
• The likely cause of her breathlessness is atelectasis, probably with some superadded pulmonary infection

Table 9 Mrs Aaronson's blood test results.

	Hb (g/dL)	WCC (× 10⁹/L)	Neutrophils (× 10⁹/L)	Platelets (× 10⁹/L)	Na (mmol/L)	K (mmol/L)	Urea (mmol/L)	Creatinine (μmol/L)	CRP (mg/L)
Normal	12–16	4–11	2–7.5	150–400	135–145	3.5–5	2.5–8	60–110	<8
Preop	13.2	6.2	4.3	230	141	4.1	4	76	2
Postop day 1	9.8	11.5	7.0	410	143	3.6	7	90	26
Postop day 2	10.1	13.0	9.2	460	146	3.6	10	94	55

Hb, haemoglobin; CRP, C-reactive protein; WCC, white cell count.

• Postoperative anaemia and previously undiagnosed COPD may also be contributing to her symptoms

How would you manage her breathlessness?

Mrs Aaronson needs treatment of her lung atelectasis and infection, control of abdominal pain to facilitate breathing and coughing, optimization of probable COPD and improvement in fluid balance.

Atelectasis

Atelectasis can be improved by increasing lung expansion and clearance of secretions with:
• Physiotherapy to increase deep breathing and coughing
• Nebulized saline or mucolytics to make secretions easier to clear
• Continuous positive airway pressure (CPAP). This can reduce postoperative lung atelectasis by maintaining lung expansion, but should only be used if other treatment fails as it has complications including discomfort, gastric distension and pressure-related lung trauma

Infection

Mrs Aaronson's pulmonary infection has developed around 72 h after hospital admission. Hospital-acquired pneumonia occurs most commonly in the first 5 postoperative days and is most likely to be caused by multiple organisms including:
• Gram-negative bacteria, particularly:
  ○ *Pseudomonas aeruginosa*
  ○ *Haemophilus influenzae*
• *Staphylococcus aureus*
• *Streptococcus pneumoniae*

Organisms acquired in hospital may be multidrug-resistant. Hospital-acquired pneumonia is therefore usually treated with broad-spectrum antibiotics that are effective against drug-resistant bacteria (Box 95).

Control of abdominal pain

Postoperative pain can be controlled with opiate analgesia; however, opiates can cause respiratory depression and worsen respiratory complications. An alternative is epidural anaesthesia, which reduces postoperative pulmonary complications significantly compared to opiate analgesia. Physical measures including supporting the abdominal wound during coughing may also be effective.

Box 95 Example antibiotic treatment regime for hospital-acquired pneumonia

Early onset infection (came on <5 days from admission)
• Start with cefuroxime IV or co-amoxiclav IV
• Switch to oral co-amoxiclav if the patient is responding after 48 h
• Give antibiotics for a total of 7 days

Late onset infection (came on ≥5 days from admission)
• ceftazidime IV ± gentamicin IV
• The patient should be reassessed for consideration of ongoing treatment after 7 days
Once sputum culture results are available the treatment regime may need to be modified depending on the findings:

Pseudomonas aeruginosa	treat as for late onset infection
Methicillin-resistant *S. aureus*	add IV vancomycin
Legionella pneumophila	add erythromycin
Evidence of aspiration	add metronidazole

Optimization of COPD

She should be given bronchodilators (e.g. nebulized salbutamol and ipratropium). If her COPD fails to improve or deteriorates, oral prednisolone could be added to treatment, but this should be done cautiously as corticosteroids impair wound healing.

Improve fluid balance

Systemic dehydration can make respiratory secretions more difficult to clear and cause other important effects such as renal impairment. Reasons for her dehydration may include:
• Increased insensible loss because of pyrexia and tachypnoea
• Inability to regulate her own fluid intake as she is nil by mouth following abdominal surgery

Her fluid requirements should be calculated by adding:
• Usual daily requirement (2–3 L)
• Estimated fluid deficit (estimated by looking for negative fluid balance (output > input) on fluid balance charts or from clinical evidence of low venous pressure, urine output and blood pressure)

Box 96 Risk factors for postoperative pulmonary complications

Patient factors
- Age >50 years
- Poor general health or functional dependence
- Underlying lung or heart disease
- Recent cigarette use
- Current upper respiratory tract infection
- Morbid obesity

Surgical factors
- Surgery to brain, face, thorax or upper abdomen
- Emergency surgery
- General anaesthesia
- Prolonged operation/anaesthesia
- Use of long-acting neuromuscular blocker during anaesthesia

Box 97 Prevention of postoperative pulmonary complications

Preoperative strategies
- Stop smoking at least 8 weeks before surgery
- Optimize treatment of underlying lung (or cardiac) disease
- Delay elective surgery in patients with upper respiratory tract infection

Intraoperative strategies
- Minimize operating time
- Use alternative approaches (e.g. keyhole surgery where possible)
- Anaesthesia
  - consider epidural rather than general anaesthesia
  - avoid long-acting neuromuscular blockade

Postoperative strategies
- Chest physiotherapy
- Adequate analgesia
- Early mobilization

Other strategies
- Anti-embolism stockings and prophylactic dose low molecular weight heparin to prevent deep vein thrombosis and pulmonary embolus

- Estimated daily insensible loss (usually 500 mL, may be 1 L in Mrs Aaronson's case)

The resulting volume should be given over the next 24 h as 0.9% saline or 5% dextrose.

Mrs Aaronson is treated with intravenous 0.9% saline and potassium supplementation, nebulized salbutamol and ipratropium. Her opiate analgesia is increased and she is started on intravenous co-amoxiclav. She receives chest physiotherapy.

After 48 h Mrs Aaronson is much less breathless. She is now able to walk around the ward and go to the bathroom unaided. She is apyrexial and oxygen saturations are 96% on air. Her treatment is changed to oral antibiotics and inhaled, rather than nebulized bronchodilators.

Could Mrs Aaronson's postoperative pulmonary complications have been predicted?

Risk factors for postoperative pulmonary complications are shown in Box 96. Mrs Aaronson is over 50 and probably has underlying lung disease, although this has not been formally diagnosed. People undergoing upper abdominal or thoracic surgery are considered to be at high risk of lung complications if they have one additional risk factor (Box 96). Mrs Aaronson is in that category.

Could Mrs Aaronson's postoperative respiratory complications have been prevented?

High risk patients should be identified in the preoperative clerking clinic and preventative measures implemented at this time. As Mrs Aaronson had a chronic cough and prolonged smoking history, the possibility of underlying COPD should have been recognized. She should have had diagnostic spirometry and optimization of lung function with bronchodilators before surgery. Additionally, she could have had better preoperative advice about the importance of clearing lung secretions postoperatively and more postoperative analgesia. Other measures are shown in Box 97.

Outcome. Mrs Aaronson continues to make an uneventful recovery. At outpatient review 8 weeks later in the chest clinic, spirometry confirms mild COPD. As she has already stopped smoking and feels well on short-acting bronchodilators she does not require further intervention.

CASE REVIEW

Mrs Aaronson becomes short of breath and mildly hypoxic following upper abdominal surgery. She has been unable to cough or take a deep breath because of pain from her abdominal wound. Full assessment identifies pulmonary atelectasis, infection and suggests underlying COPD. She is treated with physiotherapy, rehydration, nebulized bronchodilators and antibiotics. She makes an uneventful recovery and is found to have mild COPD at follow-up.

KEY POINTS

- Shortness of breath is a common postoperative complication
- Initial assessment of breathlessness in a postoperative patient should attempt to distinguish between respiratory, cardiac or other causes
- Important respiratory postoperative complications are:
  ○ atelectasis
  ○ infection
  ○ bronchospasm
  ○ ventilatory failure
  ○ exacerbation of underlying lung disease
- Patients at risk of postoperative respiratory complications can be identified at the preoperative clerking clinic
- Useful preoperative measures to prevent respiratory complications include:
  ○ smoking cessation
  ○ optimal treatment of underlying lung disease
- Useful postoperative measures to prevent or treat postoperative respiratory complications include:
  ○ chest physiotherapy
  ○ adequate analgesia
  ○ early mobilization
- Anti-embolism stockings and low dose low molecular weight heparin should be used to prevent postoperative deep vein thrombosis and pulmonary embolus

Case 20 A 16-year-old boy with a sore throat

Matthias Obugu is a 16-year-old boy who presents to his GP with a 3-day history of a sore throat. He tells Dr Brewster that it is very painful and difficult to swallow and he is feeling feverish.

What are the main issues the GP should address during the consultation?

Sore throat is very common and is usually a minor self-limiting illness. GPs will see many patients with this symptom and must sift the few who need investigation, treatment or even hospital referral from the majority who will get better on their own.

What causes a sore throat?

The usual cause is infection, which is most commonly viral or bacterial (Box 98). This leads to inflammation in the pharynx or tonsils which is painful.

What clinical features would reassure Dr Brewster that Matthias has a self-limiting viral illness?

It is very difficult to distinguish between viral and bacterial causes of a sore throat using clinical features. However, other symptoms of a common cold, including runny and blocked nose, sneezing, cough and recent contact with people with colds, would point to a viral upper respiratory tract infection (Box 99).

Matthias denies cough or nasal symptoms. On examination his temperature is 38°C and he has a red inflamed pharynx with large tonsils covered with exudate. He has tender swollen anterior cervical lymph nodes.

How do you interpret this new information?

The clinical findings indicate infection of the pharynx and tonsillitis. It is still not possible to distinguish clinically between a viral and bacterial cause.

What pathophysiological processes underlie changes found in his throat?

Infection of the pharynx causes increased lymph drainage from the affected area to the tonsils and anterior cervical nodes. Antigen-presenting cells carried in the lymph trigger reactive changes, including activation of B and T lymphocytes and increased blood flow, in the tonsils and nodes which become enlarged and painful. The tonsillar exudate comprises inflammatory cells, particularly neutrophils, and debris on the surface of the tonsils.

Dr Brewster is concerned that Matthias may have a bacterial throat infection. She checks his immunization history, performs a throat swab and gives him a prescription for antibiotics.

Why does Dr Brewster check Matthias's immunization history?

Sore throat and upper respiratory tract symptoms can be caused by infections with potentially serious complications, including measles, mumps, diphtheria (Box 100) and rubella. In the UK these infections are rarely seen because most children are immunized against them. However, recent reduction in the uptake of vaccination and increased immigration or travel from countries without vaccination programmes has led to re-emergence of these conditions.

Dr Brewster is reassured to find that Matthias is fully vaccinated and has not travelled abroad.

Why did Dr Brewster perform a throat swab?

Culture of a throat swab can identify bacteria present in the throat. The most common bacterial throat infection is with group A β-haemolytic streptococcus (Box 101). However, the use of throat swabs is *not* recommended

---

Box 98 Causes of a sore throat

Infection
- Viruses, including:
  - rhinovirus
  - coronavirus
  - parainfluenza virus
  - respiratory syncitial virus
  - influenza virus
  - adenovirus
  - Epstein–Barr virus
- Bacteria:
  - group A β-haemolytic streptococcus (*Streptococcus pyogenes*)
  - *Corynebacterium diphtheriae*
  - *Haemophilus influenzae*
  - *Neisseria gonorrhoea*
- Fungi
  - *Candida albicans*

Non-infective
- Allergy
- Dryness
- Pollution and irritants
- Muscle strain
- Acid reflux

Box 99 Important facts about the common cold

Impact
- Most adults get colds 2–3 times per year and symptoms resolve over about 1 week
- This may lead to lost work productivity in the general population
- Colds can have serious health effects by triggering exacerbations in people with chronic respiratory disease (e.g. COPD, asthma)

Spread
- Cold viruses are highly infectious, requiring only 1–30 viral copies to enter the nose to start an infection
- People with colds are most infectious over the first 3 days when they have the highest concentration of virus in their nasal secretions
- Spread is by respiratory droplets. Cold virus contaminates the hands of those who sneeze, use tissues or touch their noses. Virus is spread directly through human contact (e.g. handshaking) or indirectly by contact with furniture or other surfaces. The virus enters a new respiratory tract when the contaminated person touches their hands or face and will infect 95% of people it comes into contact with

Prevention
- This is particularly important for patients with chronic respiratory disease
- There is no vaccine to prevent colds because they are caused by over 100 different viruses
- To avoid contracting a cold:
  - avoid those with colds, especially during the first 3 days of their infection
  - keep a good distance from people coughing and sneezing to avoid direct contact with respiratory droplets
  - wash hands carefully with soap and water after contact with people with colds, children (a major reservoir for the cold virus) or potentially contaminated surfaces
  - avoid touching face and eyes

---

routinely in general practice for patients with sore throat (Box 102) because:

- A positive result does not necessarily indicate infection as bacteria can be carried in the throat without causing disease
- A negative result does not necessarily exclude bacterial infection as the swab may miss the causative pathogen
- Throat swab results come back over 48 h later, so tend not to alter a GP's prescribing decisions
- Throat swabs are expensive

Throat swabs may guide therapy in a few patients where the sore throat is not responding to treatment.

Matthias's throat swab is unlikely to make much difference to the management of his condition and could have been avoided to ensure efficient use of health care resources.

Should Dr Brewster have given Matthias a prescription for antibiotics?

The use of antibiotics for upper respiratory tract infections (URTI) is a difficult issue in general practice. On the one hand, GPs feel pressure to prescribe to ensure they do not undertreat serious infections and patients or parents may demand prescriptions. On the other hand, most URTIs resolve without antibiotics and prescription can increase patient reattendance, antibiotic resistance and health care costs. In the UK, the National Institute for Clinical Excellence (NICE) has issued guidelines for

PART 2: CASES

Box 100 Diphtheria

Cause
Toxin-producing *Corynebacterium diphtheriae*

Epidemiology
This disease is seen rarely in countries with a widespread vaccination programme. It is endemic with epidemic outbreaks in USSR, India, South-East Asia and South America. Immigrants or travellers from these countries could potentially develop the infection in the UK.

Transmission
Transmission is by respiratory droplet spread by close contact. Incubation period is 1–7 days

Pathogenesis
- The bacterium infects the throat and upper airway where it releases toxin. This causes necrosis of mucosal cells and growth of a membrane, which contains fibrin, epithelial cells, bacteria and neutrophils. This membrane may cause respiratory obstruction
- There is reactive lymphadenopathy and soft tissue swelling in the neck, which becomes very enlarged ('bull neck')
- The bacterium does not invade beyond the throat, but there is systemic release of the toxin which can affect the heart and nervous system, causing cardiac failure with shock and paralysis

Treatment
- Penicillin to kill the bacteria and stop toxin production
- Antitoxin to neutralize toxin in blood if systemic effects
- Supportive therapy including maintenance of patent airway, cardiac support, ventilation if required

Box 101 Group A β-haemolytic streptococcus

Group A β-haemolytic streptococci are found in approximately 30% of people with sore throats.

Infection may be complicated by:
Local suppurative complications
- Otitis media
- Sinusitis
- Peritonsillar abscess (quinsy)

Toxin production
- Scarlet fever (desquamative rash)
- Streptococcal toxic shock syndrome (rare)

Non-suppurative complications
These are now very rare in developed countries, but are still a problem in the developing world:
- Rheumatic fever
- Glomerulonephritis

Treatment
- Symptoms of sore throat caused by group A streptococci resolve spontaneously in 85% people within 1 week
- If antibiotics are required use penicillin or erythromycin if penicillin-allergic
- Antibiotics should not be used to prevent the complications of streptococcal infection as they have little clinically significant impact in the UK

Box 102 NHS funded Clinical Knowledge Summaries Service

Useful guidelines to aid clinical practice are published by the NHS as part of the UK National Library for Health. These can be found at: http://www.prodigy.nhs.uk

prescribing antibiotics in patients with sore throats (Box 103).

Dr Brewster felt that Matthias's condition fell within these guidelines as he has systemic upset with fever. She was also concerned about his difficulty swallowing. Hence her decision to prescribe antibiotics was justified.

Should patients with acute sore throats ever be referred to hospital?

Patients may need hospital care if throat swelling is causing significant airflow obstruction or preventing swallowing. Other indications for referral include a developing quinsy or underlying immunosuppression.

Box 103 NICE recommendations for antibiotics in patients with sore throat

Patients with sore throat should only receive antibiotics if there are:
- Features of marked systemic upset secondary to the acute sore throat
- Unilateral peritonsillitis
- History of rheumatic fever
- Increased risk from acute infection (e.g. diabetes mellitus or immunodeficiency)

Matthias does not need hospital referral unless his difficulty swallowing prevents drinking and causes dehydration.

Dr Brewster gives Matthias 250 mg amoxicillin t.d.s. for 5 days. He is back in her surgery 48 h later complaining of itching. On examination he has a widespread maculopapular rash.

Why might this rash have developed?

Aminopenicillins (amoxicillin, ampicillin, co-amoxiclav) should not be used as first line treatment for patients with a sore throat (Box 89, p. 153). This is because patients with sore throat caused by infectious mononucleosis (glandular fever; Box 104) almost always develop a rash if given these drugs. This unexplained reaction may lead to patients mistakenly being labelled as penicillin-allergic. Phenoxymethylpenicillin (or erythromycin if penicillin-allergic) should be the first line antibiotic for patients with a sore throat.

It is also possible that his rash may have arisen from a true penicillin allergy.

Box 104 Infectious mononucleosis

Cause
Epstein–Barr virus, a member of the herpes family.

Transmission
The virus is transmitted via respiratory secretions and saliva.

Epidemiology
Epstein–Barr virus most commonly infects young children and young adults (15–25 years) who share secretions. Hence, it is also known as 'kissing disease'.

Clinical features
Infection causes fever, sore throat, lymphadenopathy and hepatosplenomegaly. Systemic symptoms of fatigue, lethargy and debilitation may persist for months. Complications, which are relatively rare, include:
• Haemolytic anaemia and thrombocytopaenia
• Neurological involvement
• Cardiac involvement

Treatment
No specific treatment is required as the infection resolves spontaneously.

How could Dr Brewster confirm the diagnosis of infectious mononucleosis?

• *Blood film* – patients with infectious mononucleosis have a lymphocytosis with atypical activated T lymphocytes
• *Monospot or Paul–Bunnell tests* – for IgM heterophil antibodies which are able to agglutinate horse (Monospot) or sheep (Paul–Bunnell) red blood cells, indicating infection with Epstein–Barr virus.

If Dr Brewster stops Matthias's antibiotics, what other treatment options are available for sore throat?

Sore throat should be treated with paracetamol or soluble aspirin for symptomatic relief and fluid intake should be maintained. Symptoms of URTI will usually resolve in approximately 1 week, but infectious mononucleosis may take weeks or even months to resolve completely.

When Matthias is better should he have his tonsils removed?

Matthias has had one episode of tonsillitis and is unlikely to benefit from tonsillectomy. Guidelines indicate that patients should have five or more episodes of tonsillitis per year that prevent normal functioning before they should be considered for tonsillectomy.

Outcome. Matthias's Monospot test was positive and he was diagnosed with glandular fever. His rash resolved on stopping the antibiotics and his sore throat improved with rest and paracetamol. He remained tired and listless for a few weeks but gradually returned to normal activities.

CASE REVIEW

Matthias Obugu sees his GP complaining of a sore throat for the past 3 days. He is pyrexial with enlarged tonsils and lymphadenopathy. His GP treats him with amoxicillin, causing Matthias to develop a widespread maculopapular rash. His GP suspects Epstein–Barr virus infection and this is confirmed with a positive Monospot test. Matthias' condition improves over several weeks.

KEY POINTS

- Sore throat is most commonly caused by viral or bacterial infection
- Throat swabs are not generally indicated but may be useful in a few patients who are not responding to treatment
- Most sore throats will resolve with symptomatic relief irrespective of aetiology
- Antibiotics are only indicated if there are:
  - features of marked systemic upset secondary to the acute sore throat
  - unilateral peritonsillitis
  - history of rheumatic fever
  - increased risk from acute infection (e.g. diabetes mellitus or immunodeficiency)
- First line antibiotics for treatment of sore throat are phenoxymethylpenicillin or erythromycin for penicillin-allergic patients
- Aminopenicillins should not be prescribed for patients with sore throats as they will cause a rash in those with infectious mononucleosis, which may be mistaken for penicillin allergy
- Patients with sore throat rarely require hospital referral, but this may be indicated if they have:
  - airflow obstruction
  - inability to swallow
  - quinsy (tonsillar abscess)
  - immunosuppression

PART 2: CASES

Case 21 A 45-year-old woman with a chronic cough

Mrs Li is a 45-year-old woman who attends the chest clinic complaining of a 6-month history of cough occurring throughout the day and at night. She has had prolonged periods of coughing in the past, although these have usually recovered more quickly.

Mrs Li coughs up phlegm at least 20 times a day which is yellow or green and has been streaked with blood on several occasions. She gets an ache in her left side and is short of breath running for a bus. She has no nasal obstruction or bleeding, although she has been treated for sinusitis. She has not noticed heartburn or reflux. She is on no medication and has never smoked. She feels tired and has poor appetite, but has no weight loss or night sweats.

Analyse this information to produce a differential diagnosis for her cough

• The first step is to decide whether her cough is acute or chronic (see Part 1, Approach to the Patient, p. 20). Mrs Li's cough is clearly chronic as she has had it for much longer than 8 weeks

• The next step is to determine whether her chronic cough is caused by lung disease, postnasal drip, gastro-oesophageal disease or drugs (Box 18, p. 20). Mrs Li's productive cough and shortness of breath point to lung disease. She has no nasal or gastro-oesophageal symptoms and is not taking any medication

• The next step is to narrow down the respiratory differential diagnosis. Her copious sputum production indicates bronchiectasis. Haemoptysis is seen in bronchiectasis, but tuberculosis should be considered. Her age, prolonged history and non-smoker status make other causes of haemoptysis (lung cancer, pneumonia, pulmonary emboli) less likely (Box 19, p. 22).

What other information would be helpful at this point?

She should be asked about causative and risk factors to distinguish between bronchiectasis and tuberculosis and the effect of her cough on her life should be established.

Mrs Li was born in the UK, but was hospitalized for several months aged 5 with severe pneumonia. After that she often had a cough as a child and finds that colds 'go to her chest' as an adult. She had the bacille Calmette–Guérin (BCG) vaccination aged 14. On leaving school she started work in an office and is still working for the same company. She is married with two children who are well, lives in a modern house and has no pets. She has no personal or family history of asthma, hayfever or eczema and has never had family or social contacts with tuberculosis. She finds that her cough is embarrassing, causes stress incontinence of urine and restricts her social life.

How do you interpret this information?

• Her severe childhood respiratory infection could have caused bronchiectasis

• Childhood cough could also indicate asthma, although she has no personal or family history of atopic disease (some asthmatics are allergic to the fungus *Aspergillus* and develop bronchiectasis of proximal airways known as allergic bronchopulmonary aspergillosis)

• She has no history of risk factors for tuberculosis (Box 107, p. 188). She has been vaccinated against tuberculosis

• Her cough is having considerable impact on her quality of life

On examination she looks well. She has finger clubbing but no lymphadenopathy. Her oxygen saturations are 98%. She has coarse crepitations on auscultation at her left lung base.

How do you interpret her examination findings?

Mrs Li has finger clubbing, which is seen in a number of respiratory conditions (Box 21, p. 24). Patients with bronchiectasis commonly develop finger clubbing, particularly if they have extensive disease or chronic infection. However, finger clubbing has been reported in 20–30% of patients with tuberculosis.

Crepitations at her left lung base could be consistent with bronchiectasis or tuberculosis, although tuberculosis more commonly affects the lung apices. The otherwise normal findings do not exclude other diagnoses.

How would you investigate Mrs Li?

Mrs Li's main differential diagnosis is bronchiectasis or pulmonary tuberculosis. Investigation should aim to distinguish between these diagnoses and exclude unexpected diagnoses such as asthma, lung cancer or lung abscess. Initial tests should include:

- Chest X-ray to look for structural lung abnormalities
- Sputum microscopy and culture to look for *Mycobacterium tuberculosis* and other pathogens including bacteria and fungi
- Peak flow measurements and/or lung function tests to look for airways obstruction
- Full blood count:
  - neutrophils – elevation could indicate infection
  - eosinophils – may be elevated in asthma
  - white cells – immunosuppression can predispose to lung infection
- Plasma biochemistry:
  - glucose – diabetes can predispose patients to lung infections

---

KEY POINT

- The lung function department *must* be informed if there is any chance that a patient to be tested may have tuberculosis
- Patients with suspected tuberculosis are tested at the end of the day prior to disinfection of lung function equipment to prevent cross-infection via contaminated tubing

---

Mrs Li's results:

Chest X-ray – Fig. 74

Sputum microscopy – no acid-fast bacilli

Sputum culture – Haemophilus influenzae +++

Awaiting results of prolonged culture for mycobacteria

Lung function

FEV$_1$ 1.9L (68% predicted), FVC 3.0L (92% predicted), FEV$_1$/FVC 63%

Blood tests unremarkable

How do you interpret these results?
Chest X-ray

Thick-walled airways can be seen on the chest X-ray as double white lines (tramtracks) behind the heart (arrow).

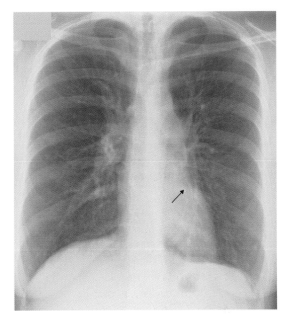

Figure 74 Chest X-ray.

This is consistent with bronchiectasis. There are no features of tuberculosis or other lung pathology.

Sputum

Her sputum has grown *Haemophilus influenzae* and this infection may be exacerbating her symptoms.

There were no acid-fast bacilli on sputum microscopy, but a single negative sputum sample does not rule out tuberculosis. Pulmonary tuberculosis can be difficult to diagnose, requiring accumulation of evidence from clinical symptoms and signs, Mantoux testing, chest X-ray and microbiology (see Case 23). Consistent lack of evidence of tuberculosis and positive evidence of bronchiectasis in this patient makes the diagnosis of tuberculosis decreasingly likely.

Lung function

Her FEV_1 is <80% predicted and FEV_1/FVC is <70% predicted. These results are consistent with airflow obstruction. This can occur in patients with bronchiectasis, asthma or chronic obstructive pulmonary disease (COPD).

There is still some diagnostic doubt. What other investigations could be useful?

- A high-resolution computed tomography (HRCT) scan of her chest is the best way of confirming a diagnosis of bronchiectasis

• Further tests to exclude tuberculosis would include two more sputum samples for microscopy and culture and a Mantoux test

• Evidence of allergy to *Aspergillus* (IgE [RAST] and skin prick testing)

One slice from Mrs Li's HRCT chest is shown in Fig. 75. Her Mantoux test and further sputum microscopy and culture for tuberculosis were negative.

What does the HRCT show?

Large dilated airways can be seen in the periphery of the lung (arrows). These have thick walls. This is consistent with bronchiectasis.

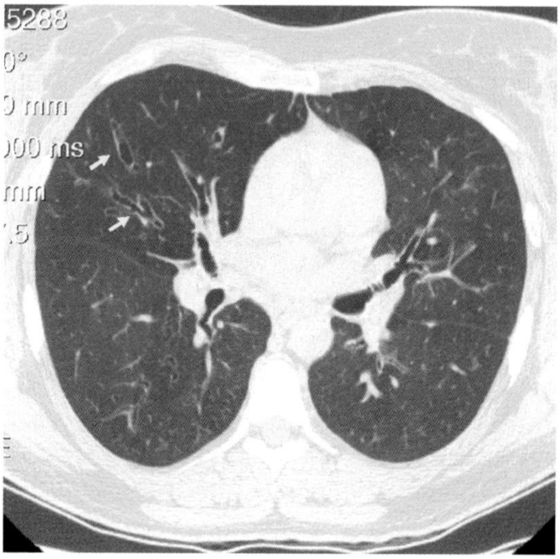

Figure 75 Computed tomography (CT) scan of chest.

What is bronchiectasis?

The term is derived from the Greek *ektasis* meaning 'expand' or 'dilate'. Bronchiectasis is abnormal and irreversible dilatation of the bronchi.

What causes bronchiectasis?

Bronchiectasis is caused by factors that impair the immune defences of the lung (Fig. 76). These causative factors and the subsequent bronchiectasis may be generalized (e.g. cystic fibrosis, dysfunctional cilia, defects of innate or acquired immunity) or localized (e.g. inhaled foreign body, pneumonia).

Mrs Li's bronchiectasis was most likely caused by her severe childhood pneumonia, causing localized damage.

How do these factors lead to the pathological findings of bronchiectasis?

Reduction in host immunity leads to pulmonary infection and inflammation, which heals with scarring. Scarring causes a permanent deficit in mucociliary clearance, increasing the risk of further infection and more damage. This sets up a vicious cycle, with progressive scarring and thickening of the bronchial walls.

Why do patients with bronchiectasis produce a lot of sputum?

Bronchiectatic airways (Fig. 77) are infiltrated with neutrophils, which produce an enzyme called elastase. This stimulates secretion of large volumes of mucus from submucosal glands. As this mucus is not cleared effectively by damaged mucociliary apparatus it pools in the lungs, increasing bacterial colonization and

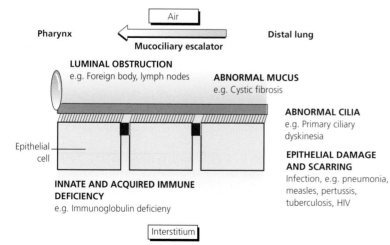

Figure 76 Some causes of bronchiectasis. Bronchiectasis can be initiated by any factor that disrupts normal lung defence, particularly the mucociliary escalator. Damage initiates a vicious cycle of infection, lung damage and more infection which causes scarring and dilatation of the bronchi. Investigation of a patient with bronchiectasis should include immunoglobulin levels and other tests for underlying defects in lung defence.

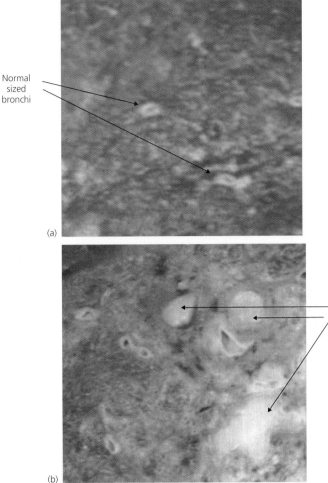

Normal sized bronchi

Dilated pus-filled bronchi

Figure 77 Pathology of bronchiectasis.
(a) Normal lung. (b) Bronchiectasis.

(a)

(b)

chronic infection. Bronchiectatic airways may bleed as a result of inflammation or abnormal vessels, causing haemoptysis.

How is bronchiectasis treated?

The aims of treatment are to relieve symptoms and prevent deterioration of disease by keeping the lungs clear of respiratory secretions as far as possible and by treating infection. The underlying cause should be identified and treated if possible.

Clearance of respiratory secretions

Physiotherapy is used to keep the lungs clear of respiratory secretions. The procedure involves:

1 Loosening of secretions by vibration of the chest (e.g. by manual percussion)

2 Clearance of loosened secretions by gravitational drainage, requiring a head down posture

Ideally, patients should do this themselves for 15–30 min 3–4 times per day. In practice, many cannot find the time or perform the technique correctly.

Pharmacological assistance for sputum clearance includes:

1 Bronchodilators to treat airflow obstruction
2 Good hydration, inhaled saline or mucolytic drugs to hydrate and thin mucus and make it easier to clear from the chest

Treatment of infection

Patients with bronchiectasis should receive antibiotics:

• To treat an acute infective exacerbation

• Chronically if they have frequent recurrent exacerbations

As patients with bronchiectasis have scarred lungs and impaired pulmonary defence against infection they are at risk of infection with unusual organisms including:

• Bacteria (e.g. *Pseudomonas aeruginosa*)
• Fungi (e.g. *Aspergillus fumigatus*)
• Atypical mycobacteria (e.g. *Mycobacterium avium intracellulare*)

These need to be identified by sputum examination and treated appropriately.

Outcome. Mrs Li was informed of her diagnosis of bronchiectasis. She was treated with 500 mg amoxicillin t.d.s. for 10 days, inhaled salbutamol and started home physiotherapy. Her GP was contacted and confirmed the diagnosis of severe childhood pneumonia and her bronchiectasis was attributed to this.

She returned to clinic for follow-up 6 weeks later. She was pleased to report that she was doing her physiotherapy regularly and had noticed a considerable improvement. Her sputum was now white following the antibiotics, her cough was less frequent and her stress incontinence had improved. She was encouraged to persist with physiotherapy and seek early antibiotic treatment for future exacerbations.

CASE REVIEW

Mrs Li presents with a chronic recurrent cough, productive of purulent sputum and blood, which is severely impairing her quality of life. Bronchiectasis is confirmed by HRCT scanning and investigations show no evidence of tuberculosis. Her bronchiectasis is attributed to scarring following childhood pneumonia. She is treated with antibiotics, bronchodilators and physiotherapy with considerable improvement in symptoms and is advised to treat future exacerbations promptly.

KEY POINTS

• Bronchiectasis is defined as chronic and irreversible dilatation of the bronchi
• Bronchiectasis occurs in patients with local or generalized impairment in lung defence against infection
• Loss of host defence triggers infection and inflammation that damage the bronchi and impair mucociliary clearance
• Bronchiectasis may present clinically with copious sputum production, recurrent chest infections or haemoptysis
• Clinical signs of bronchiectasis may be non-specific, but include finger clubbing and lung crepitations

• A firm diagnosis of bronchiectasis can be made by HRCT scanning of the chest
• Additional tests should be carried out to look for ongoing respiratory infection or underlying reduction in host immunity (e.g. immunoglobin levels)
• The mainstay of bronchiectasis treatment is physiotherapy to clear pooled lung secretions
• Additional treatment includes antibiotics, bronchodilators and prompt treatment of exacerbations

A 17-year-old girl with cystic fibrosis

Helen Gaskell is a 17-year-old girl who has recently moved into the area. She was diagnosed with cystic fibrosis aged 3 when she had the following test results:

Genotype – homozygous for ΔF508 mutation in CF gene

Sweat chloride 108 mmol/L (normal <60 mmol/L)

She has been referred to the cystic fibrosis unit for ongoing care of her disease.

What is cystic fibrosis?

Cystic fibrosis (CF) is an inherited disorder of a chloride transporter called the cystic fibrosis transmembrane regulator (CFTR). Transporter mutations cause malfunction and consequences are altered secretions in many organs including:

- Lung
- Pancreas
- Gastrointestinal tract
- Biliary tree
- Vas deferens
- Sweat ducts

Patients with cystic fibrosis currently have a life expectancy of around 30 years. Most die of chronic lung disease including infection and respiratory failure.

Is Helen's genotype consistent with cystic fibrosis?

Cystic fibrosis is an autosomal recessive condition, which means that mutations in *CFTR* genes must be inherited from both father and mother to cause the disease. As 1 in 25 Caucasian people carry the gene, approximately 1 in 2500 Caucasian children have the disease. CF is much less common but not unknown in people of African or Asian origin.

Helen is homozygous for the *CFTR* ΔF508 mutation, which means she has two copies of the abnormal gene required to develop the disease. The ΔF508 mutation prevents expression of CFTR on cell surfaces, which means the protein is unable to function. There are over 1000 mutations of the *CFTR* gene that can cause cystic fibrosis, but ΔF508 is the most common.

Why did she have an elevated sweat chloride concentration?

Water, Cl^- and Na^+ are filtered out of blood into sweat in the distal coil of the sweat duct. As fluid moves proximally up the normal duct, Cl^- is reabsorbed by CFTR and Na^+ is reabsorbed through epithelial sodium channels (Fig. 78a). Sweat leaving the top of the duct is dilute and Cl^- and Na^+ are conserved. In patients with cystic fibrosis, Cl^- reabsorption by CFTR is reduced or absent. Some Na^+ reabsorption still occurs, but the negative electric charge generated by movement of Na^+ into the cells and build up of Cl^- in the duct prevents Na^+ absorption (Fig. 78b). Thus, increased Cl^- and Na^+ are lost in the sweat.

Babies with CF often taste salty if you lick them. A sweat chloride of >60 mmol/L is strongly suggestive of CF. As CF patients have difficulty conserving Cl^- and Na^+ in their sweat they are at risk of salt and water depletion on hot days.

Is the information provided sufficient for a firm diagnosis of cystic fibrosis?

A diagnosis of CF requires two of:

- Typical clinical features
- Positive sweat test
- Genotype confirmation

Helen has a clear diagnosis of CF. In some children the sweat test is only mildly abnormal or unusual *CFTR* mutations are not detected and the diagnosis is more difficult.

Why has she been referred to the cystic fibrosis unit?

Cystic fibrosis requires intensive management by an experienced multidisciplinary team including doctors, nurses, physiotherapists, dietitians and lung function technicians to reduce complications and maximize life

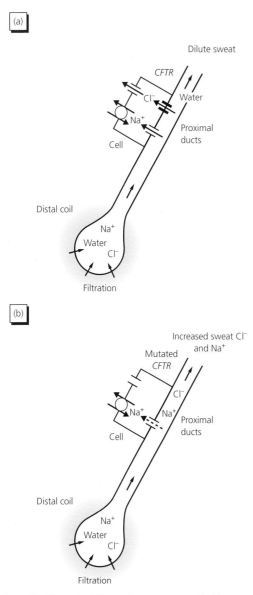

Figure 78 Effect of *CFTR* mutations on sweat chloride secretion. (a) Normal sweat duct. (b) Cystic fibrosis sweat duct.

expectancy. This expertise is concentrated in specialist centres.

Helen tells the doctor that she is studying for 'A' levels and is well enough to attend school. However, she has a blocked nose and a chronic cough, currently productive of thick yellow sputum and feels short of breath if she runs. She usually has around two chest infections per year, sometimes requiring treatment with intravenous antibiotics.

How does cystic fibrosis affect the lungs?

In CF, ion transport by respiratory epithelial cells is impaired, reducing the volume of airway surface liquid (Fig. 79). The cilia of epithelial cells are unable to beat properly in the low-volume viscous liquid, impairing mucociliary clearance. This leads to recurrent pulmonary infection which causes epithelial damage and build-up of luminal debris from dying cells which further thickens the mucus. Failing immune defences and increasing infection create a vicious cycle with progressive lung destruction, particularly of the small airways.

What types of chest infections are common in cystic fibrosis patients?

The spectrum of organisms infecting the lungs in CF patients is surprisingly limited. The reasons for this are not fully understood despite much research. Early infections in children with CF are usually with *Staphylococcus aureus* and *Haemophilus influenzae*. As patients get older their lungs become colonized and chronically infected with *Pseudomonas aeruginosa*. As lung damage increases CF patients may acquire other opportunistic pathogens including *Burkholderia cepacia*, *Aspergillus fumigatus* and non-tuberculous mycobacteria.

Why has Helen got a blocked nose?

Cystic fibrosis affects the fluid lining the nose and sinuses as well as the lungs. CF patients therefore commonly have sinusitis and nasal polyps and Helen should be checked for these conditions.

Helen also tells the doctor that she finds it difficult to put on weight and has intermittent offensive diarrhoea.

How do you explain these additional symptoms?

Cystic fibrosis gradually destroys the pancreas (Fig. 80), reducing release of pancreatic enzymes into the intestine. Without these enzymes fat is not digested or absorbed. Undigested fat in the faeces draws in water, causing steatorrhoea which is large volumes of faeces that are pale, offensive and difficult to flush away. Malabsorption of fat makes it difficult to put on weight and many CF patients have nutritional deficiencies.

How does cystic fibrosis affect the pancreas?

The pancreas is made up of acini which secrete digestive enzymes (Fig. 80). These enzymes pass from the acini

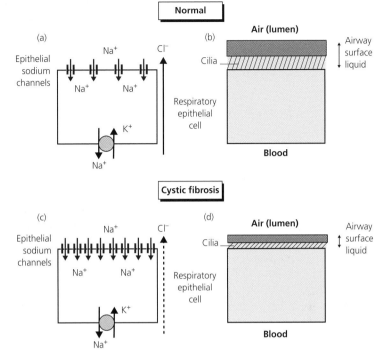

Figure 79 Effect of *CFTR* mutations on airway surface liquid. (a) In normal respiratory epithelium Na⁺ absorption through epithelial Na⁺ channels (ENaC) and Cl⁻ secretion (mostly from submucosal glands) are balanced. (b) As water follows ions, this ion transport ensures adequate airway surface liquid (ASL) volumes for normal ciliary function (see p. 9). (c) In cystic fibrosis, loss of CFTR causes reduction in Cl⁻ secretion. As CFTR normally controls ENaC activity, loss of CFTR releases ENaC from control and Na⁺ absorption is increased. (d) As water follows ions, this abnormal transport reduces the volume of ASL and ciliary function is impaired, leading to chronic infection.

along pancreatic ducts where HCO_3^-, Cl^- and water, secreted from epithelial cells, dilute and alkalinize the enzymes, washing them out into the intestine. Cl^- is secreted into the lumen by CFTR and recycled by a HCO_3^-/Cl^- exchanger, promoting the secretion of HCO_3^- (Fig. 80a).

In cystic fibrosis, *CFTR* mutations cause reduction or absence of Cl^- secretion into the pancreatic duct lumen (Fig. 80b). This results in reduced HCO_3^- secretion and reduced movement of water into the lumen. Lack of fluid in the pancreatic duct means that pancreatic enzymes cannot be carried into the intestinal lumen. Plugging of mucus in the ducts makes the situation worse. The trapped enzymes digest and destroy the pancreatic tissue.

Is insulin production by the pancreas affected?

Yes. The destruction of the pancreas also destroys islets of Langerhans which secrete insulin and insulin production falls. Diabetes mellitus is a common complication of CF and increases with age. Around 10% of 10-year-olds and 30% of 30-year-olds with CF have diabetes.

On examination Helen has a body mass index of 18 kg/m². Her oxygen saturations are 98% on air. She has finger clubbing but no lymphadenopathy.

In chest examination she has expiratory wheeze and basal crepitations.

How do you interpret her examination findings?

- She has a reduced body mass index (normal 20–25 kg/m²) consistent with poor nutrition and malabsorption
- Most patients with CF have finger clubbing resulting from chronic lung infection
- Basal crepitations are consistent with bronchiectasis that develops in patients with CF
- Expiratory wheeze indicates some airways obstruction which can occur in CF bronchiectasis and may respond to bronchodilators
- Her normal oxygen saturations on air indicate that her respiratory disease is not yet sufficient to cause respiratory failure

What investigations would you recommend to assess her disease further?

Her lung disease should be assessed by:

(a)

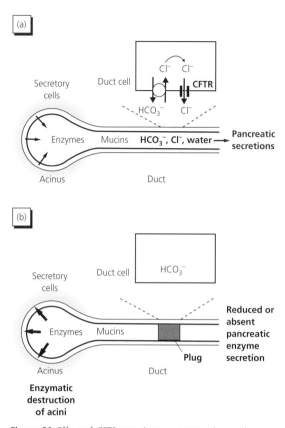

Figure 80 Effect of *CFTR* mutations on pancreatic exocrine secretion. (a) Normal. (b) Cystic fibrosis.

- Chest X-ray
- Lung function testing
- Sputum culture
  She should also have:
- Random blood glucose or oral glucose tolerance test to look for diabetes mellitus
- Blood tests to assess nutritional status, chronic inflammation and to look for other complications such as liver and bone disease including:
  ○ full blood count
  ○ C-reactive protein (CRP)
  ○ liver function tests
  ○ albumin
  ○ calcium and phosphate

Her investigations show:
Chest X-ray – Fig. 81
  Spirometry:

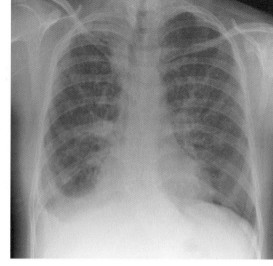

Figure 81 Chest X-ray.

Before bronchodilators:
- *FEV_1 1.7 L (52% predicted), FVC 2.8 L (74% predicted), FEV_1/FVC 61%*
After salbutamol:
- *FEV_1 2.1 L. Change of 24%*
Sputum culture
- *Pseudomonas aeruginosa*

How do you interpret these investigations?
- *Chest X-ray.* There are multiple small white patches on her chest X-ray, which are airways with thickened walls surrounded by local inflammation. At her right lung base there is loss of the costophrenic angle, consistent with old pleural inflammation, probably caused by a lung infection
- *Spirometry.* Reduced FEV_1 and FEV_1/FVC% indicate airflow obstruction caused by bronchiectasis. The finding of 24% reversibility with salbutamol indicates that her breathlessness could be improved with bronchodilators
- *Sputum.* She has respiratory infection with *P. aeruginosa* which may be driving deterioration of her lung disease

How would you summarize her clinical condition?
- Helen has an established diagnosis of CF
- Her condition is complicated by bronchiectasis with reversible airflow obstruction and pseudomonal infection

• Her low body weight and diarrhoea indicate ongoing inadequate nutrition and pancreatic insufficiency with malabsorption

What treatment would you recommend?

The aims of treatment are to optimize function and prolong survival. A multidisciplinary approach addressing physical, psychological and social needs is required to allow people with CF to live as normal a life as possible.

Lung disease

The goals of therapy are to clear secretions from the airways, reduce infective load and improve lung function.

Airways secretions

• *Physiotherapy.* Helen should have been performing chest physiotherapy with vibration and postural drainage several times daily at home ever since diagnosis. She should undergo physiotherapy review to check her technique and encourage adherence. She should also be encouraged to take as much exercise as possible, both for her lungs and her general health
• *Pharmacology.* In CF sputum there is a large amount of DNA released from degenerating neutrophils. This polymerizes and makes CF sputum more viscous. Recombinant human DNAase delivered by nebulizer degrades the concentrated DNA and reduces sputum viscosity, improving lung function and reducing infective exacerbations

Infective load

• *Treatment.* Antibiotics are used to treat infective exacerbations of CF and eradicate *Pseudomonas* from sputum if possible. Suitable first line antibiotics that can be given orally (Figs 22 & 23, pp. 39 and 40) are:
  ○ *S. aureus* – flucloxacillin
  ○ *P. aeruginosa* – ciprofloxacin

  However, as CF patients require many courses of antibiotics, they acquire resistant organisms and antibiotic sensitivity must be determined by laboratory testing. Many second line antibiotics have to be given intravenously and good nursing and pharmacy support is required to do this at home whenever possible.
• *Prevention.* Oral and nebulized antibiotics are used to prevent infection or reduce bacterial load. This strategy can reduce exacerbations and slow decline in lung function

Lung function

• Clearance of airways secretions and reduction in infection slow decline in and can improve lung function
• Bronchodilator treatment by inhaler or nebulizer can be used to treat reversible airflow obstruction

Nutrition

Good nutrition is critical for the health of CF patients as it maintains muscle, lung and immune system function and minimizes other complications including osteoporosis. Advice from a dietitian is essential:
• *Diet.* This should be high in calories and patients may require nutritional supplements
• *Pancreatic replacement.* Patients with pancreatic insufficiency take pancreatic enzymes by mouth with all meals and snacks. This helps them to digest and absorb fat and reduces unpleasant diarrhoea
• *Vitamins.* Absorption of fat soluble vitamins (A, D, E, K) is reduced in CF patients and supplements may be needed

Support

Cystic fibrosis has a huge impact on patients and families. The disease is usually diagnosed in infancy or early childhood and parents may have difficulty coming to terms with the possibility that their child may not have a normal life expectancy. Parents are essential for success of the home treatment regime including physiotherapy, medication and nutrition. This can be very time-consuming and family relationships may become strained if parents do not devote equal time to unaffected children. The illness and its treatment can impact on all aspects of life, including schooling, leisure activities, work, holidays and travel and may cause financial hardship. Teenagers may find CF particularly difficult to handle, being embarrassed by their illness and concerned that they will not be able to have a normal social life. Teenagers may rebel against their CF by stopping treatment and experimenting with cigarette smoking and this can be potentially life-threatening. Psychologists, counsellors, social workers and patient and/or family support groups therefore all have a role in helping patients and their families to live as normally as possible with CF (Box 105).

I *After review by the CF team Helen's treatment is as follows:*

• *Chest physiotherapy – at least twice daily*
• *Salbutamol inhaler 100 µg, 2 puffs as required*
• *Salmeterol inhaler 25 µg, 2 puffs twice daily*

> **Box 105 Further information about cystic fibrosis for patients and professionals**
>
> Useful information is available from the Cystic Fibrosis Trust: http://www.cftrust.org.uk

- *Inhaled fluticasone 250 µg b.d.*
- *Nebulized colistin (antibiotic)*
- *Oral ciprofloxacin for 3 weeks*
- *High calorie diet and dietary supplements*
- *Supplementation of fat-soluble vitamins (A, D, E, K)*
- *Pancreatin, variable dose with meals and snacks*

Several months later Helen returns for routine review. She is feeling well but is concerned because she has read on the Internet that patients with CF are infertile. She asks you if she will ever be able to have children and if so whether they will have CF.

How would you answer her questions?

Nearly all men with CF are infertile because the disease affects the vas deferens, which become blocked very early in life. Thus, although men with CF can make sperm, the sperm are unable to reach the ejaculate. Specialized techniques can be used to harvest sperm from the testicles by needle if male CF patients wish to have children. This condition does not affect the fallopian tubes, so women with CF can be fertile, although the chance of pregnancy may be reduced by low body mass index and chronic infection.

Helen will be able to have children but pregnancy is likely to cause deterioration in her health and she should consider using contraception to prevent this. If she does become pregnant she will pass a defective *CFTR* gene on to her children. However, as the condition is autosomal recessive her partner would also have to donate a defective *CFTR* gene for the child to be affected.

Helen remains under the care of the CF unit. She passes her 'A' levels and goes to university. Over the next 10 years she develops chronic Pseudomonas infection and her lung function deteriorates. At the age of 27 she develops respiratory failure, requiring treatment with oxygen and frequent hospitalization. She is listed for lung transplantation.

Why does cystic fibrosis cause respiratory failure?

Infection and inflammation in CF lungs causes gradual destruction of the small airways and impairment of gas exchange.

What other pulmonary complications of cystic fibrosis can occur?

- Pneumothorax
- Massive haemoptysis

What types of transplant operations are performed in cystic fibrosis patients?

- In the early days of transplantation, CF patients received heart–lung transplants, where their heart and both diseased lungs were replaced by donor heart and lungs. The CF patient's heart was then donated to a second recipient if healthy
- Subsequently, lung-only transplants have been performed, where both diseased lungs are removed and replaced by donor lungs. The patient is either put onto cardiopulmonary bypass so both lungs can be replaced at once, or one lung is replaced at a time, avoiding the need for bypass
- Donor organs are very scarce, so transplants of two lobes from different living donors have also been used

What is the likelihood of Helen receiving a lung transplant?

In the UK, over half of CF patients on the transplant waiting list die before transplantation.

Does transplantation increase life expectancy for cystic fibrosis patients?

Survival after lung transplant is around 70–80% at 1 year and 30–45% after 5 years. Early deaths are usually because of overwhelming infection following immunosuppression. Later deaths result from transplant rejection (e.g. from bronchiolitis obliterans). Transplantation increases life expectancy in CF patients with a prognosis of <2 years and can improve quality of life.

Outcome. Helen was on the transplant list for 18 months without success. During that time her condition deteriorated despite optimal care. As her respiratory failure became terminal she asked to be removed from the transplant list and to be made comfortable. Morphine and benzodiazepines were used to relieve her breathlessness. Two weeks later she died peacefully in her sleep.

CASE REVIEW

Helen Gaskell was diagnosed with CF aged 3 on the basis of a genotype homozygous for the ΔF508 mutation and elevated sweat chloride. She is referred to a new CF unit aged 17 when she moves areas. On assessment she has respiratory infection with *Pseudomonas aeruginosa*, nasal symptoms, is underweight and has diarrhoea. Helen is treated with regular home chest physiotherapy, bronchodilators and antibiotics. She is given a high calorie diet, vitamin supplementation and replacement pancreatic enzymes with food. Despite treatment she develops chronic pseudomonal infection and her lung function deteriorates over the next 10 years. She is listed for lung transplantation, but waits 18 months without success. Her condition deteriorates further and she dies comfortably with palliative care support.

KEY POINTS

- Cystic fibrosis is an autosomal recessive inherited condition caused by mutations in the *CFTR* gene
- ΔF508 is the most common *CFTR* mutation causing disease, but there are over 1000 others
- In the UK, 1 in 25 Caucasians carry *CFTR* mutations, hence 1 in 2500 Caucasian children have CF
- *CFTR* mutations alter secretions in many organs. Most of the morbidity and mortality of the disease occurs because of lung and pancreatic abnormalities:
  - in the lung, thickened secretions impair mucociliary clearance, resulting in recurrent lung infection and inflammation, bronchiectasis and respiratory failure
  - in the pancreas, thickened secretions block the pancreatic duct, resulting in pancreatic autodigestion. Reduction in exocrine secretions causes malabsorption and low body weight. Loss of endocrine tissue reduces insulin secretion, resulting in diabetes
- The mainstays of CF treatment are:
  - *lung* – daily home physiotherapy, prompt treatment of infection and bronchodilators
  - *pancreas* – high calorie diet, vitamin supplements, replacement of pancreatic enzymes to aid digestion
- People with CF should be managed in a specialist centre by a multidisciplinary team. Optimal management will both prolong life and allow support around specialist issues including:
  - fertility and pregnancy
  - unusual complications and infections
  - lung transplantation
  - end of life issues in young people

PART 2: CASES

A 25-year-old woman with cough and weight loss

Mrs Jamila Ahmed is a 25-year-old woman who is referred to the medical assessment unit by her GP. Mrs Ahmed does not speak English, but her husband acts as an interpreter. She gives a 1-month history of a cough productive of clear sputum which has now become green with streaks of blood. She also complains of fevers and drenching night sweats and has lost approximately 10 lb in weight. She has no significant past medical history, is not on any regular medication and does not smoke or drink alcohol.

What are your main differential diagnoses at this stage?

• *Pulmonary tuberculosis (TB)*. Cough, haemoptysis, night sweats and weight loss are classic features of TB
• *Other lower respiratory tract infection:*
  ○ *pneumonia* – this is an important cause of haemoptysis, purulent sputum and fevers. A 1-month history is probably too long for acute bacterial pneumonia. However, viral infection complicated by bacterial pneumonia could have a more prolonged course
  ○ *bronchiectasis* – clinical features are consistent with bronchiectasis, although the normal past medical history and relatively short (1 month) onset of symptoms make this less likely
• *Underlying malignancy*. Haematological malignancies, such as lymphoma and leukaemia, cause 'B' symptoms of weight loss and night sweats. These conditions could cause chest symptoms by suppressing normal immunity and predisposing to infection
• *Underlying HIV infection*. This could cause systemic symptoms of weight loss and predispose to opportunistic respiratory infection

If you suspect tuberculosis what should you do next?

Tuberculosis is caused by the bacterium *Mycobacterium tuberculosis*. This can be caught from a person with active pulmonary TB who has *M. tuberculosis* aerosolized in respiratory droplets expelled from their lungs. These droplets are released when the person coughs, speaks or spits. Tuberculosis is difficult to treat and can be fatal, therefore infection should be prevented whenever possible.

If she has TB, it is important to ensure that Mrs Ahmed does not infect other hospital patients or staff, particularly patients who are immunocompromised. UK guidelines (www.nice.org.uk/page.aspx?o=CG033) state that patients with suspected pulmonary TB admitted to hospital should be isolated in a side room to reduce the risk of spread. If they leave the room they should wear a surgical mask. People entering the room should wear a mask if there is suspicion of drug-resistant TB or if the patient is generating respiratory droplets (cough, sputum induction or bronchoscopy).

Mrs Ahmed should be isolated until the diagnosis has been proved and treatment commenced, or until active TB has been excluded with three negative sputum samples examined for *M. tuberculosis* by microscopy.

> **!RED FLAG**
>
> Have a low threshold for suspecting TB in patients with pulmonary illness
>
> If you have any suspicion of pulmonary TB, isolate the patient first and ask questions afterwards.

How infectious is tuberculosis?

According to the World Health Organization (WHO), a person with active pulmonary TB can infect 10–15 people per year. The risk is greatest in family members or other people who have close and frequent contact with the infected person. Health care workers are also at risk of contracting TB as they can be exposed to the infection many times throughout their career.

For more information see the WHO TB fact sheet: www.who.int/mediacentre/factsheets/fs104/en

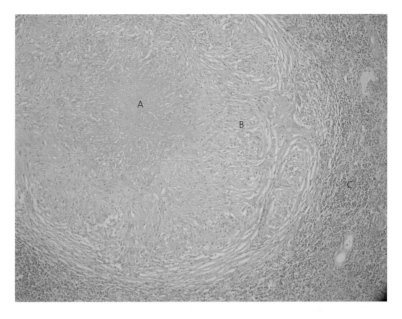

Figure 82 Caseating granuloma from a patient with tuberculosis. (A) Central necrosis or caseation. (B) Epithelioid macrophages. (C) Lymphocyte and fibroblast cuff.

What happens when a patient is infected with *Mycobacterium tuberculosis*?

Primary tuberculosis

When *M. tuberculosis* reaches the pulmonary alveoli it:

• Invades alveolar macrophages and replicates

• Is taken up by (but does not replicate in) dendritic cells and is transported to local lymph nodes

• A few bacteria may 'escape' into the blood stream

Infection by *M. tuberculosis* causes a local inflammatory reaction at infected sites, resulting in formation of granulomas (Box 106; Figs 82–84) which contain the infection. Possible outcomes at this stage include:

• Eradication of infection and healing, sometimes with calcification

• Latent infection

• Failure of the immune process, resulting in widespread dissemination of *M. tuberculosis* throughout the body, causing miliary TB

In the lung, the site of primary infection is usually the periphery of the lung (subpleural) in the mid or upper zones. The small area of granulomatous inflammation seen on chest X-ray is known as a Ghon's focus or complex in conjunction with hilar lymphadenopathy.

A patient with primary TB is usually not unwell and may not know they have been infected until they have a chest X-ray or develop postprimary TB. They are *not* infectious.

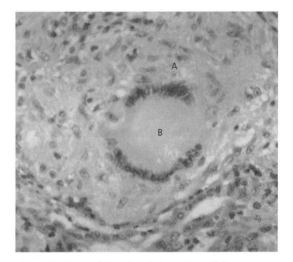

Figure 83 Giant cell. Langhans' giant cells result from merging of multiple activated macrophages during the granulomatous response to tuberculosis. They have (A) multiple nuclei seen around the periphery of (B) a large area of cytoplasm.

Postprimary tuberculosis

A total of 5–10% of people infected with *M. tuberculosis* will go on to develop active disease at some point in their life, with the greatest period of risk being in the first 2 years after infection. The risk of developing active TB is

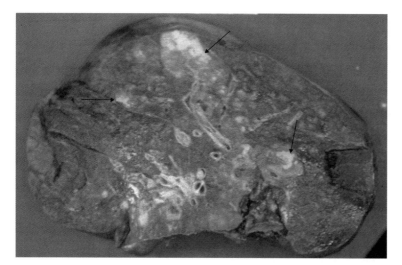

Figure 84 Caseation. Arrows indicate areas of caseation in response to *M. tuberculosis* infection (Box 106).

Box 106 Formation of caseating granulomas

- Invasion of alveolar macrophages by *Mycobacterium tuberculosis* stimulates an inflammatory reaction
- The infected macrophages become surrounded by T and B lymphocytes and fibroblasts (Fig. 82)
- Within the aggregate of cells (granuloma), T lymphocytes (CD4+) secrete cytokines. This activates infected macrophages to destroy their invading bacteria. CD8+ T lymphocytes also kill infected cells
- Activated macrophages may fuse together to form giant cells (Fig. 83)
- Dead macrophages and giant cells accumulate as necrosis at the centre of the granuloma
- With the naked eye the necrotic material generated by tuberculous granulomas looks like cheese (Fig. 84) and so is called 'caseation'

Box 107 Risk factors for tuberculosis

Development of tuberculous disease usually requires exposure to *Mycobacterium tuberculosis* infection followed (or accompanied) by suppression of host defence mechanisms, allowing reactivation of infection.

Risk factors for exposure to *Mycobacterium tuberculosis*
- Overcrowded living conditions
- Homelessness
- Infected family member
- Residence in or immigration from place with high prevalence of TB
  - worldwide – Eastern Europe/Russia, Asia, Africa, South America
  - in UK – areas of cities, particularly those with high migrant population

Risk factors for reactivation or potentiation of infection
- Human immunodeficiency virus (HIV)
- Drugs (e.g. corticosteroids, chemotherapy, disease-modifying drugs for inflammatory conditions)
- Malignancy
- Diabetes mellitus
- Debilitation, especially old age
- Alcohol excess, substance abuse

NB. Neonates and young children are also susceptible to TB as a result of underdeveloped immune systems and are particularly at risk of miliary TB.

much greater in patients infected with both *M. tuberculosis* and HIV.

In postprimary TB, the immune response to *M. tuberculosis* is the main cause of tissue damage. Postprimary TB therefore only occurs once the immune response to *M. tuberculosis* has developed (2–10 weeks). It is triggered by:
- Reactivation of latent infection resulting from a reduction in host immunity (most common; Box 107)
- Re-infection with *M. tuberculosis*

In the lung, the main pathological processes are:

• *Consolidation or cavitation.* This usually occurs in the lung apices or superior segments of the lower lobes as these have higher oxygen tension which supports bacterial growth. Processes include:
  ◦ further formation of granulomas
  ◦ necrosis and caseation, causing lung cavities
  ◦ fibrosis
• *Pleural infection.* This may cause a pleural effusion and/or thickening
• *Bronchiectasis.* Obstruction of large airways by enlarged lymph nodes can cause pulmonary collapse and bronchiectasis
• *Miliary tuberculosis.* This affects the whole body. In the lung it may be seen on chest X-ray as multiple small nodules throughout both lung fields. This form of TB is particularly serious and needs urgent treatment as it carries 20% mortality even with urgent treatment

Patients with consolidation, cavitation or bronchiectasis may have cough or haemoptysis. Patients with extensive parenchymal disease or a large pleural effusion may be breathless. Patients may also have systemic features of disease such as lethargy, fevers, sweats and weight loss.

Patients with active pulmonary disease may shed *M. tuberculosis* into their lung secretions. *These patients are infectious.*

KEY POINT

There is a crucial difference between TB infection and tuberculous disease:
• *Tuberculosis infection.* The patient has live *M. tuberculosis* organisms somewhere in their body but their immune system is controlling the infection effectively and they are not unwell or infectious
• *Tuberculous disease.* This usually occurs when the immune system becomes weakened and latent infection is reactivated. This results in tissue destruction and the patient becomes unwell. If the lung is affected they may be infectious

---

Armed with this information, what other features would you ask about in the history to support your diagnosis of pulmonary tuberculosis?

You now need to determine whether Mrs Ahmed may have been exposed to TB and whether she has any risk factors for reactivation of infection (Box 107).

Mrs Ahmed is originally from Somalia and came to the UK 3 years ago shortly after marrying. She now has a 2-year-old child. She is not aware of any previous exposure to TB or possible immunodeficiency.

What are your concerns when taking a full history from Mrs Ahmed?

Patients have a right to confidentiality. Mrs Ahmed is unable to speak English and her husband is acting as an interpreter. There may be information relating to her condition that she does not wish to share with him. This is highlighted by the difficulty of taking a history of possible HIV exposure in these circumstances.

How might you address these difficulties?

One option is to speak to Mrs Ahmed at a separate time without her husband present. An independent Somali interpreter could be used who is either present in person or on a three-way phone line using a service such as Language Line.

Mrs Ahmed agrees to be examined. Her temperature is 37.6°C. There is no evidence of lymphadenopathy. On auscultation there are crepitations over the right upper zone of her chest. No other abnormalities are identified.

Does her examination yield any new information?

The pyrexia fits with a diagnosis of TB or other respiratory infection. Right upper zone crepitations would be consistent with consolidation or other pathology at this site.

What initial investigations would you perform?

The aim of initial investigation is to look for evidence to support your clinical diagnosis of pulmonary TB and rule out other diagnoses including pneumonia, bronchiectasis or malignancy.
• *Chest X-ray.* This would be particularly useful to look for features of TB or other lung disease
• *Full blood count and inflammatory markers.* These would be carried out to look for:
  ◦ raised neutrophil count and C-reactive protein (CRP) consistent with bacterial infection
  ◦ anaemia and raised inflammatory markers of chronic disease such as TB

○ abnormal cell counts consistent with haematological malignancy or immunosuppression
• *Biochemical profile.* To look for abnormalities in renal, hepatic or bone profiles – sites that might be affected by TB

Mrs Ahmed's chest X-ray is shown in Fig. 85.
 Her blood test results were as follow:

		Normal range
Haemoglobin	9.8 g/dL	(12–16 g/dL)
Mean cell volume (MCV)	84 fl	(80–96 fl)
White cell count	10.8×10^9/L	$(4–11 \times 10^9$/L)
Neutrophils	8.2×10^9/L	$(3.5–7.5 \times 10^9$/L)
Lymphocytes	0.8×10^9/L	$(1.5–4 \times 10^9$/L)
Platelets	220×10^9/L	$(150–400 \times 10^9$/L)
Erythrocyte sedimentation rate (ESR)	57 mm/h	(1–20 mm/h)
CRP	77 mg/L	(<10 mg/L)
Sodium	131 mmol/L	(135–145 mmol/L)
Potassium	4.1 mmol/L	(3.5–4.8 mmol/L)
Liver/bone/renal profiles	Normal	

How do you interpret these investigations?
Chest X-ray
The striking abnormalities are:
• Consolidation, which is dense white shadowing containing black air bronchograms
• Cavitation of the lung within the consolidation, seen as a large black hole
• The abnormality is in the right upper lobe, defined at the bottom of the shadow by the horizontal fissure

Blood tests
Abnormalities identified are:
• Normocytic anaemia which can be caused by chronic disease such as TB
• Mildly elevated neutrophil count but low lymphocyte count, which could indicate suppression of cell-mediated immunity
• Mildly elevated CRP and ESR, indicating underlying inflammation
• Hyponatraemia (low sodium). Tuberculosis, pneumonia and lung abscess can cause syndrome of inappropriate antidiuretic hormone secretion (SIADH), with dilution of plasma sodium by retention of excess water

How do these results affect your differential diagnosis?
Cavitating upper lobe consolidation on chest X-ray is highly suspicious for TB.
 Other causes of cavitation (Box 108) are less likely as staphylococcal or klebsiella pneumonia would cause more systemic upset, lung cancer is unlikely in a 25-year-old non-smoker and purulent sputum and weight loss point away from a pulmonary embolus.

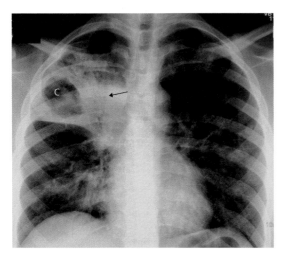

Figure 85 Chest X-ray. The arrow indicates air bronchograms within consolidation of the right upper lobe. (C) indicates a cavity within the consolidated right upper lobe.

> ### Box 108 Causes of cavitating lung disease
>
> A lung cavity is an abnormal hole in the lung tissue where lung parenchyma has been destroyed. Causes include the following.
>
> **Cancer**
> • Primary lung cancer
> • Lung metastases
>
> **Infection**
> • Tuberculosis
> • Bacterial pneumonias (*Staphylococcus* spp., *Klebsiella* spp.)
>
> **Infarction**
> • Pulmonary embolus
> Lung cavities can become infected with bacteria (abscess), or with *Aspergillus*, which can grow into a fungal ball called a mycetoma.

What tests could confirm the diagnosis of pulmonary tuberculosis?

Sputum analysis

Three morning sputum samples should be sent for:

• *Direct microscopy with specific staining*. The sample can be stained with Ziehl–Neelsen stain (red) or auramine (fluorescent). The bacteria have lipid-rich cell walls, which require phenol to make them permeable to dyes. This means that once they are stained the colour cannot be removed by acidic or alcohol washes. If these acid-fast bacilli (AFB) are seen on microscopy the sample is designated 'smear positive', which indicates high infectivity

• *Culture*. All samples are sent for culture:

  ○ smear-positive samples are cultured to determine whether the mycobacterium is tuberculosis or an atypical form and to determine antibiotic sensitivities to guide treatment

  ○ smear-negative samples may still contain AFB in numbers too small to be seen. The absence of *M. tuberculosis* needs to be confirmed by prolonged culture

• *Microscopy, culture and sensitivity* to detect the presence of other organisms that could cause pneumonia with cavitation (Box 108)

Tuberculosis skin test

This is also known as the tuberculin test and detects immunological evidence of infection with *M. tuberculosis*. The antigen used is tuberculin, a glycerine extract of the tubercle bacillus which is prepared as a purified protein derivative. The test is performed by:

• Intradermal injection of a standard dose of tuberculin into the forearm away from visible blood vessels using one of two methods:

  ○ *Mantoux test* (named after the French physician who developed it). A single needle is used to inject tuberculin

  ○ *Heaf test* (named after a British physician). Six tiny needles in a circle are used to inject tuberculin

• Measurement of the delayed-type hypersensitivity reaction to tuberculin:

  ○ Mantoux test is read 48–72 h after tuberculin injection

  ○ if there has been previous exposure to bacterial protein, an immune response will be mounted around the injection site

  ○ the reaction is quantified by measuring the diameter of induration (palpable raised hardened area) across the forearm (perpendicular to the long axis) in millimeters. Absence of induration should be recorded as '0 mm'. Erythema (redness) should not be measured.

  ○ the tuberculin skin test detects an immune response to TB antigen. It is therefore positive in those with active disease, latent infection, treated (cured) TB or those who have received vaccination against TB. The results must therefore be interpreted with care (Table 10).

Mrs Ahmed gives three early morning sputum samples and they are all smear-negative for AFB on microscopy. She was not sure whether she had previously had a BCG vaccination, but on examination she did not have a scar on the upper arm or lateral thigh region. Her Mantoux test was read at 48 h and measured as having produced induration of 2 mm.

What is BCG vaccination?

BCG stands for bacille Calmette–Guérin which is a live attenuated vaccine against TB. The vaccine was developed to confer immunity to infection with *M. tuberculosis* and prevent tuberculous disease. It is usually given into the upper arm around the insertion of the deltoid muscle. However, the vaccine is not universally effective:

Table 10 Interpreting the tuberculin skin test (Mantoux).

Mantoux induration*	<4 mm	4–15 mm	>15 mm
Result	Negative	Positive	Strongly positive
Possible interpretations	No TB exposure or vaccination	Previous vaccination	Likely infection
	Lack of immune response despite TB exposure or vaccination (e.g. HIV)	If no vaccination indicates TB infection	

*Using 10 tuberculin units (0.1 mL 100 TU/mL [i.e. 1 : 1000 concentration]).

• Not everyone who is vaccinated develops an immune response to tuberculin
• Those who do develop an immune response to tuberculin are not all protected against TB
• Even where there is an effect, the duration is not known
• There is no evidence it is effective in people >35 years

Vaccination also interferes with the use of tuberculin skin tests to look for TB infection.

In view of the limitations of BCG vaccination it is no longer given to everyone in the UK, but is used selectively in:
• Tuberculin-negative new immigrants from high prevalence countries aged ≤35 years
• Tuberculin-negative household contacts of pulmonary TB
• Neonates of ethnic minority groups (e.g. Indian Subcontinent or Black African)
• Tuberculin-negative, previously unvaccinated health care workers
• Neonates born in areas of the UK with high TB prevalence (>40/100,000 cases per year)

How do you interpret Mrs Ahmed's test results?

So far tests have not confirmed the diagnosis of TB as her three sputum samples are smear-negative and her Mantoux test is negative.

Are these test results surprising?

Her history and chest X-ray are strongly indicative of TB. The results are surprising but TB still remains the most likely diagnosis. False negative sputum microscopy can occur if the bacterial load is low or the sample is taken poorly. A false negative Mantoux test could indicate underlying immunosuppression (e.g. HIV).

What other investigations would help to make a diagnosis?

• Computed tomography (CT) scan of her chest to characterize the abnormality seen on X-ray and exclude less likely diagnoses including cancer and pulmonary embolus
• Sputum induction, i.e. physiotherapy to induce coughing after inhalation of hypertonic saline to obtain samples from deep in the lung

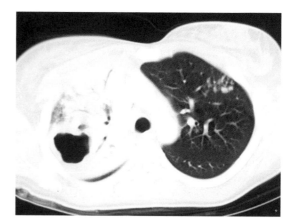

Figure 86 Chest CT.

• Flexible bronchoscopy to sample lower airway secretions if sputum induction is unhelpful in a further attempt to isolate AFB
• HIV test

Mrs Ahmed's chest CT confirms consolidation and cavitation in the right upper lobe (Fig. 86), consistent with pulmonary TB. She also has mediastinal lymph node enlargement. Sputum induction was unsuccessful. Bronchoscopic appearances were unremarkable, but microscopy of washings from the right upper lobe identified M. tuberculosis, which was fully sensitive to antituberculous treatment when cultured.

After bronchoscopy Mrs Ahmed commences quadruple antituberculous therapy with rifampicin, isoniazid, pyrazinamide and ethambutol.

What else must be done now a diagnosis of tuberculosis has been made?

• Tuberculosis is a notifiable disease, which means that there is a statutory requirement to inform the local 'proper officer', usually the Consultant in Communicable Disease Control, of any cases that have occurred. This information is collected by the Health Protection Agency and allows detection of TB outbreaks and monitoring of TB management
• People close to Mrs Ahmed may have become infected with *M. tuberculosis*. Her contacts must now be identified, traced, tested and treated as necessary

Mrs Ahmed is counselled for and consents to an HIV test which is found to be positive.

What is the significance of a positive HIV test?

A positive HIV test indicates that Mrs Ahmed has antibodies to and is infected with the human immunodeficiency virus (HIV).

HIV is a retrovirus that infects immune cells, particularly the CD4 (or T helper) lymphocyte. It replicates in and damages these cells:

- Directly during the release of virus from the cell
- By inducing apoptosis
- By marking the cell for destruction by other immune cells

As a consequence of HIV the CD4 count is reduced and this impairs cell-mediated immunity, increasing susceptibility of the affected person to infection with opportunistic pathogens and to tumour growth. Mrs Ahmed may have reactivated latent TB as her cell-mediated immunity became impaired by HIV.

How might Mrs Ahmed have contracted HIV?

HIV infection is very common in sub-Saharan Africa, although prevalence rates in Somalia, where Mrs Ahmed comes from, are relatively low. HIV is spread from person to person by contact with body fluids. The most common modes of transmission are:

- Sexual contact
- Parenteral exposure to infected needles or blood products
- Vertical transmission from mother to infant during delivery or breastfeeding

Why was Mrs Ahmed counselled before undergoing an HIV test?

When HIV was first discovered in the 1980s it was untreatable and the only benefit in knowing the diagnosis was reduced risk of transmission of virus to others. By contrast, there were many disadvantages to testing including concerns around confidentiality, insurance and legal issues as well as the negative emotional and social consequences of a positive result.

Testing has become more important since the development of highly active antiretroviral therapy (HAART), which prolongs survival and reduces morbidity from HIV. However, a positive HIV test can still have considerable physical, emotional and social implications and counselling before testing is still practiced.

How does HIV affect the respiratory system?

The effects of HIV on the respiratory system depend on the stage of the illness (Table 11). Once decline in cell-mediated immunity has begun the major respiratory infections associated with HIV are TB and pneumocystis pneumonia (Box 109).

> *Outcome. Mrs Ahmed is referred to an infectious diseases consultant who takes over her care. Her TB is treated first before she is given HAART for her HIV because of potential drug interactions. She improves rapidly on antituberculosis quadruple therapy and is discharged home to continue treatment. Contact and family testing for TB and HIV are planned.*

Box 109 Pneumocystis pneumonia

Cause

Pneumocystis pneumonia is caused by the fungal organism *Pneumocystis jirovecii* (not *P. carinii*, a similar organism which affects rats). Despite this it is usually known as *Pneumocystis carinii* pneumonia (PCP). *Pneumocystis* is widespread in the environment and is not a pathogen to healthy individuals, but causes lung infection in people who are immunocompromised.

Pathology

Infection causes thickening of the alveoli and alveolar septae. This causes severe hypoxia which can be fatal if untreated.

Clinical features

Patients experience fever, cough and breathlessness. On examination they may be extremely hypoxic without chest signs or with inspiratory crepitations and wheezes.

Diagnosis

Successful diagnosis is more likely if clinicians maintain a high index of suspicion for PCP in immunocompromised patients.

A chest X-ray may show perihilar haziness resulting from alveolar thickening (Fig. 87).

Diagnosis is confirmed by visualization of the organism by microscopy of induced sputum or bronchial washings.

Treatment

PCP is treated with co-trimoxazole, a combination of trimethoprim and sulfamethoxazole antibiotics. Alternative drugs include pentamidine, trimethoprim-dapsone, clindamycin, primaquine and atovaquone.

Patients with hypoxia and moderate to severe PCP are given corticosteroids to reduce alveolar inflammation and hasten recovery.

Table 11 Respiratory effects of HIV infection.

Illness stage	Respiratory effect
Acute HIV infection Initial infection with seroconversion	Flu-like illness with pharyngitis, lymphadenopathy and fever
Latency Stage I*	
Stable CD4 count and HIV viral load	No effect
Stage II*	Recurrent upper respiratory tract infections including sinusitis, pharyngitis, bronchitis
Stage III*	Pulmonary tuberculosis
	Bacterial pneumonia
Stage IV*	AIDS
	Opportunistic lung infections including candidiasis, pneumocystis pneumonia
	Kaposi's sarcoma

Stages II*, III*, IV*: Progressive decline in CD4 count and increase in HIV load

*World Health Organization (WHO) classification.

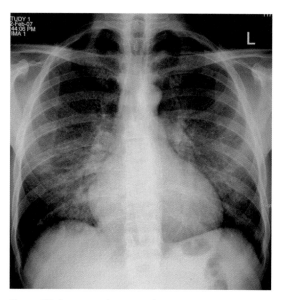

Figure 87 *Pneumocystis* pneumonia.

CASE REVIEW

Mrs Ahmed is referred for urgent assessment of fever, weight loss and haemoptysis. Her chest X-ray demonstrates consolidation and cavitation in the right upper lobe. As TB seems likely she is admitted to a side room to avoid spread of infection. Initial investigations do not confirm TB and her negative tuberculin test raises the possibility of a false negative result because of coexistent HIV infection. Subsequently, *M. tuberculosis* is seen in bronchial washings and she is started on quadruple antituberculous treatment. She is also found to be HIV positive and is referred to the infectious diseases consultant for consideration of HAART.

KEY POINTS

- Tuberculosis should be suspected in all patients presenting with night sweats, weight loss or haemoptysis
- If a patient is suspected of having active pulmonary TB they should be cared for in a side room to prevent cross-infection
- Risk factors for TB include:
  - previous exposure
  - impaired immunity, reactivating previous infection
- Initial diagnostic tests for pulmonary TB should include:
  - chest X-ray
  - three early morning sputum samples for microscopy and culture
  - tuberculin skin testing
- If these are unhelpful other useful tests for pulmonary TB include:
  - induced sputum for microscopy and culture
  - fibreoptic bronchoscopy with bronchial washings for microscopy and culture
- Once the diagnosis of pulmonary TB has been made:
  - the patient should be started on appropriate treatment
  - the case must be notified to the Health Protection Agency via the local officer
  - contact tracing should be performed to identify, screen and treat close contacts as necessary
- Co-infection with HIV and *M. tuberculosis* is common and HIV testing should be considered in all patients with TB
- HAART prolongs life and reduces morbidity in patients with HIV
- The most common pulmonary manifestations of AIDS are TB and pneumocystis pneumonia

Case 24 A 44-year-old man commencing treatment for tuberculosis

Mr Stanislav Bulovski is a 44-year-old man who has posterior cervical lymphadenopathy. Histological examination of a fine needle aspirate from a lymph node revealed acid-fast bacilli (Fig. 88). Mycobacterial culture is not yet available. His chest X-ray showed an old granuloma, consistent with tuberculosis (TB) infection. Fibreoptic bronchoscopy was unremarkable and mycobacteria were not seen on bronchial washing microscopy. He is HIV negative and is not immunosuppressed.

How do you interpret this information?

Mr Bulovski has evidence of previous primary TB infection on chest X-ray. He now has postprimary TB involving his posterior cervical nodes, but no evidence of pulmonary TB. This is extrapulmonary TB (Box 110).

If acid-fast bacilli were seen on histology why was the lymph node also sent for culture?

Culture allows differentiation of *Mycobacterium tuberculosis* from other members of the *Mycobacterium* species (Box 111) and takes 20–56 days. Once the *Mycobacterium* has been formally identified, the organism can be tested for sensitivity to antimycobacterial drugs which may take a further 4–6 weeks. The process can be speeded up using polymerase chain reaction (PCR) amplification to detect mycobacteria and identify gene mutations associated with antibiotic resistance.

Should the doctors wait for culture results before starting treatment?

A presumptive diagnosis of TB can be made from the clinical features and investigation results and treatment should be started promptly. Treatment can then be modified once culture and sensitivity results are available.

Is Mr Bulovski likely to infect his family with tuberculosis?

Tuberculosis is usually spread by respiratory droplets and patients with extrapulmonary TB are rarely infectious.

However, care should be taken with any suppurating extrapulmonary TB as TB can be spread from these secretions. Mr Bulovski has no evidence of pulmonary TB and bronchial washings are negative for mycobacteria, so he is unlikely to infect his family. However, contact tracing should still be performed as he may have acquired his infection from another family member.

In clinic the TB specialist explains the diagnosis and need for prolonged therapy to cure his TB. Mr Bulovski is anxious to start therapy and confident that he will be able to stick to the treatment regime unaided. In clinic he has blood taken to test his liver and renal function and is sent for eye tests. He is then started on:

Rifater (rifampicin, isoniazid and pyrazinamide), 6 tablets daily

Ethambutol 1050 mg/day

Why is he treated with multiple antituberculous drugs?

The aims of treatment are to:
• Eradicate mycobacteria, curing the patient
• Prevent transmission of infection

Metabolic states

Mycobacterium tuberculosis exists in several metabolic states:
• Rapid growth – this form is responsible for active infection
• Intermittent growth
• Slow growth – this form is responsible for latent infection

Different drugs are effective against bacteria in different metabolic states. At least two different drugs must be used to kill all bacteria and eradicate infection.

Emergence of resistance

Mycobacteria resistant to antituberculosis drugs arise spontaneously during treatment. If a single drug is used,

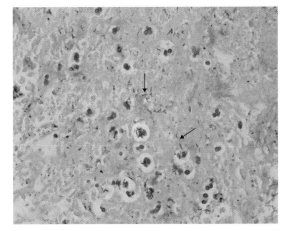

Figure 88 Acid-fast bacilli. Arrows indicate multiple small dark rods which are the bacilli.

> **Box 111 *Mycobacterium* species**
>
> Mycobacteria are a family of slow growing, acid-fast, aerobic bacilli, classified into three groups according to their capacity to cause disease:
> 1 *Mycobacterium tuberculosis* complex – cause TB
>   ○ *Mycobacterium tuberculosis*
>   ○ *Mycobacterium bovis* (cattle and can infect humans)
> 2 Non-tuberculous mycobacteria. Environmental pathogens found in soil and water that cause a lung disease resembling TB in immunocompromised patients and those with chronic lung disease such as bronchiectasis:
>   ○ *Mycobacterium avium intracellulare*
>   ○ *Mycobacterium kansasii*
> 3 *Mycobacterium leprae* – causes leprosy

> **Box 110 Extrapulmonary tuberculosis**
>
> Tuberculosis spreads via the blood stream and/or lymphatics to any extrapulmonary organ or body system, most commonly the lymph nodes and bones:
> • *Bones and joints.* TB osteomyelitis or arthritis can occur
> • *Heart.* TB can cause constrictive pericarditis
> • *Gastrointestinal tract.* TB of the small intestine can cause malabsorption. Peritoneal infection can cause ascites
> • *Genitourinary system.* There may be a tuberculous mass in the kidney. TB can cause epididymitis (men) or salpingitis (women)
> • *Central nervous system.* Tuberculous meningitis or intracranial tuberculomas
> • *Other.* Infections of the skin, eyes and adrenal glands are described

resistant organisms survive and vulnerable tubercle bacilli are killed. The use of multiple drugs ensures that bacilli emerging with resistance to one drug are killed by other drugs in the regimen, ensuring that all tubercle bacilli are eradicated.

What is the role of each drug in the treatment regimen?

• Isoniazid is bacteriocidal against (kills) rapidly dividing bacteria and makes the patient non-infectious within days of starting treatment
• Rifampicin is bacteriocidal against rapidly growing and slowly dividing bacteria (persisters) and can cause complete eradication of tubercle bacilli (sterilization)

• Pyrazinamide eradicates slowly dividing and intracellular bacteria, also contributing to sterilization
• Ethambutol is not particularly effective at killing tubercle bacilli; however, it prevents emergence of resistance during therapy

Why are three drugs given together as a combination pill?

• To aid adherence to the treatment regime by reducing number of pills taken
• To ensure that three active drugs are taken together, as separate use could lead to mycobacterial resistance

Why does he have blood taken for liver and renal function testing?

Isoniazid, rifampicin and pyrazinamide

These cause hepatic toxicity (Boxes 112–114) and are eliminated by the liver. Liver function testing before treatment is essential to:
• Establish a baseline to allow detection of drug-related hepatotoxicity
• Identify underlying liver disease, necessitating reduction in dosage of drug used or frequent monitoring of liver function

Ethambutol

Ethambutol (Box 115) is renally excreted, therefore renal function should be checked to:
• Identify underlying renal disease, necessitating reduction in ethambutol dose or use of an alternative drug

Box 112 Pharmacology of isoniazid

Mechanism of action
- Inhibits synthesis of mycolic acid, essential for formation of mycobacterial cell walls and is bacteriocidal

Uses
- As part of a multidrug regimen for the treatment of active TB
- Alone or with rifampicin in patients with latent TB who are at risk of developing active TB (e.g. patients taking steroids)

Pharmacokinetics
- Metabolized in the liver by acetylation
- Co-administration with anti-epileptic drugs raises plasma level (e.g. of phenytoin)

Major side-effects
- Hepatic toxicity
- Neuropathy – this can be prevented by co-administration of pyridoxine, particularly in patients who are malnourished (e.g. <50 kg)

Box 113 Pharmacology of rifampicin

Mechanism of action
- Interferes with the synthesis of bacterial RNA

Uses
- Part of a multidrug regimen for the treatment of active TB
- Used with isoniazid in patients with latent TB to prevent development of active TB
- Also active against *Legionella pneumophila, Neisseria meningitides, Staphylococcus aureus* and *Haemophilus influenzae*

Pharmacokinetics
- Induces liver enzymes, increasing metabolism of many drugs including anti-epileptic drugs, the oral contraceptive pill and warfarin

Major side-effects
- Turns body fluids orange and can stain soft contact lenses
- Hepatic toxicity
- 'Flu-like' syndrome (drug fever)

Box 114 Pharmacology of pyrazinamide

Mechanism of action
- Bacteriocidal to mycobacteria

Uses
- Part of a multidrug regimen for the treatment of active TB

Pharmacokinetics
- Pro-drug taken up by mycobacteria and converted by pyrazinamidases to pyrazinoic acid which is bacteriocidal
- Metabolized in the liver but little potential to interact with other drugs

Major side-effects
- Hepatotoxicity
- Hyperuricaemia and gout

Box 115 Pharmacology of ethambutol

Mechanism of action
- Bacteriostatic (stops the growth of bacteria), possibly acts by inhibiting bacterial RNA synthesis

Uses
- Part of a multidrug regimen for the treatment of active TB

Pharmacokinetics
- Renally excreted

Major side-effects
- Optic neuritis
- Peripheral neuritis

KEY POINTS

- Drugs used for the treatment of TB have great potential to interact with other drugs given at the same time because they alter the activity of liver enzymes
- Appendix 1 of the *British National Formulary* should always be checked for potential drug interactions when antituberculous medication is given with other drugs: http://www.bnf.org/bnf/registration.htm

What type of eye tests should Mr Bulovski have?

Ethambutol can cause optic neuritis which first presents as red–green colour blindness then loss of visual acuity.

He should therefore have testing of his colour vision (Ishihara testing) as well as visual acuity testing with a Snellen chart.

What advice would you give him before sending him home to start treatment?

He should look out for any:
- Signs of hepatic toxicity (e.g. fever, malaise, vomiting or jaundice)
- Change in his vision
- Other unexpected effects

If these occur he should discontinue therapy and seek immediate medical advice.

He should be given a contact number for emergencies and a follow-up appointment for 2 weeks' time.

Mr Bulovski returns for follow-up 2 weeks later. He finds he is able to tolerate his medication and is not aware of any side-effects apart from nausea. He has no problems with his eyesight. He asks the TB nurse how long he must stay on treatment for.

What assessment is required at follow-up during treatment for tuberculosis?

It is important to establish:
- *Treatment efficacy.* This can be monitored by checking symptoms and resolution of active disease. In Mr Bulovski's case his lymphadenopathy would be expected to resolve
- *Adherence to treatment regime* (Box 116):
  - this is indicated by clinical improvement in TB symptoms and signs
  - it can be checked by asking the patient and performing tablet counts
  - other checks include examination of urine (should be orange with rifampicin) or measurement of plasma drug levels
- *Drug side-effects.* Patients should be asked about changes in eyesight and liver function should be checked

How would you answer his question?

- *Initial phase.* Patients take four drugs until culture and sensitivities are available, which usually takes about 2 months
- *Continuation phase.* If sensitivity testing shows no bacterial resistance to isoniazid or rifampicin, treatment is continued with these two drugs alone for a further 4 months and pyrazinamide and ethambutol are stopped

> **Box 116 Definitions of compliance, concordance and adherence**
>
> These terms refer to the prescriber–patient interaction around the prescribing of medicines.
>
> **Compliance** implies an old fashioned consultation model, sometimes referred to as 'paternalistic' (fatherly), where the prescriber tells the patient what to do. The patient then does what they are told (complies) or does not (non-compliant).
>
> **Concordance** indicates an alternative consultation model. The prescriber and patient both come to the consultation with valid knowledge, attitude and beliefs. They discuss treatment options and come to an agreement (concordance) on the way forward.
>
> **Adherence** is a measure of whether the patient sticks to the agreed treatment regimen. These days patients are 'adherent' or 'non-adherent' to treatment, rather than 'compliant' or 'non-compliant'.

Is the duration of treatment the same for all tuberculosis infections?

Treatment duration may be affected by:
- Drug resistance
- Site of TB (e.g. prolonged treatment is required for CNS disease)

Outcome. Mr Bulovski tolerated antituberculous therapy. After 2 months lymph node culture grew M. tuberculosis fully sensitive to therapy. His four-drug regime was reduced to rifampicin and isoniazid and he completed the course of treatment without significant toxicity. His family were screened and were all negative for TB. At the completion of treatment his lymphadenopathy had resolved and he was discharged.

CASE REVIEW

Mr Bulovski presented with postprimary TB affecting his posterior cervical lymph nodes. Prior to treatment his liver and renal function were checked and he underwent eye tests for red–green colour vision and visual acuity. He was started on rifampicin, isoniazid, pyrazinamide and ethambutol. He did not have severe side-effects of treatment and was able to complete 2 months on these four drugs, before reducing treatment to rifampicin and isoniazid for a further 4 months. At the end of treatment his lymphadenopathy had resolved and he was discharged.

KEY POINTS

- *Mycobacterium tuberculosis* may spread from the site of primary infection in the lung to other sites by blood or lymphatics
- The most common sites for extrapulmonary TB infection are lymph nodes and bone
- A diagnosis of TB is likely if acid-fast bacilli and caseating granuloma are seen on microscopy of fine needle aspirates
- Culture is required to:
  - confirm that acid-fast bacilli are *M. tuberculosis* and not another member of the species
  - test the bacilli for sensitivity to antimycobacterial drugs
- TB culture takes several weeks, therefore treatment should be started while results are awaited
- In the initial phase (first 2 months) four drugs are used for treatment (mnemonic RIPE):
  - rifampicin, isoniazid, pyrazinamide, ethambutol

- In the continuation phase (further 4 months), rifampicin and isoniazid are continued to complete treatment
- Multiple drugs are required to ensure eradication of bacteria in different growth phases and to prevent emergence of resistance
- Major side-effects of treatment are hepatic toxicity (rifampicin, isoniazid, pyrazinamide), visual disturbance (ethambutol) and neuropathy (isoniazid, ethambutol)
- Liver and renal function, red–green colour vision and visual acuity are checked prior to starting treatment
- Patients are monitored for disease response, treatment adherence and drug side-effects during treatment
- Treatment for TB is usually for 6 months, but may be given for longer if it is infecting non-pulmonary sites or is multidrug resistant

A 32-year-old man who absconds from directly observed therapy for tuberculosis

Mr Ewan Evans, a 32-year-old man, is admitted to hospital with fevers and a cough productive of brown sputum. His chest X-ray (Fig. 89) shows right upper lobe shadowing (A) and hilar lymphadenopathy (B) and his sputum is smear-positive for acid-fast bacilli. The sample rapidly cultures Mycobacterium tuberculosis which is fully sensitive to treatment. He undergoes an HIV test which is negative. His case is notified and he is commenced on quadruple antituberculosis therapy with rifampicin, isoniazid, pyrazinamide and ethambutol.

How can you find out whether he has infected other people with tuberculosis?

When a diagnosis of tuberculosis (TB) is made, contact tracing is performed, usually by nurse specialists in TB, with the aims to identify people with:

• Active disease who require treatment
• Latent infection, who may require prophylactic treatment to prevent active disease
• No evidence of infection but who may benefit from bacille Calmette–Guérin (BCG) vaccination

The infected person is referred to as the index case. The 'index case' is most likely to have infected people they are very close to (e.g. those they share accommodation with). These people are traced and contacted first and offered screening. If more than 10% of these close contacts are positive for TB, the next 'ripple' of less frequent contacts is screened (e.g. people who work with the index case; Fig. 90). If more than 10% of these contacts are positive, the tracing and screening is extended further into more casual contacts. This can be referred to as a 'stone in the pond' or patient-centred model. Tracing and screening stop at the level of contacts where <10% have been infected.

How is contact tracing coordinated?

Specialist nurses performing contact tracing usually work as part of an NHS TB service in a local hospital,

primary care or a local Health Protection Unit (HPU; Fig. 91). Services are organized differently depending on local needs and expertise throughout the country. The NHS team notifies each clinical case to the Consultant in Communicable Disease Control in the local Health Protection Unit (HPU). The involvement of the HPU allows coordination of individual NHS providers (hospitals and primary care) at local, regional or national level as appropriate to investigate and manage disease outbreaks.

How are contacts screened?

Screening is performed with tuberculin skin testing (Mantoux) and chest X-ray. The results can be interpreted as follows:

• Positive Mantoux and abnormal chest X-ray and/or clinical features of TB – possible active disease
• Positive Mantoux and normal chest X-ray and/or no clinical features of TB – possible latent disease or previous BCG vaccine
• Negative Mantoux and normal clinical assessment – not infected with TB

Although this appears clear-cut it can be more difficult in practice. Mantoux results can be falsely positive as a result of BCG vaccination or exposure to environmental mycobacteria or falsely negative because of immunosuppression. New γ-interferon (IFN-γ) immunological tests aim to be more specific for *Mycobacterium tuberculosis* infection (Box 117) and have been used to diagnose latent TB.

How are the results of screening used?

• Contacts with possible active disease require further investigation and are likely to need antituberculous treatment
• Patients with latent disease have a 10–15% chance of developing active disease. Treatment with isoniazid for 6 months or isoniazid and rifampicin for 3 months has been shown to reduce the risk of developing active disease

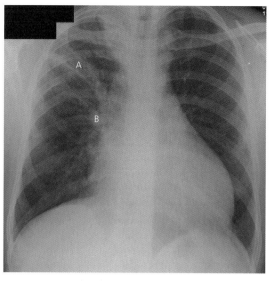

Figure 89 Chest X-ray.

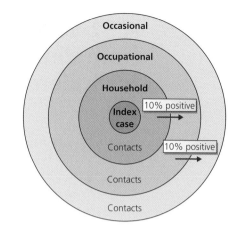

Figure 90 'Stone in the pond' model used for contact tracing.

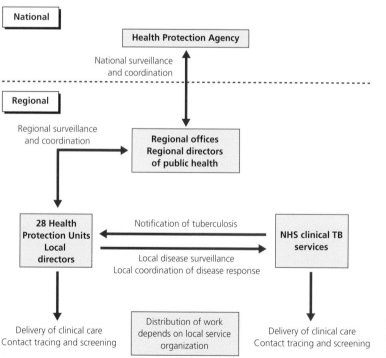

Figure 91 Organization of services for management and control of tuberculosis.

in the future. As hepatotoxicity of drugs increases with age, the risk of treatment of latent TB begins to outweigh the benefits in older patients, so only those ≤35 years are usually treated

• Contacts who have not been infected with TB should be offered the BCG vaccine. There is no evidence of BCG efficacy for people over 35 years, therefore vaccination is usually limited to people who are ≤35 years

Mr Evans is interviewed by the TB specialist nurse. He has a past history of intravenous drug use, has recently been homeless and is currently staying in a hostel.

Box 117 γ-Interferon immunological tests for *Mycobacterium tuberculosis*

Principles
- The test determines the immunological response to 'early secretion antigen target 6' (ESAT-6) and culture filtrate protein (CFP-10)
- ESAT-6 and CFP-10 are used because they are expressed by *M. tuberculosis* and not by most environmental mycobacteria or the live attenuated bacillus used in the BCG vaccine

Methods
- A sample of whole blood is taken from the patient
- The antigens (ESAT-6 and CFP-10) are added to the blood
- Immunological response is measured either by release of IFN-γ from the whole sample (QuantiFERON-TB Gold) or by counting individual activated T cells (T.SPOT-*TB*)
- Research has shown that positive responses to these immunological tests correlate with degree of exposure to *M. tuberculosis* and are much less influenced by previous BCG vaccination

What concerns do his social circumstances raise?

- He lives in a hostel where he has come into contact with a large number of people who may have become infected. Some of these may be particularly susceptible to infection because of immunosuppression (e.g. with HIV)
- His lifestyle is unstable and he will not reliably be able to complete the 6-month course of antituberculous treatment required to cure his disease

What should be done to prevent him from infecting other people?

As his social circumstances will not permit some form of 'home isolation', he needs to remain in hospital until he is unlikely to infect others. The minimum treatment time for fully sensitive acid-fast bacilli in the lungs to be killed and for the patient to become non-infectious is generally accepted as 2 weeks. Where it is essential (as in this case) to ensure the patient is non-infectious, three smear-negative sputum samples produced on separate occasions may be required before discharge.

How will his circumstances affect contact tracing?

He is likely to have come into contact with many people when homeless or living in the hostel who will now be hard to trace. The National Institute for Clinical Excellence (NICE) recommends active case finding for TB in homeless people using chest X-rays taken opportunistically and in symptomatic patients. Contact tracing is likely to be difficult and may require input from the Health Protection Agency.

The TB nurses arrange contact tracing at the hostel. They screen 20 staff and find that six have possible evidence of M. tuberculosis infection, although none have active disease. The six staff with possible M. tuberculosis infection undergo IFN-γ testing, which identifies four who receive treatment for latent infection to prevent active disease. On discussion with the local HPU, the clinical team decide to offer chest X-rays to all hostel residents, irrespective of contact with Mr Evans. Two cases of active disease are identified and treated.

Why is it important that Mr Evans receives adequate antituberculosis treatment?

Completion of antituberculosis therapy is very important for two main reasons:

1 Incomplete treatment may allow tubercle bacilli to mutate and become multidrug-resistant. This is much more difficult to treat than fully sensitive TB
2 Relapse of the disease can lead to a resurgence of infectivity which may become a public health concern

How could you ensure Mr Evans receives the full course of antituberculosis treatment?

Mr Evans could receive directly observed therapy (DOT). DOT is used when the clinical team are concerned that a patient may have difficulty adhering to a treatment regimen and completing the full course of antituberculous medication. DOT involves a TB nurse specialist administering the tablets and watching the patient swallow them in a hospital clinic. Alternatively, a responsible individual outside the hospital, such as a school teacher, can perform DOT at a location more convenient to the patient. Hospital visits for DOT can be minimized by using treatment regimens where tablets are taken three times per week.

What other ways are there to ensure that patients take their treatment?

- Education, regular support and reminders from health care workers are important

- Medication is given as combination tablets (e.g. Rifater contains rifampicin, isoniazid and pyrazinamide) to make treatment adherence easier
- Patients should be seen and monitored regularly:
  - tablet counts can be performed to assess whether medication has been taken
  - rifampicin stains the urine red, which can be assessed
  - blood levels of some antituberculosis drugs can be checked

Mr Evans remains in hospital for the first 2 weeks of antituberculosis treatment. His cough improves and he becomes apyrexial. Once three smear-negative sputum samples are obtained he is discharged from hospital to receive DOT as an outpatient. After discharge he attends for treatment twice, then absconds and is lost to follow-up.

Three months later, the TB nurse specialists are contacted by staff from a nearby hospital informing them that Mr Evans has been admitted to one of their negative pressure rooms. He is unwell with fevers, weight loss and a productive cough. His chest X-ray shows multilobar shadowing. He has informed them that he received some treatment for TB, but stopped this as he had felt better. They now suspect that he may have drug-resistant TB.

What is drug-resistant tuberculosis?

When bacteria multiply they develop mutations that may confer resistance to one or more drugs used to treat TB:

- Resistant organisms are defined as those that need four or more times the usual drug concentration to kill them or inhibit their growth
- Multidrug-resistant TB (MDR-TB) is infection with *M. tuberculosis* resistant to isoniazid and rifampicin, which are the two most important drugs used in the treatment of TB
- Extreme drug-resistant TB (XDR-TB) is infection with *M. tuberculosis* resistant to usual antituberculous treatment and to three out of six available second line drugs used for MDR-TB

How do patients acquire drug-resistant tuberculosis?

- Fully sensitive TB may become drug-resistant if:
  - clinicians prescribe inadequate treatment (e.g. do not use multiple drugs)
  - patients do not adhere to the treatment regimen, as in Mr Evans' case
- Patients may become infected by a drug-resistant strain of *M. tuberculosis*

Why is multidrug-resistant tuberculosis a major concern?

Multidrug-resistant TB is difficult to treat because some or all of the drugs usually used in quadruple therapy are ineffective. This means that patients:

- Remain infectious for longer
- Are more likely to die and less likely to be cured
- Need alternative drugs that:
  - are much more expensive and more difficult to use than usual therapy
  - may be associated with greater toxicity than usual treatment

The problems are magnified further in XDR-TB, which may be untreatable.

The treatment of MDR-TB is specialized and complex and should only be undertaken at recognized centres with experience of managing such patients.

What is a negative pressure room?

This is a room where the ventilation system is designed to remove air from the room to the outside of the building, creating a negative pressure inside the room. Air is thus drawn into the room. This prevents infectious particles escaping from the room into the corridor and reduces or prevents cross-infection. Any patient with suspected MDR-TB should be isolated in a negative pressure room to prevent spread of this infection which is difficult to treat. Staff and visitors entering the room also need to wear face masks that meet health and safety criteria.

> **!RED FLAG**
>
> Patients with suspected MDR-TB should immediately be isolated in a negative pressure room until MDR-TB is ruled out or confirmed and treated.

Why did the nearby hospital suspect that Mr Evans had multidrug-resistant tuberculosis?

Mr Evans had previous inadequate treatment for TB, which could have resulted in emergence of drug-resistant organisms. Other factors in the history associated with an increased risk of drug-resistant disease include:

1 Contact with another patient known to have drug-resistant disease
2 Birth in foreign country, particularly sub-Saharan Africa and the Indian Subcontinent
3 HIV infection
4 Residence in London
5 Age 25–44
6 Male gender

How can multidrug-resistant tuberculosis be treated?

Treatment should be started before drug sensitivities are available. A detailed history and information from other organizations should be sought to find out what drugs the patient has already been exposed to. The clinicians should then start treatment with 3–4 alternative antituberculosis drugs that the patient has not received previously. When the results of drug resistance testing are known the regimen can be tailored accordingly. Treatment for MDR-TB is usually longer than for fully sensitive TB and less likely to be successful. Surgery may sometimes have a place in MDR-TB treatment. For example, if disease is confined to one or two lobes, lobectomy may offer a better chance of cure than continued drug treatment.

Mr Evans is started on treatment with six antituberculosis drugs (rifampicin, isoniazid, pyrazinamide, amikacin, clarithromycin and ciprofloxacin). On sensitivity testing he has a strain of M. tuberculosis that is resistant to rifampicin

and isoniazid, but sensitive to the other four drugs, which are continued. He is advised that he must stay in isolation until his sputum is culture negative. At this point he attempts to leave the ward.

What are your concerns around him leaving the ward?

He has MDR-TB, is infectious and may spread the disease to others. He thus poses a public health risk and should not leave the ward until he is no longer infectious.

Is there any way he can be prevented from leaving?

Discussion and reasoning should be tried first. If all else fails, Section 38 of the Public Health (control of disease) Act 1984 can be used to detain him. Section 38 authorizes the 'detention for a period specified in the order' of a person with TB (or other named contagious diseases). The hospital has to apply for an order to a local magistrate. There is a time limit set against the order but it can be extended as often as is necessary. If a patient leaves hospital the court may order that he is brought back to the hospital. The act does not, however, allow treatment to be enforced upon the patient.

Outcome. Mr Evans is eventually persuaded to remain in hospital and continue with treatment. After 2 months his sputum is culture negative for M. tuberculosis and he is discharged. He remains under close supervision and this time successfully completes 9 months of treatment, which results in cure of his TB, although his chest X-ray shows residual pulmonary scarring.

CASE REVIEW

Mr Evans is admitted to hospital with smear-positive pulmonary TB and commences quadruple antituberculosis therapy. He has a past history of intravenous drug use and homelessness and is living in a hostel. In view of his unstable social circumstances he remains in hospital until his sputum is smear-negative for acid-fast bacilli, then is discharged to receive DOT in the community. He absconds before completing treatment, but re-presents 3 months later with MDR-TB. This time he is required to stay in hospital until his sputum is culture negative for TB as he is considered to be a public health risk. He is treated with second line antituberculosis medication for 9 months and is cured of his MDR-TB.

KEY POINTS

- Patients with active pulmonary disease are likely to have infected close contacts
- Contact tracing should be used to identify contacts of the 'index case', who should be invited for screening
- The aims of screening are to identify those:
  - with active tuberculous disease who require treatment
  - with latent *M. tuberculosis* infection who require prophylactic treatment to reduce the risk of developing active disease
  - who are not infected with *M. tuberculosis* but who require BCG vaccination
- The core components of contact screening are clinical assessment, Mantoux testing and chest X-ray. IFN-γ testing may be used to detect latent TB
- Patients with TB must receive a full course of treatment with multiple drugs to prevent the emergence of drug-resistant strains of *M. tuberculosis*
- MDR-TB is defined as resistance to rifampicin and isoniazid
- Patients with MDR-TB are infectious for longer, more likely to die and less likely to be cured than patients with fully sensitive TB
- Patients recognized as being at risk of MDR-TB on admission to hospital should be isolated in a negative pressure facility to prevent transmission
- MDR-TB should be treated in recognized centres with experience in treating this condition
- Section 38 of the Public Health Act 1984 can be used to detain a patient with TB against their wishes if they are considered to be a risk to public health, but cannot be used to enforce treatment

A 32-year-old woman with a skin rash and abnormal chest X-ray

Mrs Elaine Manson is a 32-year-old woman who is referred for assessment of a painful rash over both shins. The rash has been present for the last week and she has felt unwell, achy and feverish. On examination she has large raised lumps on the front of her calves.

What is this rash?
This is erythema nodosum, crops of painful red nodules up to 5 cm in diameter which fade to leave bruising and staining of the skin.

What causes erythema nodosum?
It appears to be an immunological reaction which can occur in response to a range of antigenic stimuli (Box 118). Immune complexes are found deposited in the dermal vessels.

How would you distinguish clinically between these causes?
- History of:
  - associated respiratory or gastrointestinal symptoms
  - infection contacts or travel
  - medication use
- Examination:
  - evidence of lymphadenopathy, respiratory disease
- Investigations:
  - chest X-ray
  - full blood count

On questioning Mrs Manson admits to a persistent dry cough over the past 2 months. She is not aware of any exposure to tuberculosis or other infections and had the BCG vaccination aged 14. She does not take any medication and uses condoms for contraception. Examination was unremarkable apart from her erythema nodosum.
Chest X-ray. See Fig. 92

Full blood count:

		Normal range
Haemoglobin (Hb)	13.6 g/dL	(12–16 g/dL)
White cell count (WCC)	4.6×10^9/L	$(4–11 \times 10^9$/L)
Neutrophils	3.8×10^9/L	$(3.5–7.5 \times 10^9$/L)
Lymphocytes	0.6×10^9/L	$(1.5–4 \times 10^9$/L)
Platelets	270×10^9/L	$(150–400 \times 10^9$/L)

What is the differential diagnosis?
- The history of chronic cough would be consistent with sarcoidosis or tuberculosis
- Her chest X-ray shows hilar lymphadenopathy (Box 119), which is bilateral, and some reticular nodular shadowing
- The association of bilateral hilar lymphadenopathy and erythema nodosum is almost always caused by sarcoidosis
- Tuberculosis is less likely, particularly as she has been vaccinated against it and has no known contacts with the disease

What is sarcoidosis?
Sarcoidosis is a condition characterized by the appearance of non-caseating granuloma in multiple tissues and organs. These granulomas can interfere with the normal function of affected organs, causing ill health. Any organ can be affected by sarcoidosis but it most commonly involves the lungs, skin and eyes.

What are granulomas?
Granulomas are small foci of chronic inflammation, involving collections of epithelioid cells, macrophages and T lymphocytes (Fig. 93). They occur in response to chronic antigens or irritants and are found in a number of diseases including sarcoidosis, tuberculosis, fungal infections, Crohn's disease and autoimmune disorders. In sarcoidosis the trigger for formation of granulomas has not been identified.

> **Box 118 Causes of erythema nodosum**
>
> **Infective, e.g.**
> - Streptococcus
> - Tuberculosis
> - Viral
>
> **Inflammatory**
> - Sarcoidosis
> - Inflammatory bowel disease
>
> **Drugs**
> - Sulphonamide antibiotics
> - Oral contraceptive pill

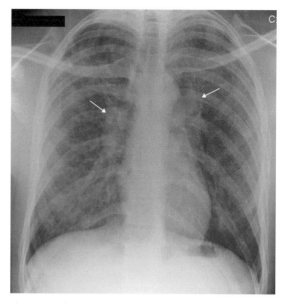

Figure 92 Chest X-ray. Arrows indicate the hila, which are bulky due to lymphadenopathy. There is patchy 'reticulonodular' shadowing throughout both lung fields due to parenchymal lung disease. This is seen as multiple small specks.

> **Box 119 Causes of hilar lymphadenopathy**
>
> - Sarcoidosis (most common cause if bilateral)
> - Tuberculosis
> - Lymphoma
> - Bronchogenic carcinoma

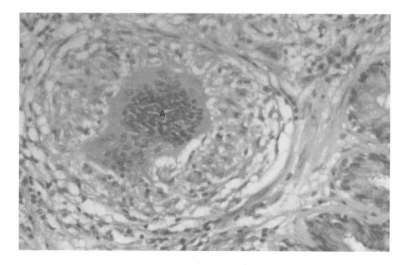

Figure 93 Non-caseating granuloma. Compare this non-caseating granuloma of sarcoidosis to the caseating granuloma caused by tuberculosis shown in Fig. 82, p. 187. The centre of this non-caseating granuloma is cellular (A), containing epithelioid cells, macrophages and T lymphocytes. There is no evidence of central necrosis, seen as (A) amorphous material in Fig. 82.

What is caseation?

If necrosis occurs in the centre of the granuloma this looks soft and cheese-like, so is called caseation (from the Latin '*caseus*' for cheese). Caseation is the hallmark of granulomas caused by tuberculosis. There is little or no necrosis in the centre of a sarcoid granuloma, so this is called a non-caseating granuloma.

How do you interpret her full blood count?

The major abnormality is a low blood lymphocyte count. This probably occurs because lymphocytes are concentrated in the lungs. It does not appear to cause immunosuppression in sarcoidosis patients, as they have no evidence of increased risk of infection or neoplasms.

What further investigations would you arrange?

The diagnosis is most likely to be sarcoidosis, but tuberculosis remains a possibility and should be excluded. Two useful tests can help to distinguish between these diagnoses:

• Tuberculin skin testing (Mantoux or Heaf). This should be positive in tuberculosis, but is negative in sarcoidosis, probably because T lymphocytes are sequestered in the lung, interfering with this cell-mediated immune response

• Fibreoptic bronchoscopy with bronchoalveolar lavage and biopsies for pathological and microbiological examination (see Part 1, Approach to the Patient, p. 33)

Mrs Manson's Mantoux test is negative. At fibreoptic bronchoscopy her airways looked normal, but bronchoalveolar lavage, endobronchial and transbronchial biopsies were performed.

Three days later her pathology results were available. Bronchoalveolar lavage showed a lymphocytosis and was smear-negative for acid-fast bacilli. Non-caseating granulomas, but no acid-fast bacilli, were found in endobronchial and transbronchial biopsies.

How do you explain the lymphocytosis in her lavage?

Increased cell numbers are seen in bronchoalveolar lavage samples from sarcoidosis patients. There is a predominance of T lymphocytes (Box 120), particularly CD4 type, and there is an increased CD4:CD8 ratio.

Why were both endobronchial and transbronchial biopsies taken?

Sarcoidosis can involve the mucosa of the large airways, sampled by endobronchial biopsy, or the lung parenchyma, sampled by transbronchial biopsy. If both types of biopsy are taken this increases the chance of making a positive diagnosis of sarcoidosis at fibreoptic bronchoscopy.

How do you interpret her results?

Her results are strongly suggestive of sarcoidosis and consistently negative for tuberculosis. Her lavage and biopsies should be cultured for mycobacteria and this will take around 8 weeks. Negative cultures will provide further reassurance that she does not have tuberculosis.

Box 120 T lymphocytes

T lymphocytes arise from stem cells in the bone marrow and migrate to the thymus where they mature.

Mature T lymphocytes are found in the circulation and lymphatic tissue, including spleen and lymph nodes. They survey the body for pathogens and if they find these they differentiate further.

• *T lymphocytes differentiated into the CD4 subtype* become T helper cells that regulate the function of other immune cells through release of cytokines and growth factors

• *T lymphocytes differentiated into the CD8 subtype* become cytotoxic T cells whose role is to destroy infected cells or tumour cells

In sarcoidosis, T lymphocytes in the lung are predominantly CD4 type T helper cells. The reason for this is unclear.

Mrs Manson returns to clinic and the diagnosis of sarcoidosis is explained to her. Further investigations are booked and the results are as follows:

Blood tests:

		Normal range
CRP	26 mg/L	(<8 mg/L)
ESR	42 mm/h	(<20 mm/h)
Serum calcium	2.48 mmol/L	
Albumin	40 g/L	(34–48 g/L)
Corrected calcium	2.48 mmol/L	(2.20–2.67 mmol/L)
Serum ACE	126 IU/L	(<80 IU/L)
24-h urine		
Calcium excretion	3 mmol/day	(2.5–7.5 mmol/day)
ECG	Normal	

Lung function

FEV_1 1.9 L (60% predicted), FVC 2.1 L (57% predicted), FEV_1/FVC 90%

Gas transfer 61% predicted

HRCT scan. See Fig. 94

Why did the doctor request all these investigations?

Sarcoidosis can involve any tissue or organ (Box 121). These investigations were performed to look for metabolic or cardiac abnormalities associated with sarcoid. Inflammatory markers, serum angiotensin converting enzyme (ACE) level (see below), lung function tests and high-resolution computed tomography (HRCT) scan assess the severity of sarcoidosis and establish baseline

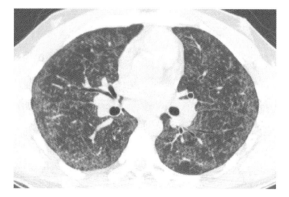

Figure 94 High-resolution CT scan.

values for monitoring of progression or treatment efficacy.

How do you interpret her blood, urine and ECG results?

- Her inflammatory markers are mildly raised. This can be attributed to her sarcoidosis
- Her serum calcium and urinary calcium excretion are reassuringly normal (Box 121)
- Her serum ACE concentrations are raised. This is common, but not invariable, in patients with sarcoidosis, especially if the disease is active as there is some evidence that ACE is synthesized by lung granulomas. Elevated serum ACE levels are supportive but not conclusive evidence of sarcoidosis, as serum ACE is also raised in other conditions (e.g. connective tissue disease). If elevated at diagnosis, changes in serum ACE can be useful in monitoring disease progression or response to treatment
- Her electrocardiogram (ECG) is normal and there is no evidence of cardiac sarcoidosis

How do you interpret her lung function?

- Her FEV_1 is reduced below levels predicted for her age, gender and height. In general, a reduction in FEV_1 can be caused by either obstructive or restrictive lung disease
- Her FVC is reduced by a similar amount to FEV_1 and her FEV_1/FVC ratio is 90%. She thus has a restrictive defect in her lung function
- Her gas transfer between alveoli and capillaries is also reduced
- Taken together these results suggest an abnormality in the lung parenchyma, which is preventing full lung expansion and causing thickening of the alveolar–capillary membrane, interfering with gas transfer. This

Box 121 Tissues and organs affected by sarcoidosis

Any tissue can be affected by sarcoidosis. Apart from lung disease and erythema nodosum manifestations of sarcoidosis include:

Eyes
- Anterior uveitis causes painful red eyes and disturbed vision. Posterior uveitis causes progressive loss of vision

Metabolism
- Abnormal macrophages increase activation of vitamin D, causing hypercalcaemia. Symptoms of this include constipation, depression and increased urinary calcium excretion with kidney stone formation

Bones
- Sarcoidosis affecting the bones can cause cysts and swelling

Skin
- Infiltration of the skin causes chilblain-like lesions called lupus pernio

Spleen
- Splenomegaly may occur with sequestration of blood cells, thrombocytopenia and anaemia

Bone marrow
- Involvement may exacerbate haematological abnormalities

Heart
- Cardiac involvement is rare but may lead to heart block, arrhythmias and myocardial dysfunction

Nervous system
- Involvement is also rare but includes meningoencephalitis, peripheral neuropathy and cranial nerve palsies

abnormality could be caused by infiltration of alveolar walls and interstitium with chronic inflammatory cells, leading to the formation of sarcoid granulomas

Do the HRCT findings fit with the abnormal lung function results?

Her HRCT shows multiple small nodules consistent with chronic inflammatory cells in the interstitium. She also has hilar lymphadenopathy.

Summarize Mrs Manson's clinical condition

It is useful to do this before deciding on a management plan.

> Mrs Manson has a firm diagnosis of sarcoidosis with evidence of:
> - Erythema nodosum
> - Symptomatic (cough) stage II lung disease – hilar lymphadenopathy with non-fibrotic parenchymal disease (Box 122)
>
> There is no evidence of other organ involvement.

How should her sarcoidosis be treated?

The treatment of sarcoidosis is difficult and controversial. As the cause of sarcoidosis is not fully understood, treatment comprises immunosuppression for active disease causing functional impairment. The treatment that works best is corticosteroids, although these potentially have serious side-effects, especially if used long term. Steroid-sparing agents may also be used to minimize the dosage of steroids required (Box 123). The decision to treat should be a joint one between the doctor and patient, weighing up the pros of symptomatic and functional improvement against the cons of treatment side-effects and potential lack of effectiveness.

Box 122 Staging of sarcoidosis

This staging system has some practical use as it may guide treatment:
Stage I. Bilateral hilar lymphadenopathy without evidence of parenchymal disease
Stage II. Bilateral hilar lymphadenopathy with non-fibrotic parenchymal disease
Stage III. Non-fibrotic parenchymal lung disease alone (hilar nodes are shrinking, therefore not seen)
Stage IV. Fibrosis and distortion of the lung

Box 123 Some immunosuppressant drugs used as steroid-sparing agents in the treatment of sarcoidosis

- Azathioprine
- Methotrexate
- Cyclophosphamide
- Chlorambucil

> After a long discussion the doctor and Mrs Manson agree that she should have a trial of steroid treatment as she has:
> - Symptoms
> - Evidence of functional impairment of her lungs
>   She commences 30 mg/day prednisolone. Before starting treatment she asks the doctor what the chances are of her being cured.

How should the doctor answer Mrs Manson's question?

There is a good chance that her sarcoidosis could resolve. Studies have shown that:
- 30–50% patients remit spontaneously over a period of up to 3 years
- 20–30% patients remain stable over 5–10 years
- Around 30% progress over 5–10 years

However, sarcoidosis that comes on acutely with erythema nodosum is more likely to resolve spontaneously than disease with a more insidious onset.

How should the doctor monitor her sarcoidosis to determine whether treatment is successful?

The aims of prednisolone are to reduce disease activity, hence reducing symptoms and improving function. Treatment could therefore be monitored by:
- *Disease activity:*
  - levels of inflammatory markers (CRP and ESR) and serum ACE would be expected to fall in response to treatment
  - chronic inflammation seen as reticulonodular shadowing on the chest X-ray and HRCT should reduce or resolve. This can be monitored radiologically, ideally by chest X-ray rather than HRCT to minimize radiation dose
- *Symptoms.* These can be monitored by patient reporting at follow-up visits
- *Function.* Repeat measures of lung function should indicate reduction in restrictive defect and improvement in gas transfer as parenchymal changes are reduced

> Outcome. Mrs Manson took 30 mg/day prednisolone for 1 month, at which time she reported that her cough was much less and she had no further erythema nodosum. Her prednisolone dosage was gradually reduced by 5 mg every 4 weeks. At 4 months, on 10 mg/day prednisolone, her lung function abnormalities had resolved and her chest X-ray appeared normal. After 6 months she was able to stop prednisolone altogether with no ill effects. Two years later she remained asymptomatic with stable lung function and a normal chest X-ray.

CASE REVIEW

Elaine Manson presents with a painful rash over both shins and a 2-month history of dry cough. Endobronchial and transbronchial biopsies show non-caseating granulomas consistent with sarcoidosis. The major differential diagnosis for her presentation is tuberculosis, but this is excluded as her Mantoux test is negative and there is no evidence of infection with acid-fast bacilli. HRCT scanning shows that she has stage II sarcoidosis with bilateral hilar lymphadenopathy and non-fibrotic parenchymal disease. As she has symptoms and impairment of lung function on testing she is treated with a reducing course of prednisolone over 6 months. Her symptoms and chest X-ray abnormalities resolve and 2 years later she remains asymptomatic with stable lung function and a normal chest X-ray.

KEY POINTS

- Sarcoidosis is a condition characterized by the appearance of non-caseating granulomas in multiple tissues and organs. The cause is not fully understood
- Tissues and organs affected by sarcoidosis include:
  - lungs
  - skin
  - eyes
  - bones
  - bone marrow and spleen
  - heart
  - CNS
- Non-caseating granulomas in affected organs can interfere with normal function, causing ill health
- Sarcoidosis usually presents with respiratory symptoms, erythema nodosum, rheumatological or ophthalmological complaints or hypercalcaemia, or may be asymptomatic
- Sarcoidosis is diagnosed by a combination of:
  - clinical features
  - demonstration of non-caseating granulomas in biopsies of affected tissues
  - radiological appearance
- Pulmonary sarcoidosis is staged radiologically:
  - *Stage I.* Bilateral hilar lymphadenopathy without evidence of parenchymal disease
  - *Stage II.* Bilateral hilar lymphadenopathy with non-fibrotic parenchymal disease
  - *Stage III.* Non-fibrotic parenchymal lung disease alone (hilar nodes are shrinking, therefore not seen)
  - *Stage IV.* Fibrosis and distortion of the lung
- Sarcoidosis should be treated with immunosuppression if there is evidence of active disease causing functional impairment or symptoms
- The treatment of sarcoidosis is glucocorticoids. However, these have side-effects including:
  - metabolic effects such as diabetes mellitus, osteoporosis, weight gain and hypertension
  - increased susceptibility to infection
  - adrenal suppression
- Steroid-sparing agents may be used to reduce the dose of glucocorticoids required
- The prognosis for patients with sarcoidosis is:
  - 30–50% remit spontaneously over a period of up to 3 years
  - 20–30% remain stable over 5–10 years
  - around 30% progress over 5–10 years

A 68-year-old woman with worsening breathlessness on exertion

Mrs Borg is a 68-year-old woman who presents to her GP complaining of shortness of breath. This has been coming on for several months and she is now panting when going up a slight incline or doing housework. She is not breathless at rest or at night. She denies other symptoms including cough, chest pain, palpitations or ankle swelling.

She has no significant past medical history or significant family history.

She is not on any medication.

She has never smoked, has spent her life bringing up her family and has no pets.

Summarize the main features of her history

Isolated shortness of breath on exertion in a 68-year-old woman.

What is your differential diagnosis so far?

• *Respiratory or cardiac disease.* These are the most common causes of shortness of breath. However, she has no associated features or risk factors to point to either of these systems as the source of her breathlessness

• *Anaemia.* This could account for shortness of breath with no other cardiorespiratory symptoms

• *Other diagnoses.* In the absence of cardiac or respiratory features other diagnoses that should be considered include:
   ○ renal failure
   ○ thyroid disease
   ○ breast disease with pulmonary involvement (pleural effusion, lymphatic involvement)

The GP examines Mrs Borg.

She has no pallor or cyanosis. She has finger clubbing. Breast, thyroid and lymph node examination are normal.

Pulse 68 beats/min, regular, jugular venous pressure (JVP) not elevated, blood pressure 112/72 mmHg.

Heart sounds normal, no murmurs, no ankle oedema.

Chest. Trachea midline, expansion and percussion normal, auscultation – bilateral basal end-inspiratory crepitations.

Abdominal examination is normal and there is no hepatomegaly.

How do you interpret these findings?

Inspiratory crepitations indicate a pathological process involving the alveoli or airways (Box 124). As Mrs Borg's crepitations are bilateral they are most likely caused by pulmonary oedema or fibrosis.

At this stage, pulmonary fibrosis appears more likely than oedema as the cause of her crepitations as:

• She has finger clubbing, which is seen with fibrosis

• She does not have any other signs of heart failure (her JVP is normal and she has no peripheral oedema or hepatomegaly)

There is no evidence of anaemia, thyroid or breast disease on examination.

What should Mrs Borg's GP do next?

Mrs Borg's GP should order some basic investigations to:

• Distinguish between her differential diagnoses

• Determine whether Mrs Borg can be managed in the community or needs a specialist opinion

• Decide which specialist service Mrs Borg should be referred to if required (respiratory, cardiac or other)

What investigations should the GP order?

• Chest X-ray – to look for the cause of her crepitations and assess heart size

• ECG – to look for heart disease that might be causing pulmonary oedema

• Blood tests to look for anaemia, thyroid or renal disease

Mrs Borg returned 1 week later for the results of her investigations. Her GP checked the results, which were as follows.

Chest X-ray report: 'There is volume loss bilaterally with areas of reticular shadowing at both bases' (Fig. 95)

ECG: normal.

Blood tests: normal.

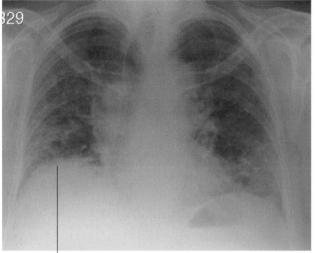

(a)

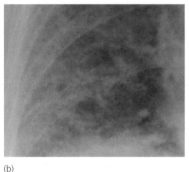

(b)

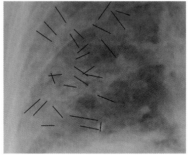

(c)

Figure 95 (a) Chest X-ray.
(b) Enlargement of the right lower lung field shows multiple fine white lines and nodules which as emphasized in (c) with drawn lines.

Box 124 Causes of crepitations

Crepitations can originate in the alveoli or airways

Alveolar causes
Alveolar crepitations are often fine, like crumpling an empty crisp packet
• Fluid in the alveoli:
  ○ pulmonary oedema
  ○ pneumonia (inflammatory exudate)
• Inflammation or fibrosis in or around the alveoli:
  ○ pulmonary fibrosis
  ○ extrinsic allergic alveolitis

Airways
Crepitations can be caused by secretions in the airway. These crepitations are usually coarser and lower pitched:
• Bronchitis
• Bronchiectasis
• Bronchiolitis

What is reticular shadowing?

The word reticular comes from the Latin 'reticulum' which is the diminutive of 'rete', meaning a net. Reticular shadowing on a chest X-ray is a term used to describe 'netlike' shadowing, caused by multiple fine white lines crossing over each other. These fine white lines are caused by thickening of the interstitium resulting from inflammation or fibrosis.

How does this information affect your differential diagnosis?

The chest X-ray findings support the diagnosis of pulmonary fibrosis, which was considered most likely after examining Mrs Borg. The investigation results rule out anaemia, renal and thyroid disease and make cardiac disease less likely.

What should the GP do now?

Mrs Borg should be referred for a specialist opinion from a hospital respiratory physician to:

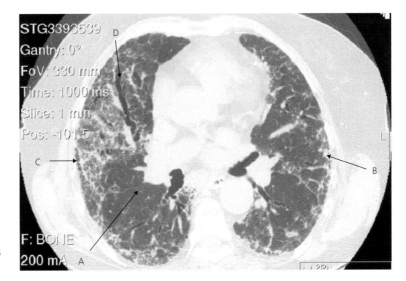

Figure 96 High-resolution CT scan.
(A) Relatively normal area of lung tissue. (B) The dense white tissue, particularly seen towards the edge of the lung, is caused by fibrosis.
(C) Fibrosis replaces normal lung tissue and causes holes to appear surrounded by thick white lines. This is called 'honeycombing'. An early example is seen in this scan.
(D) Fibrosis pulls on the walls of the airways, making them baggy and dilated. This is called 'traction bronchiectasis' and a good example is seen in this scan.

- Confirm the diagnosis
- Look for underlying causes
- Establish the type of condition and prognosis
- Consider treatment options

Mrs Borg was referred for a respiratory opinion. The consultant agreed with the GP's examination findings and arranged a high-resolution CT scan to look for interstitial lung disease (Fig. 96).

What does the high-resolution CT scan show?

Lung tissue normally looks light grey and is 'homogeneous', which means it looks the same throughout the lung fields. In this CT scan patches of the lung look normal (A), but other patches have been replaced by dense white tissue (B) which is fibrosis. The fibrosis contracts the lung, pulling other parts of the lung out of place. This can be seen as honeycombing (C) and traction bronchiectasis (D).

What type of disease is this?

The terminology of this type of disease is very complicated as it has a number of names:

• It is often referred to as pulmonary fibrosis or fibrosing alveolitis, particularly in older text books
• It is a type of 'interstitial lung disease' or 'interstitial pneumonia', so-called because the pathological changes appear to start in or involve the interstitium (i.e. the space in between the cells)

• Another term for this group of lung diseases is 'diffuse parenchymal lung diseases' (DPLD). The lung parenchyma refers to the alveoli, capillaries and supporting tissue. As can be seen from the CT scan, this disease affects the alveoli and capillaries as well as the lung interstitium, hence the use of this more inclusive term

For the rest of the case this group of diseases will be referred to as DPLD.

What causes DPLD?

This term encompasses over 200 different conditions, which present with related clinical features and have a wide range of causes. The simplest classification of DPLD is:

• DPLD of known cause or association (Box 125)
• DPLD of unknown cause (Box 126)

How should the consultant proceed with Mrs Borg's assessment?

It is important to establish:

• Whether there is an identifiable cause for her DPLD
• How the lung disease is affecting her lung function

KEY POINT

The cause of DPLD is assessed primarily by taking a meticulous history, including asking about occupational and environmental exposure in detail, then by examination.

Box 125 Diffuse parenchymal lung disease of known cause or association

Occupation or environmental exposure
- Inorganic chemicals, e.g.
  - asbestos
  - coal
  - silica
- Organic agents:
  - causes of extrinsic allergic alveolitis (Box 129, p. 222)

Drugs and toxins
- Oral drugs, e.g.
  - amiodarone
  - methotrexate
- Illicit drugs, e.g.
  - heroin
  - crack cocaine
- Radiation

Associated with systemic disease
- Connective tissue disease, e.g.
  - systemic sclerosis
  - rheumatoid arthritis
  - systemic lupus erythematosus
- Vasculitis
- Cancer

Box 126 Diffuse parenchymal lung disease of unknown cause

- Idiopathic interstitial pneumonias
- Granulomatous disease, including sarcoidosis
- Other forms

Patients should also have the following investigations:
- Full blood count and eosinophils (hypersensitivity), erythrocyte sedimentation rate (ESR)
- Renal and hepatic function
- Rheumatoid factor and antinuclear antibodies (connective tissue disease)

Other investigations will depend on history and examination findings and could include:
- Other autoantibodies if the history or examination are indicative of connective tissue disease or vasculitis
- Serum precipitins if there is a history of environmental exposure
- Serum angiotensin converting enzyme (ACE) if there is any suggestion of sarcoidosis

The effect of DPLD on her lungs should be assessed by:
- Full lung function testing
- Oxygen saturations, followed by arterial blood gases if abnormal

Mrs Borg had no features on history, examination or investigation to indicate an identifiable underlying cause for her DPLD.

Lung function:

FEV$_1$	*1.25 L (58% predicted)*
FVC	*1.45 L (57% predicted)*
FEV$_1$ % FVC	*86%*
Transfer factor	*43% predicted*
Residual volume	*1.55 L (86% predicted)*
Total lung capacity	*3.0 L (65% predicted)*

Oxygen saturations were 94% on air

How do you explain her lung function results?
Spirometry
Her FEV_1 and FVC are reduced proportionately. This is a restrictive lung defect and indicates reduced lung expansion. This is the usual finding in patients with DPLD as inflammation and fibrosis replace some alveoli and restrict expansion of others. The airways are largely spared apart from some traction bronchiectasis; hence there is no evidence of airflow obstruction.

Lung volumes
The reduction in lung volumes is also shown as a reduction in total lung capacity (TLC), which is a measure of lung volume at maximum inspiration.

The residual volume (air left in the 'dead space' of the lungs on maximum expiration) is unaffected by parenchymal changes and is normal.

Gas transfer
Loss of alveoli and capillaries resulting from fibrosis reduces the surface area available for gas transfer. This also explains the slight hypoxia measured on pulse oximetry.

What is the diagnosis?
Mrs Borg has DPLD of unknown cause, also known as idiopathic interstitial pneumonia.

Are there different types of idiopathic interstitial pneumonia?
The most common type is idiopathic pulmonary fibrosis, previously known as cryptogenic fibrosing alveolitis. The

Box 127 Classification of idiopathic interstitial pneumonias

- Idiopathic pulmonary fibrosis
- Other interstitial pneumonias, e.g.
  - desquamative interstitial pneumonia
  - non-specific interstitial pneumonia
  - respiratory bronchiolitis-associated interstitial lung disease
  - cryptogenic organizing pneumonia
  - lymphoid interstitial pneumonia

histological findings seen on lung biopsy from patients with this clinical diagnosis are referred to as usual interstitial pneumonia. Other types are listed in Box 127.

Is it important to tell between these types?

The different types of idiopathic interstitial pneumonia each have different natural history, prognosis and treatment response; therefore it is useful to distinguish between them.

How can you tell between the types of idiopathic interstitial pneumonia?

The different types of idiopathic interstitial pneumonia are defined by clinical and pathological behaviour. Clinicians, radiologists and pathologists therefore must work as a team to combine information from history and examination, radiology and pathology to make a final diagnosis. The diagnosis can often be made from clinical information and using the CT scans. Sometimes a lung biopsy is required.

How are lung biopsies taken?

There are three main methods, all of which can be complicated by haemorrhage, pneumothorax and are associated with a small risk of death.

Open lung biopsy

- A surgical incision is made in the chest wall (thoracotomy) and a piece of lung is removed
- A general anaesthetic is required and the complication (7%) and mortality (<1%) rates are the highest for any form of lung biopsy
- The diagnostic yield is good

Video assisted thoracoscopic (VATS) lung biopsy

- A fibreoptic endoscope and operating instruments are inserted into the thorax through small holes in the chest wall and used to take biopsies from the periphery of the lung
- This has similar diagnostic yield but probably less complications than open lung biopsy

Transbronchial lung biopsy

- A biopsy forceps is inserted as deep as possible into the lungs through a bronchoscope and a biopsy taken of the airway wall and associated lung parenchyma
- This has the advantages of being a relatively safe outpatient procedure which does not require a general anaesthetic. However, it has lower diagnostic yield than open or VATS lung biopsies

Mrs Borg's case was reviewed at the multidisciplinary team meeting. The radiologists felt that her CT findings were consistent with idiopathic pulmonary fibrosis. On discussion the team agreed that this was a firm diagnosis and there was no need for a lung biopsy.

What is the natural history of idiopathic pulmonary fibrosis?

Idiopathic pulmonary fibrosis (IPF) is a progressive disease with a poor prognosis. The median survival for a patient with this diagnosis is less than 3 years.

Is there any treatment available for idiopathic pulmonary fibrosis?

Immunosuppression is used in an attempt to stop inflammation of the lung progressing to fibrosis. However, this treatment is not very effective, possibly because the fibrosis occurs without prior inflammation. Additionally, treatment may have considerable adverse effects. Patients may receive a treatment trial with:

- Corticosteroids
- A second immunosuppressive agent such as azathioprine (Box 128)

Disease is monitored using symptoms, radiology and lung function. If there is improvement treatment may continue; if there is no improvement or deterioration treatment is usually discontinued.

What should the consultant discuss with Mrs Borg when she returns to clinic?

It will be a difficult consultation for them both. Ethical principles governing the consultation should include the following.

> **Box 128 Pharmacology of azathioprine**
>
> **Mechanism of action**
> Metabolized to mercaptopurine which interferes with nucleic acid metabolism during white cell proliferation after antigen stimulation. Particularly active against T cells.
>
> **Uses in respiratory disease**
> As a steroid-sparing agent for immunosuppression in diffuse parenchymal lung disease resulting from known and unknown causes.
>
> **Pharmacokinetics**
> Precursor of mercaptopurine, which is the active molecule.
>
> **Major side-effects**
> • Hepatitis
> • Bone marrow suppression
> • Hair loss

Autonomy

Mrs Borg is entitled to understand her diagnosis and prognosis to allow her to plan her future. She also needs to be given full information about the likely benefits and possible harm of treatment so she can decide whether to go ahead with therapy.

Non-malifience (do no harm)

The diagnosis and prognosis must be discussed realistically but compassionately so as not to destroy hope. As available treatment is not very effective, it is particularly important that Mrs Borg is aware of the risks of treatment and supported if she chooses not to go ahead.

Mrs Borg is concerned about her diagnosis and keen to try any treatment available, whatever the side-effects. She is started on prednisolone and azathioprine and returns to clinic regularly for monitoring. However, she deteriorates despite therapy and at her 12-month review she is found to be short of breath at rest with oxygen saturations of 88%. She is very distressed by her rapid decline and asks you whether she might be a candidate for a lung transplant.

How would you answer her question?

Transplantation of solid organs is usually not offered to patients over 60 years of age because of comorbidities that affect the success of transplantation and lack of available organs. However, patients with IPF who are otherwise well should be discussed with the transplant centre up to the age of 65. Unfortunately, Mrs Borg is now 69 years old and is not a candidate for transplantation.

Lung transplantation has a 1 year survival of approximately 80% and 3-year survival of approximately 55%, therefore it is worth considering in younger patients with severe IPF.

What management plan would you recommend?

• Corticosteroids and azathioprine are not preventing deterioration of her IPF and should be stopped as they potentially have severe side-effects and may cause more harm than good
• Her hypoxia should be treated with continuous oxygen both at home and when she is out (ambulatory oxygen). Oxygen may:
  ○ improve symptoms and increase activity
  ○ prevent secondary pulmonary hypertension and cor pulmonale
• Palliative care

Outcome. Mrs Borg remains extremely distressed at her condition and lack of treatment options. She requests a second opinion and although the diagnosis and prognosis are the same at the second hospital she is entered into a clinical trial. Despite the trial therapy she deteriorates and is started on oxygen therapy. She is referred to her local hospice and therapy including relaxation, benzodiazepines and opiates are used to control her anxiety. Several months later she has lost weight and is unable to care for herself at home. She is admitted to the hospice, where she dies peacefully.

CASE REVIEW

Mrs Borg presents with worsening shortness of breath over several months. On examination she has finger clubbing and bilateral basal end-inspiratory crepitations. High-resolution CT scanning indicates pulmonary fibrosis and, as clinical assessment and investigation fail to identify an underlying cause, a diagnosis of idiopathic pulmonary fibrosis is made. Mrs Borg has a trial of treatment with prednisolone and azathioprine, but deteriorates despite therapy. At this stage she has no further therapeutic options as she does not meet criteria for consideration for lung transplantation. She is commenced on home oxygen and referred to her local hospice for palliative support.

KEY POINTS

- The term 'lung parenchyma' refers to the lung alveoli, capillaries and supporting tissue
- The term 'diffuse parenchymal lung diseases' encompasses a group of conditions where the pathology (inflammation and fibrosis) affects the lung parenchyma
- The cause of DPLD may be unknown (idiopathic pulmonary fibrosis) or of known cause or association, e.g.
  - occupational or environmental exposure
  - drugs or toxins
  - associated with systemic disease (e.g. connective tissue disease)
- Patients with DPLD usually present with shortness of breath or cough and may have finger clubbing and end-inspiratory bibasal crepitations on auscultation of the lung bases
- Structural changes of DPLD are best identified by a high-resolution CT scan of the thorax

- Patients with radiological evidence of DPLD require meticulous review of history and investigation to look for an underlying cause
- A lung biopsy may be performed to make a histological diagnosis of DPLD type. The benefits of lung biopsy in determining treatment and prognosis should be weighed against the risks of haemorrhage, pneumothorax and small risk of death
- Idiopathic pulmonary fibrosis is a progressive disease with median survival of less than 3 years from diagnosis
- Treatment of IPF with immunosuppression (prednisolone and azathioprine) is not very effective
- Transplantation may be considered for patients with IPF who are otherwise well up to the age of 65 years
- Patients with end-stage IPF may require home oxygen and palliative care support

Case 28 A 35-year-old man with chronic shortness of breath

A 35-year-old man, Robert Stephens, is referred for a respiratory opinion. He has noticed increased shortness of breath over the last 6–8 months. He now finds he is breathless when hurrying and cannot keep up with his girlfriend when they shop together. At night he is able to lie flat and sleeps well without waking. His breathlessness is associated with a dry cough which has also been present for several months and occurs more during the day than at night. He has not noticed chest pain, palpitations, ankle swelling or wheeze. He has no night sweats and feels he has put on 1–2 stone in weight over the past year. He has no significant past medical history.

How would you summarize the information available so far?

Chronic shortness of breath and cough in a young man (under 40) with associated weight gain.

What is your differential diagnosis for this presentation?

Breathlessness is most commonly caused by respiratory disease, cardiac disease or anaemia. Other diagnoses including renal failure, thyroid disease and anxiety should also be considered. In Mr Stephen's case the following should be considered.

Respiratory disease

• The associated chronic cough makes respiratory disease the most likely cause of his breathlessness
• Asthma is a common cause of breathlessness and cough in young people. However, the lack of nocturnal symptoms and onset at age 35 are less typical features of this disease
• Chronic obstructive pulmonary disease (COPD) is unlikely in a man of 35 years, but possible if he has had heavy cigarette smoke exposure or a genetic predisposition (α_1-antitrypsin deficiency).
• Most other respiratory diseases could cause this presentation including:

○ tuberculosis (TB)
○ interstitial lung disease and alveolitis
○ chronic thromboembolic disease

None of these seem particularly likely so far in a previously well young man with associated weight gain.

Cardiac disease

There are no clinical features to indicate a cardiac cause.

Anaemia

This is unusual in a young man.

Other

• Hypothyroidism could cause weight gain with deconditioning and breathlessness
• Anxiety is a possible cause of his symptoms, but he needs further assessment before this should be considered

What other questions would you ask to help make a diagnosis?

The differential diagnosis is still very broad at this stage. It would be helpful to ask about risk factors and associated features relating to the possible diagnoses.

Respiratory disease

• *Asthma.* A personal or family history of atopy (asthma, eczema, hayfever) or seasonal variation in symptoms, with exacerbations in the pollen (spring) or fungal spore (autumn) season could support this diagnosis
• *COPD.* A smoking history of at least 20 pack years or a history of emphysema in young family members might point to COPD as a cause for his symptoms
• *Tuberculosis.* Risk factors for TB include recent immigration, homelessness, overcrowded living conditions, immunosuppression including HIV infection or diabetes or known contacts with TB
• *Interstitial lung disease and alveolitis.* Possible precipitants for interstitial lung disease and alveolitis include occupational exposure, associated connective tissue

disease and exposure to organic antigens from animals, birds or fungi. You should also ask about associated features of sarcoidosis (skin, eye, bone involvement)

• *Chronic thromboembolic disease.* You should ask about immobility, travel history and family history of thromboembolic disease

Other

• *Hypothyroidism.* Associated symptoms could include cold intolerance, constipation, altered appearance and depression.

> Mr Stephens has never smoked and has no personal or family history of respiratory or thromboembolic disease or atopy. He is otherwise well and has no joint, skin or eye symptoms. He was born in the UK, has worked as an accountant since completing his training and is not aware of any occupational exposure to toxins or allergens or exposure to TB infection. Twelve months ago he moved into his girlfriend's flat where she keeps a budgerigar.
>
> On examination he looked well. Oxygen saturations were 97% on air and pulse was 84 beats/min, regular. He had a body mass index of 32 kg/m². There were no abnormal examination findings.

How does this information affect the differential diagnosis?

• The only positive finding in his history is 1 year of contact with a budgerigar, with exposure starting around 4 months before his symptoms commenced. His symptoms could be caused by respiratory allergy to this bird, either:
  ○ asthma; or
  ○ extrinsic allergic alveolitis
• His body mass index is elevated and obesity and deconditioning could also account for his symptoms
• Lack of any smoking history makes COPD very unlikely
• Normal pulse rate and lack of other symptoms make hypothyroidism less likely, although weight gain could be brought about by an underactive thyroid gland
• There is no history to support TB or thromboembolic disease

---

KEY POINT

Patients often do not mention that they keep birds when asked about pets. It pays to ask specifically and repeatedly about bird exposure to jog their memories and to ask family members.

What investigations would you do at this clinic visit?

Investigations that could be performed immediately and would give useful information to guide further management are:
• Spirometry to look for obstructive or restrictive lung disease
• Chest X-ray to look for parenchymal lung disease
• To exclude other diagnoses:
  ○ electrocardiogram (ECG) to exclude cardiac disease
  ○ full blood count to exclude anaemia
  ○ thyroid function tests to rule out hypothyroidism

> Investigation results were as follows:
> Spirometry: FEV_1 2.2 L (62% predicted), FVC 2.8 L (67% predicted), FEV_1/FVC 79%
> Chest X-ray report: there is diffuse shadowing throughout the lungs with a nodular quality
> ECG, full blood count and thyroid function tests: normal.

How do you interpret these results?

Spirometry shows an equal reduction in both FEV_1 and FVC with an FEV_1/FVC ratio >70%. This is consistent with restrictive lung disease.

The chest X-ray shows some diffuse shadowing, which needs further imaging by high-resolution CT (HRCT) scanning.

Other tests reassuringly show no evidence of cardiac disease, anaemia or hypothyroidism.

How do these results modify your differential diagnosis?

Mr Stephens appears to have a restrictive lung disease (Box 129) to account for his chronic cough and breathlessness. As he is a young man and has exposure to bird antigens the most likely diagnosis is extrinsic allergic alveolitis.

Asthma is now less likely because he has no evidence of airflow obstruction and he has an abnormal chest X-ray.

Obesity can cause restrictive lung function, but should not cause an abnormal chest X-ray (Box 129).

What is extrinsic allergic alveolitis?

'Alveolitis' means inflammation of the alveoli. The inflammation actually also affects the small airways, hence this disease is also called 'hypersensitivity pneumonitis'. Extrinsic allergic alveolitis (EAA) is caused by inhalation of organic antigens (Box 130). Susceptible patients develop a hypersensitivity reaction, leading to alveolar

---

> **Box 129 Causes of restrictive lung function (reduction in lung volumes)**
>
> **Pulmonary**
> Lung disease in the interstitium or alveoli restricts expansion of the alveoli, e.g.
> - Interstitial lung disease
> - Alveolitis
>
> **Pleural or chest wall**
> Abnormalities of the pleural or chest wall can constrict the lungs, preventing expansion, e.g.
> - Diffuse bilateral pleural thickening or pleural effusions, e.g. caused by asbestos (benign pleural thickening or mesothelioma) or infection (empyema)
> - Severe obesity (Pickwick's syndrome)
>
> **Neuromuscular disorders**
> Diseases of the nerves or muscles prevent full lung expansion during breathing, e.g.
> - Motor neurone disease
> - Guillain–Barré syndrome
> - Myasthenia gravis
> - Muscular dystrophy

> **Box 130 Causes of extrinsic allergic alveolitis**
>
> Allergens causing EAA come from organic material or organisms growing on organic material. Some examples are:
> - *Bird fancier's lung.* This is caused by antigens secreted by birds that are associated with feather dust (bloom) or found in bird droppings
> - *Farmer's lung.* This is caused by organisms (thermoactinomycetes) growing on hay stored in damp conditions
> - *Humidifier fever.* This is caused by organisms (protozoa – *Naegleria gruberi*, *Thermoactinomyces vulgaris*) growing in contaminated water, which is aerosolized by air conditioners
> - *Maltworker's lung.* This is caused by mouldy barley growing *Aspergillus fumigatus* or *A. clavatus*

and small airway inflammation that impairs gas transfer and causes breathlessness and cough (Fig. 97).

How does extrinsic allergic alveolitis differ from asthma and allergic rhinitis?

These three conditions are all allergic diseases of the respiratory tract. They have a number of important differences.

Anatomy
- Extrinsic allergic alveolitis affects the alveoli and small airways
- Asthma affects the bronchi and larger bronchioles
- Rhinitis affects the nasal epithelium

Allergens
- Extrinsic allergic alveolitis is most commonly caused by bird proteins, fungal and protozoal allergens. Allergens must be small enough (approximately 1 μm) to be deposited in the distal lung
- Asthma and rhinitis are caused by:
  - seasonal allergens – tree and grass pollen (spring), fungal spores (autumn)
  - perennial (year round) allergens – animal and bird proteins, house dust mites

Pathology
- Extrinsic allergic alveolitis is caused by a *type III hypersensitivity* reaction. Inhaled antigens become bound to circulating IgG (precipitins) to that antigen. The resulting immune complexes trigger minor mast cell degranulation and inflammatory cell infiltration, initially with neutrophils then with lymphocytes and macrophages which form granulomas. The reaction and development of symptoms takes 4–12 h after antigen exposure
- Asthma and rhinitis are caused by a *type I hypersensitivity* reaction. Inhaled antigens bind to immunoglobulin E (IgE) on the surface of mast cells, causing mast cell degranulation and release of inflammatory mediators. Increased vascular permeability with oedema, inflammatory infiltrate and bronchoconstriction can come on over 5–10 min

Effect on lung function
- Extrinsic allergic alveolitis causes alveolar and interstitial inflammation which limits lung inflation, causing a restrictive picture on spirometry. As small airways are also involved there may be a component of obstruction
- Asthma causes oedema and constriction of the larger airways, obstructing airflow and causing an obstructive picture on spirometry

How would you investigate Mr Stephens to confirm the diagnosis of extrinsic allergic alveolitis?

Tests should be arranged to look at his lung structure and function and identify histological evidence of alveolitis and immunological evidence of hypersensitivity. The

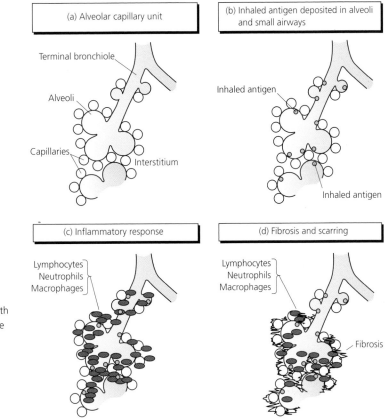

Figure 97 Pathogenesis of extrinsic allergic alveolitis. Inhaled antigens (b) trigger an inflammatory response with cellular inflammation and oedema in the small airways, alveoli and interstitium (c) which impairs gas exchange. If inflammation is chronic, fibrosis and thickening of the alveolar septae and basement membrane occurs causing permanent impairment.

doctor arranged the following tests, which are shown with their results.

> *Transbronchial biopsy: pieces of lung tissue showing non-caseating granulomas with an associated prominent lymphocytic infiltrate and foamy macrophages consistent with EAA.*
>
> *HRCT scan (Fig. 98): demonstrated diffuse ground glass change and mosaicism.*
>
> *Gas transfer: 63% of predicted values.*
>
> *Avian precipitins:*

		Normal range
Budgerigar serum (IgG abs)	*8.1 mg/L*	*(0–40 mg/L)*
Budgerigar feathers (IgG abs)	*72.1 mg/L*	*(0–40 mg/L)*
Budgerigar droppings (IgG abs)	*48 mg/L*	*(0–40 mg/L)*

How do you interpret these results?

• A transbronchial lung biopsy showed inflammatory changes characteristic of the type III hypersensitivity reaction that causes EAA. However, this result is unusually informative as biopsy results are often non-diagnostic

• The inflammatory infiltrate in the alveoli and interstitium looks grey on CT scan images, like ground glass, and replaces air which normally looks black. Mosaicism means that there are some grey patches (A) and some black patches (B) on the images. The black patches are caused by pockets of air trapped in some alveoli by small airway inflammation

• His gas transfer is reduced. This is not surprising because there is inflammation of the alveoli and interstitium which impairs diffusion of oxygen between alveoli and capillaries

• He has elevated avian precipitins (IgG) for budgerigar feathers and droppings. This indicates that he has been exposed to and has an immunological reaction to these antigens. In the context of the other investigation results it is likely that he has subacute EAA (Box 131) caused by chronic inhalation of budgerigar antigens

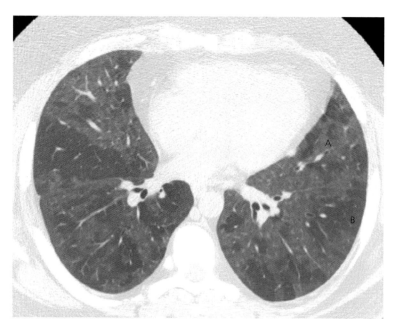

Figure 98 High-resolution CT scan.

Box 131 Classification of extrinsic allergic alveolitis

Acute extrinsic allergic alveolitis
- Acute episodes occur 4–12 h after exposure to antigen
- Reaction proportional to exposure
- Respiratory and systemic symptoms occur, including fever and chills
- Symptoms usually resolve on removal of antigen

Subacute extrinsic allergic alveolitis
- Onset of symptoms more insidious than the acute form, probably because of ongoing antigen exposure

Chronic extrinsic allergic alveolitis
- Fibrosis of the lung secondary to acute or subacute EAA

How should Mr Stephen's subacute extrinsic allergic alveolitis be treated?
Antigen avoidance
This is very important, but can be extremely difficult. In Mr Stephen's case he would be advised to find a new home for the budgerigar. However, people may be reluctant to get rid of their (or their partner's) pets, and even if they do, bird antigens can persist in the home for a long time. In other cases of EAA a change of job may be required.

Immunosuppression
Prednisolone can suppress the type III hypersensitivity reaction and speed recovery of symptoms. However, symptoms may reoccur when steroids are stopped if antigen exposure continues.

Mr Stephens was advised to get rid of the budgerigar and take 30 mg prednisolone for 2 weeks, followed by a reducing dose of steroids to stop after a total of 6 weeks of treatment. Before agreeing to follow this plan he asks how much improvement he can expect in his condition.

How would you answer his question?
If he is able to avoid bird antigens he is likely to make a full recovery. This is likely as he has had a relatively short exposure to the budgerigar, there is no evidence of irreversible fibrosis on his investigations and he is young. The outlook for older patients with more chronic exposure or fibrosis is worse.

Outcome. Mr Stephens takes the prescribed course of steroids and feels much better. He is no longer breathless and his cough disappears. On review in clinic his chest X-ray is now normal and his gas transfer has increased to 92% predicted. His girlfriend agrees to get rid of the budgerigar and they decide to take the opportunity to move from their flat to a larger house. With this antigen avoidance strategy he has no further symptoms.

CASE REVIEW

Robert Stephens presents with a 6–8 month history of shortness of breath and dry cough. Twelve months ago he moved into his girlfriend's flat where she keeps a budgerigar. A combination of insidious onset of symptoms, restrictive lung function abnormality, diffuse ground glass change on HRCT, lymphocytic infiltrate on transbronchial biopsy and positive avian precipitins gives a diagnosis of subacute EAA. He is treated with a course of prednisolone and advised to get rid of the budgerigar. After moving house he has no further symptoms.

KEY POINTS

- Extrinsic allergic alveolitis is inflammation of the alveoli and small airways that occurs as a hypersensitivity reaction to the inhalation of organic antigens
- Organic antigens causing EAA include:
  - bird antigens
  - moulds and other microorganisms (growing on material, e.g. damp hay, contaminated water, mouldy barley)
- Extrinsic allergic alveolitis may be:
  - acute with symptoms immediately following exposure
  - subacute with insidious symptoms probably caused by ongoing antigen exposure
  - chronic with fibrosis of the lung secondary to acute or subacute EAA
- Symptoms of EAA may be respiratory (cough, shortness of breath) and/or systemic (fever and chills)

- Investigation of EAA may show:
  - restrictive defect in lung function with reduced gas transfer
  - patchy ground glass shadowing on HRCT scanning
  - lymphocytic infiltration on pathological examination of transbronchial lung biopsy or bronchoalveolar lavage
  - elevated IgG (precipitins) to the causative antigen
- Treatment of EAA requires avoidance of the causative antigen. This should be permanent if possible to prevent recurrence of alveolitis and development of irreversible fibrosis
- A course of prednisolone can be given to speed recovery of symptoms

Case 29 An overweight 52-year-old man who snores

Mr Callum Campbell is a 52-year-old man who is referred to the sleep clinic by his GP for investigation of his snoring. He is a heavy goods vehicle driver and over the last 10 years he has put on around 4 stones in weight. His wife reports that over a similar time period his snoring has become louder. She has also noticed that he quite frequently stops breathing for several seconds during sleep when he either stirs or she has to shake him awake.

What do you suspect the diagnosis may be?

Obstructive sleep apnoea.

What is obstructive sleep apnoea?

The Scottish Intercollegiate Guidelines Network (www.sign.ac.uk/pdf/sign73.pdf) define obstructive sleep apnoea/hypopnoea syndrome (OSAHS) as 'A condition where the upper airway collapses intermittently and repeatedly during sleep causing either total obstruction of the airway lumen with no respiratory flow (apnoea), or partial obstruction with reduction in the cross-sectional area of the upper airway lumen causing hypoventilation (hypopnoea).'

How does this syndrome account for his wife's observations?

The following cycle occurs:
- As the person falls into a deep sleep, the muscle tone of the upper airway decreases leading to upper airway narrowing:
  - if the narrowing is complete, the patient stops breathing
  - if the narrowing is partial, the patient snores
- Airway narrowing stimulates an increase in inspiratory effort in an attempt to overcome the narrowing
- This causes transient arousal from deep sleep to wakefulness or a lighter sleep phase during which the muscle tone is restored. This arousal may be triggered by

pharyngeal or pleural receptors detecting increased inspiratory effort
- The cycle is completed when the patient then falls back into a deep sleep and muscle tone decreases once again
- The cycle can occur many times throughout the night, disrupting sleep
- The daytime consequences include sleepiness and uncreased risk of cardiovascular disease (Box 136, p. 229)

Why do you think his condition has become worse over the past 10 years?

Mr Campbell has put on 4 stones in weight because of his sedentary occupation and it is likely that his collar size has also increased. Obesity is a major risk factor for obstructive sleep apnoea. The mechanisms underlying this are not fully understood; however, it is likely that the weight of soft tissues in a large neck compresses the pharynx and causes narrowing of the upper airway.

What features in his history would further support your provisional diagnosis of obstructive sleep apnoea?

The main features of obstructive sleep apnoea include:
- History of poor sleep:
  - restless sleep
  - unrefreshing sleep
  - nocturia
- Evidence of upper airways collapse during sleep:
  - choking episodes during sleep
  - witnessed apnoeas
  - snoring
- Daytime problems resulting from poor sleep:
  - excessive daytime sleepiness
  - impaired concentration
  - irritability and personality change
  - decreased libido

Collateral history from a family member is often required to obtain this history as patients may not notice or admit to many of these features.

On further questioning Mr Campbell admits that he does not feel refreshed when waking from sleep and often falls asleep in the evening when watching television. He has never fallen asleep at the wheel when driving. His wife complains that he is restless at night and has become difficult to talk to. He is irritable and forgetful and she feels he has lost interest in sex. Mr Campbell has a 40 pack year smoking history and continues to smoke around 20 cigarettes per day. He drinks 2–3 bottles of beer every night and more at weekends. His Epworth Sleepiness Score (ESS) is 16/24.

How do you interpret this new information?

Mr Campbell has features of disturbed sleep as well as daytime problems resulting from poor sleep. His use of cigarettes and alcohol may be exacerbating his condition (Box 132).

What is the Epworth Sleepiness Score (ESS)?

This is a validated scoring system for assessing the level of daytime sleepiness (Box 133).

How do you interpret Mr Campbell's Epworth Sleepiness Score?

Mr Campbell's ESS is clearly abnormal at 16, reflecting moderate subjective daytime sleepiness. Patients with abnormal ESS require further assessment and possible investigation for obstructive sleep apnoea.

What should Mr Campbell be advised regarding his driving at this stage?

This is very important as people with daytime sleepiness are at increased risk of falling asleep at the wheel and can cause road traffic accidents. At this stage he should be informed that he must not drive if he feels sleepy and that falling asleep at the wheel is a criminal offence that can

potentially lead to a prison sentence. He may require further advice about his driving if the diagnosis of obstructive sleep apnoea is confirmed.

Are there any other causes of daytime sleepiness?

Many other factors can cause daytime sleepiness (Box 134) and should be considered in the differential diagnosis of obstructive sleep apnoea. It is important to clarify whether there is adequate sleep 'opportunity', as inadequate quality or quantity of sleep may cause sleepiness. Common everyday factors that can interfere with sleep include:
- Shift work
- Poor sleep environment:

> **Box 132 Factors predisposing to obstructive sleep apnoea and hypopnoea**
>
> - Increasing age
> - Male gender
> - Obesity
> - Sedative drugs
> - Smoking (causes nasal and pharyngeal congestion)
> - Alcohol consumption (reduces tone in pharyngeal muscles)

> **Box 133 Epworth Sleepiness Score**
>
> The following questionnaire should be completed independently by both the patient and their partner to improve accuracy. Patients are particularly unlikely to admit to falling asleep in a car as they may be anxious about being told not to drive.
>
> 'How likely are you to doze off or fall asleep in the following situations in contrast to just feeling tired? Use the following scale to choose the most appropriate number for each situation.'
>
> 1 would never doze
> 2 slight chance of dozing
> 3 moderate chance of dozing
> 4 high chance of dozing
>
> **Situation**
> 1 Sitting and reading
> 2 Watching TV
> 3 Sitting inactive in a public place (e.g. a theatre or a meeting)
> 4 As a passenger in a car for an hour without a break
> 5 Lying down to rest in the afternoon when circumstances permit
> 6 Sitting and talking to someone
> 7 Sitting quietly after a lunch without alcohol
> 8 In a car, while stopped for a few minutes in traffic
>
> **Interpretation**
> The maximum score is 24 points:
>
> | | |
> |---|---|
> | Normal | ESS <11 |
> | Mild subjective daytime sleepiness | ESS 11–14 |
> | Moderate subjective daytime sleepiness | ESS 15–18 |
> | Severe subjective sleepiness | ESS >18 |

> **Box 134 Pathological causes of daytime sleepiness**
>
> - Depression
> - Hypothyroidism
> - Drugs causing sleep disturbance and subsequent daytime sleepiness:
>   ◦ nicotine replacement
>   ◦ amphetamines
>   ◦ theophyllines
>   ◦ serotonin reuptake inhibitors
> - Drugs causing somnolence:
>   ◦ sedatives
>   ◦ β-blockers
> - Neurological conditions:
>   ◦ previous encephalitis
>   ◦ previous head injury
>   ◦ parkinsonism
> - Narcolepsy

> **Box 135 Assessment of body mass index**
>
> Body mass index (BMI) is calculated as follows:
>
> $$\text{Body mass index} = \frac{\text{weight in kg}}{(\text{height in m})^2}$$
>
> Normal range is 20–25 kg/m^2. Patients are considered obese if BMI >30 kg/m^2.

◦ too noisy
◦ too light
◦ television or other distractions in bedroom
◦ uncomfortable bed
- Poor preparation for sleep:
  ◦ recent strenuous exercise
  ◦ recent caffeine or other stimulation
- Stress, anxiety or pain

On examination Mr Campbell has a body mass index (BMI) of 33 kg/m², collar size 19 in, normal mandibular size, patent upper airway and no pharyngeal obstruction. His blood pressure is 160/95 mmHg and routine examination of all systems is normal. Spirometry is also normal and there are no features to suggest other underlying medical conditions.

How do you interpret his examination findings?

- Mr Campbell's BMI is 33 kg/m^2, which classifies him as obese (Box 135). This is a major risk factor for obstructive sleep apnoea
- His collar size is 19 in. Patients with obstructive sleep apnoea often have a neck circumference greater than 17 in (43 cm). The large amount of soft tissue around the neck appears to compress the upper airway during sleep
- He has no abnormal facial or upper airways features that might predispose to obstructive sleep apnoea. Features to look for include:

◦ an abnormally small mandible which can reduce airway calibre
◦ nasal obstruction – this can be detected visually using a speculum or by asking the patient to sniff while occluding each nostril in turn. When the nose is blocked the pressures in the pharynx are more negative during inspiration (compare breathing in when your nose is pinched to breathing in through a clear nose), which may increase upper airways collapse
◦ mouth – look for a large tongue (macroglossia) and 'crowded' pharynx with large ('kissing') tonsils or uvula that may increase obstruction of the airway
- He is hypertensive. Hypertension is associated with obstructive sleep apnoea, although the mechanism is not fully understood (Box 136) (NB a large cuff should be used when measuring blood pressure in obese patients as an inappropriately small cuff will lead to overestimation of blood pressure.)
- No other abnormalities were detected on examination:
  ◦ respiratory, cardiovascular and neurological examinations should be performed to detect any coexisting disease as clinically indicated
  ◦ spirometry should be checked to look for associated chronic obstructive pulmonary disease (COPD). This is particularly important as a combination of severe obstructive sleep apnoea and COPD can lead to decompensated respiratory failure and right heart strain

What tests would you perform to determine whether Mr Campbell has obstructive sleep apnoea?

He should undergo a sleep study to confirm the diagnosis of obstructive sleep apnoea and to determine the severity of the condition. Essential components of a sleep study include detection of:
- Ventilation
- Disruption of ventilation by upper airways obstruction
- Effect of disruption on sleep quality

Limited sleep studies can be performed at home, allowing the patient to sleep in their own bed, reducing costs and increasing the number of studies that can be performed. These should be sufficient to diagnose obstructive sleep apnoea but the information provided may be too limited to identify other disorders. More complex sleep studies (polysomnography) provide in-depth assessment of sleep but require hospital admission, which is more costly and itself may disrupt the patient's sleep.

<hr>

Box 136 Cardiovascular risk and obstructive sleep apnoea

Patients with obstructive sleep apnoea commonly have other cardiovascular risk factors such as hypertension, insulin resistance and diabetes mellitus. This association may be partly caused by underlying obesity and lack of exercise. However, obstructive sleep apnoea appears to be an independent risk factor for hypertension and possibly for other cardiovascular disease. Putative mechanisms underlying the causal association include:
• Chronic sympathetic activation
• Chronic inflammation
• Endothelial dysfunction
• Hypercoagulability
• Metabolic dysregulation (e.g. activation of the renin–angiotensin system)

There is increasing evidence that obstructive sleep apnoea is an independent risk factor for development of and morbidity and mortality from cardiovascular and cerebrovascular disease.

<hr>

Mr Campbell has a home sleep study. On the day of the test he spends some time with the lung function technician and is trained to set up the equipment and use a pulse oximeter, nasal probe and chest and abdominal straps. That night he puts on the equipment and attaches the instruments to a sleep monitor. After a night's sleep he returns the sleep monitor to the hospital for analysis. The results of his sleep study are shown in Fig. 99.

What does each instrument measure?
• The pulse oximeter provides continuous measurements of oxygen saturation and pulse rate
• The nasal probe comprises a thermistor, which records airflow from the nose and a room microphone to record the level of snoring
• Movement sensors (straps) attached to the patient's ribcage or abdomen are used to measure respiratory effort

How can his sleep study results be interpreted?
Nasal flow
This determines how much air he is moving in and out of his nose. In Fig. 99 at (A) nasal flow changes continuously throughout inspiration and expiration, which shows his airway is not obstructed. At (B) the nasal flow line becomes flat because there is no movement of air. This is an apnoea. In analysis of the study a breathing pause must last for at least 10s to count as an apnoea. The breathing pause marked lasts for 20s until airflow resumes at (C). Hypopnoeas are 10-s events where airflow continues but is reduced by at least 50% from the

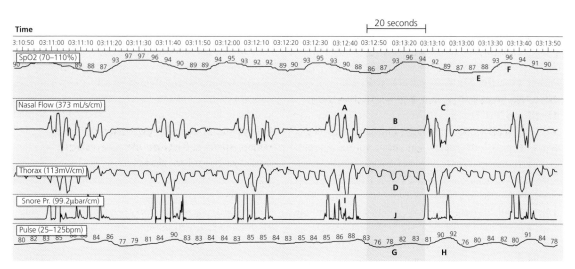

Figure 99 Sleep study.

previous baseline, but are not seen in Mr Campbell's sleep study.

Thoracic movements

During the apnoea, movement of thoracic muscles continues (D). This indicates that Mr Campbell has stopped breathing because his airway is blocked (obstructive sleep apnoea), rather than because of lack of signal from the respiratory centre to his respiratory muscles (central sleep apnoea).

Pulse oximetry

Oxygen saturations can be seen to fall from 96% to 88% (E). This desaturation lags behind the apnoea, as does recovery of oxygenation (F) following restoration of airflow. The pulse oximeter also shows relative bradycardia during the apnoea (G) with an increase in pulse rate when airflow is restored (H). These transient rises in heart rate are an indirect marker of arousal from sleep.

Microphone

This detects the volume of snoring which can be seen to be loud when there is airflow (I) and silenced during apnoea (J). This indicates that there is continuous partial airflow obstruction during sleep which worsens intermittently to complete apnoea.

How bad is his obstructive sleep apnoea?

The severity of obstructive sleep apnoea is determined by the hourly frequency of apnoeas or hypopnoeas (Table 12) and is known as the apnoea/hypopnoea index (AHI) or respiratory disturbance index. In this part of his study Mr Campbell can be seen to have six apnoeas in 3 min. Over the whole night his AHI is 60 per hour (i.e. he has severe obstructive sleep apnoea).

What should Mr Campbell now be advised regarding his driving?

In the UK, the Driver and Vehicle Licensing Agency (DVLA) regulations state that driving must cease if the driver is excessively sleepy (from any cause). Group 1 drivers (ordinary licence holders) with a diagnosis of sleep apnoea should notify the DVLA but can drive provided their sleepiness is controlled by treatment. Group 2 drivers (public service and heavy goods vehicles) should cease driving until it has been confirmed by a specialist that their condition is adequately treated. The doctor should now advise Mr Campbell to stop driving and to inform the DVLA about his condition. If Mr Campbell

Table 12 Severity of obstructive sleep apnoea.

Severity	Apnoea/hypopnoea rate (per hour)	Treatment strategies
Borderline	5–14	Behavioural
Mild	15–30	Behavioural unless severe symptoms
Moderate	30–50	CPAP
Severe	>50	CPAP

CPAP, continuous positive airway pressure.

fails to inform the DVLA it is the duty of the doctor to do so. In this situation the public interest overrides individual patient confidentiality.

How can Mr Campbell retain his heavy goods vehicle licence?

He needs to commence treatment for his obstructive sleep apnoea.

What treatment options are available?

All patients should receive advice, education and support to improve their lifestyle and health and reduce their weight. While the health benefits of these behavioural interventions are taking effect, the main treatments for moderate to severe obstructive sleep apnoea are nocturnal continuous positive airways pressure (CPAP) and mandibular advancement devices.

What behavioural advice should Mr Campbell receive?

Mr Campbell should be advised to:
• Lose weight. This improves obstructive sleep apnoea and helps with control of other obesity-related disorders such as hypertension and diabetes. Weight loss is difficult to achieve but may be assisted by referral to a dietitian and starting an exercise programme
• Stop smoking. This can improve nasal patency and reduce pharyngeal congestion
• Avoid alcohol and sedatives in the evenings, which will improve his pharyngeal tone
• Avoid sleeping on his back. A tennis ball sewn into a pyjama top can help remind him to do this during the night
• Elevate the head of his bed. This also can help to maintain nasal patency

How does continuous positive airway pressure work?

Continuous positive airway pressure delivered by a nasal or full face mask splints open the patient's upper airways, preventing them from collapsing when the pharyngeal muscles relax during sleep. This prevents apnoea and hence breaks the cycle of apnoea and arousal. The patient is provided with a home machine and trained to put themselves on CPAP to continue throughout the night when they go to bed. Expected benefits in treatment are reduction in daytime sleepiness, improved driving performance and reduced risk of accidents, improved mood and quality of life and reduction in blood pressure. Despite these benefits some patients are unable to accept the need for CPAP or tolerate the noise or discomfort of the treatment.

What are mandibular advancement devices?

These are dental appliances designed to alter upper airway patency. They pull the jaw forwards, thus increasing the diameter of the upper airway. They are used to treat snorers, patients with mild obstructive sleep apnoea and patients with moderate to severe sleep apnoea who are unable to tolerate CPAP.

Is surgery an option?

Tonsillectomy could be considered for patients with obstructive sleep apnoea if indicated. Other surgical treatments remain experimental with no current convincing evidence for benefit.

Outcome. Mr Campbell is given a trial of CPAP treatment. He is reviewed after 6 weeks and reports feeling much less sleepy during the day with more refreshing sleep at night. He has joined a gym and managed to lose 4 kg in weight. Three months later his ESS has fallen to 8/24 and his blood pressure is 140/85 mmHg. As he needs to retain his HGV licence his sleep study is repeated on CPAP. His AHI has dropped to 3 per hour and he has no desaturation events. He is therefore allowed to drive his truck once more. He continues to use his CPAP machine at night and remains under review in the sleep clinic.

CASE REVIEW

Mr Campbell is referred to the sleep clinic for investigation of snoring. His ESS indicates significant daytime sleepiness and his history suggests airflow obstruction occurring during sleep. He has a home sleep study which shows frequent apnoeas (60 per hour) and other features characteristic of obstructive sleep apnoea. He is advised not to drive and to inform the DVLA of his diagnosis. He starts treatment with CPAP and gains control of his obstructive sleep apnoea, experiencing considerable improvement in his daytime symptoms. Once his condition is controlled his heavy goods vehicle licence is restored. He makes lifestyle changes, including increasing exercise and losing weight, to maintain his clinical improvement.

KEY POINTS

- Obstructive sleep apnoea is caused by intermittent upper airway collapse during sleep
- This disrupts sleep by causing transient wakefulness
- Detrimental effects of obstructive sleep apnoea include:
  - daytime sleepiness and change in mood
  - increased blood pressure
  - possible increase in risk of cardiovascular and cerebrovascular disease
- Obstructive sleep apnoea should be suspected in people who snore or have daytime sleepiness
- The diagnosis is confirmed by a sleep study which measures:
  - ventilation
  - disruption of ventilation by upper airways obstruction
  - effect of disruption on sleep quality

- Severity of obstructive sleep apnoea can be assessed on sleep study by the number of recorded apnoeas per hour
- Obstructive sleep apnoea increases the risk of patients falling asleep at the wheel and causing road traffic accidents:
  - sleepy patients should be told not to drive
  - patients with a diagnosis of obstructive sleep apnoea must inform the DVLA and must not drive until their condition is controlled
- Obstructive sleep apnoea is treated by:
  - behavioural intervention
  - CPAP
  - mandibular advancement devices

MCQs

1 *A 28-year-old man complains of a 3-month history of a cough productive of occasional yellow sputum. The cough occurs predominantly at night and is triggered by exercise and smoky atmospheres. He has previously had sinusitis but is otherwise in good health.*

Which of the following is the most likely diagnosis?
a. Asthma
b. Bronchiectasis
c. Chronic obstructive pulmonary disease (COPD)
d. Gastro-oesophageal reflux
e. Postnasal drip

2 *A 78-year-old woman develops new shortness of breath on exercise 3 weeks after a right knee replacement. She is not breathless at rest and sleeps comfortably using one pillow at night. She has a cough which causes a shooting pain in the right side of her chest. She produces clear sputum which contains occasional specks of blood. Her right leg remains swollen after surgery.*

What is the most likely cause of her breathlessness?
a. Atelectasis
b. Bronchospasm
c. Hospital-acquired pneumonia
d. Pulmonary embolus
e. Pulmonary oedema

3 *A 32-year-old man is referred to the chest clinic as his GP wonders whether he might have bronchiectasis.*

Which of the following features in his history would be most indicative of this diagnosis?
a. Cough every day for 3 months in 2 consecutive years
b. Expectoration of sputum plugs

c. Problematic night cough
d. Production of a teacupful of sputum per day
e. Weight loss and night sweats

4 *A 65-year-old man is found collapsed in the ward. On examination there is no evidence of stridor, respiratory rate is 4 breaths/min and oxygen saturations are 82% on air. His pulse is 120 beats/min and regular, blood pressure (BP) 90/60 mmHg, Glasgow Coma Scale is 3/15 and he has bilateral pupillary constriction and no focal neurological deficit.*

What is the most likely diagnosis?
a. Anaphylaxis
b. Myocardial infarction
c. Opiate toxicity
d. Pulmonary embolus
e. Raised intracranial pressure

5 *A 37-year-old man is short of breath 4 h after major abdominal surgery. Observations show: pulse 108 beats/min regular, jugular venous pressure (JVP) +1 cm, BP 98/66 mmHg. Chest examination reveals trachea midline, expansion poor bilaterally, percussion resonant right = left, auscultation vesicular breath sounds with bilateral expiratory wheeze, no ankle oedema.*

What is the most likely cause of his breathlessness?
a. Atelectasis
b. Bronchospasm
c. Hospital-acquired pneumonia
d. Pulmonary embolus
e. Pulmonary oedema

6 *A 66-year-old man is found on examination to have pulse 84 beats/min, JVP +6 cm, BP 126/84 mmHg. On chest examination he has cricosternal distance 1 cm, a tracheal tug, is using accessory muscles and has bilateral expiratory wheeze. His liver is palpable and he has bilateral pitting ankle oedema.*

What is the most likely diagnosis?
a. Congestive cardiac failure
b. Cor pulmonale
c. Deep vein thrombosis and pulmonary embolus
d. Hepatic failure
e. Nephrotic syndrome

7 *A 72-year-old woman was admitted with reduced consciousness and required invasive ventilation. Five days later she is deteriorating and is found to have new bilateral patchy consolidation on her chest X-ray.*

Which one of the following organisms is most likely to be causing her deterioration?
a. *Legionella pneumophila*
b. *Mycobacterium tuberculosis*
c. *Mycoplasma pneumoniae*
d. *Pneumocystis jirovecii*
e. *Staphylococcus aureus*

8 *A 49-year-old man was referred to the chest clinic with breathlessness and wheeze. The GP's referral letter asked the hospital consultant for help in distinguishing between asthma and COPD.*

Which one of the following would most indicate a diagnosis of COPD rather than asthma?
a. Breathlessness persistent and progressive
b. Family history of atopy
c. Nocturnal symptoms
d. Ten pack year smoking history
e. Variable breathlessness

9 *An 88-year-old man has the following blood results:*

		Normal range
Sodium	108 mmol/L	(135–145 mmol/L)
Potassium	4.0 mmol/L	(3.5–5.0 mmol/L)
Urea	4.8 mmol/L	(2.5–8 mmol/L)
Creatinine	92 μmol/L	(60–110 μmol/L)

Which of the following is most likely to have caused these abnormalities?
a. Chronic hypoxia
b. COPD
c. Prednisolone and salbutamol treatment
d. Pulmonary hypertension
e. Small cell lung cancer

10 *An 81-year-old woman has enlargement of the left supraclavicular nodes and undergoes fine needle aspiration.*

Which of the following is the most likely diagnosis?
a. Breast cancer
b. Epstein–Barr infection
c. HIV infection
d. Stomach cancer
e. Tuberculosis

11 *A 57-year-old woman has just undergone fibreoptic bronchoscopy. Monitoring shows her oxygen saturations to have fallen to 86% on 2 L/min oxygen. On examination her pulse is 88 beats/min, BP 146/84 mmHg, respiratory rate 5 breaths/min. Chest examination reveals trachea – midline, expansion right = left, percussion right = left, breath sounds vesicular, nil added.*

Which of the following is the most likely complication that has occurred following bronchoscopy?
a. Bleeding
b. Bronchospasm
c. Infection
d. Oversedation
e. Pneumothorax

12 *A 21-year-old woman is thought to have undiagnosed cystic fibrosis.*

Which of the following would be *least* suggestive of this diagnosis in her case?
a. Bronchiectasis
b. Infertility
c. *Pseudomonas aeruginosa* isolated from her sputum
d. Recent onset of diabetes mellitus
e. Steatorrhoea and body mass index (BMI) 18 kg/m^2

13 *A 23-year-old woman complains of mild chest tightness and has a provisional diagnosis of asthma.*

Which one of the following investigations would be most likely to confirm the diagnosis?
a. Antineutrophil cytoplasmic antibodies
b. IgE measurement
c. Peak flow diary
d. Skin prick testing
e. Spirometry

14 *A 72-year-old man is admitted with a chest X-ray showing a peripheral lung mass.*

Which one of the following investigations is most likely to yield a histological diagnosis?
a. Endobronchial biopsy
b. Percutaneous computed tomography (CT) guided lung biopsy
c. Positron emission tomography (PET) scan
d. Staging CT scan
e. Transbronchial needle aspiration of mediastinal lymph nodes

15 *Which one of the following is not a feature of a normal chest X-ray?*

a. The diameter of the heart is <0.5 times the cardiothoracic diameter
b. The left hemidiaphragm is lower than the right hemidiaphragm
c. The left main bronchus is more vertical than the right main bronchus
d. The right hilum is lower than the left hilum
e. The top of the right hemidiaphragm is at the 5th intercostal space in the midclavicular line

16 *A 56-year-old woman is found to have diffuse parenchymal lung disease.*

Which one of the following investigations would be most likely to reveal an underlying cause for her condition?
a. *Aspergillus* precipitins
b. Autoantibody screen

c. Retroviral test
d. Skin prick testing
e. Thrombophilia screen

17 *A 73-year-old woman has collapsed on the ward with a respiratory arrest and has vomited.*

Which one of the following pieces of equipment would be most useful to prevent aspiration?
a. Endotracheal tube
b. Guedel airway
c. Laryngeal mask
d. Mouth guard
e. Nasopharyngeal airway

18 *A 61-year-old man has an Epworth Sleepiness Score of 18/24, BP 174/98mmHg, BMI 37kg/m² and is diagnosed on a home sleep study as having obstructive sleep apnoea.*

Which one of the following statements about his treatment is most true?
a. A mandibular advancement device should be tried before continuous positive airways pressure (CPAP)
b. As he is starting treatment he does not need to inform the Driver and Vehicle Licensing Agency (DVLA) about his condition
c. He should not drive a car until he has lost weight
d. Night sedation will improve sleep quality and reduce daytime somnolence
e. Nocturnal CPAP is likely to lower his blood pressure

19 *A 35-year-old woman commences treatment with rifampicin, isoniazid, ethambutol and pyrazinamide for tuberculosis.*

Which one of the following methods should be used to monitor her for side-effects of treatment?
a. Audiometry
b. Full blood count
c. Liver function tests
d. Plasma drug levels
e. Transfer factor

20 *A 68-year-old man has moderate COPD, causing shortness of breath on exercise.*

Which one of the following treatments will best prevent progression of his lung disease?
a. Inhaled steroids
b. Pulmonary rehabilitation
c. Salmeterol
d. Smoking cessation
e. Tiotropium

21 *A 77-year-old man with known COPD is admitted to hospital with an exacerbation.*

Which one of the following is the most useful indicator in determining whether antibiotics will be effective in the treatment of his exacerbation?
a. FEV_1 <50% predicted
b. Hyperinflated lungs on chest X-ray
c. PaO_2 <8 kPa
d. Purulent sputum
e. Respiratory rate >25 breaths/min

22 *A 65-year-old woman is discharged from hospital following an exacerbation of COPD.*

Which of the following treatments is *least* likely to reduce her risk of hospitalization from future exacerbations?
a. Early self-management of exacerbations with antibiotics and steroids
b. Annual influenza vaccination
c. Regular long acting β_2-agonists and tiotropium
d. Smoking cessation
e. Twice daily inhaled steroids

23 *A 38-year-old woman has taken antituberculous treatment for 1 week and now feels so nauseated that she refuses to take any more drugs.*

Which of the following statements is most correct?
a. Partial treatment of tuberculosis increases the risk of drug resistance
b. She can be forced to take treatment in the public interest

c. She has capacity to make this decision and so should be allowed to make it
d. Treatment should be stopped under the ethical principle of non-malifience (do no harm)
e. Treatment so far is sufficient to have rendered her non-infectious

24 *A 32-year-old woman is admitted with a pulmonary embolus.*

Which one of the following is an indication for thrombolysis?
a. Bilateral emboli on computed tomography pulmonary angiography (CTPA) scan
b. Blood pressure 72/44 mmHg
c. D-dimers 4.9 mg/L (normal <0.3 mg/L)
d. PO_2 9.4 kPa (normal 10–13.1 kPa)
e. Recent surgery

25 *Which one of the following statements about lung cancer is most correct?*

a. Compression of the left recurrent laryngeal nerve by mediastinal lymph nodes causes Horner's syndrome
b. Distant metastases preclude patients from curative surgery
c. Hypernatraemia is a presenting feature of small cell lung cancer
d. Secondary tumour deposits in the lung most commonly originate from prostate
e. Squamous cell lung cancer is more likely than small cell lung cancer to have metastasized at presentation.

26 *Which one of the following respiratory infections is not correctly paired with its anatomical site?*

a. Community acquired pneumonia – alveoli
b. Diphtheria – pharynx
c. Empyema – pleural cavity
d. Infective exacerbation of COPD – lung parenchyma
e. Acute rhinitis – nasal mucosa

27 *Which one of the following respiratory diseases is not correctly paired with a relevant occupational risk factor?*

a. Asthma and working as a baker
b. Lung cancer and working as a publican
c. Mesothelioma and working with isocyanates
d. Extrinsic allergic alveolitis and working in an aviary
e. Pulmonary tuberculosis and working in a hospital

28 *A 56-year-old man complains of excessive day time sleepiness. His wife is concerned that he snores and often stops breathing when he is asleep.*

Which one of the following is most likely to have caused his condition?
a. BMI 43 kg/m^2
b. Diabetes mellitus
c. Hypertension
d. Hypothyroidism
e. Previous tonsillectomy

29 *A 39-year-old woman plans to stop smoking. Her risk of developing which of the following conditions will be least reduced by smoking cessation?*

a. Carcinoma of the bronchus
b. COPD
c. Ischaemic heart disease
d. Laryngeal carcinoma
e. Pulmonary fibrosis

30 *A 28-year-old man has nasal obstruction that makes it difficult to breathe. This has been present most days for the past 15 months. He has a postnasal drip and intermittent cough.*

Exposure to which of the following allergens is most likely to be causing his symptoms?
a. Grass pollens
b. House dust mite
c. Mould spores
d. Pigeon bloom
e. Tree pollen

EMQs

1 Microorganisms causing respiratory infection

a. Anaerobic bacteria
b. *Chlamydia psittaci*
c. *Corynebacterium diphtheriae*
d. Epstein–Barr virus
e. *Haemophilus influenzae*
f. Influenza A virus
g. *Legionella pneumophila*
h. *Moraxella catarrhalis*
i. *Mycobacterium tuberculosis*
j. *Mycoplasma pneumoniae*
k. *Pneumocystis jirovecii*
l. *Pseudomonas aeruginosa*
m. *Rhinovirus*
n. *Streptococcus pneumonia*
o. *Streptococcus pyogenes*

For each of the patients described below choose the organism most likely to be causing their respiratory infection from the list above. Each organism may be chosen once, more than once or not at all.

1. A 22-year-old woman complains to her GP of a sore throat. On examination she has mild jaundice and an enlarged liver and spleen.
2. A 17-year-old man with cystic fibrosis has increased shortness of breath and a cough newly productive of thick dark green sputum.
3. A 36-year-old man with a 2-day history of shortness of breath comes to hospital complaining of haemoptysis. On examination he has crepitations and bronchial breathing at the right lung base, which is dull to percussion.
4. A 72-year-old woman with a 2-month history of a productive cough is sent to hospital by her GP for a chest X-ray which shows consolidation with cavitation at the right lung apex.
5. A 29-year-old man with known HIV disease is admitted with increasing shortness of breath.

On examination his oxygen saturations are 89% on air. His chest X-ray shows bilateral midzone shadowing.

2 Examination

a. Asthma
b. Bronchopneumonia
c. Chronic obstructive pulmonary disease (COPD)
d. Cystic fibrosis
e. Idiopathic pulmonary fibrosis
f. Lobar pneumonia
g. Lung cancer
h. Non-tension pneumothorax
i. Obstructive sleep apnoea
j. Pleural effusion
k. Pulmonary collapse
l. Pulmonary embolus
m. Pulmonary tuberculosis
n. Sarcoidosis
o. Tension pneumothorax

For each of the patients whose examination findings are described below choose the most likely diagnosis from the list above. Each diagnosis may be chosen once, more than once or not at all.

1. A 65-year-old man with finger clubbing and bibasal end-inspiratory crepitations on auscultation.
2. A 16-year-old man with finger clubbing and widespread coarse inspiratory crepitations on auscultation.
3. A 75-year-old woman who has a cricosternal distance of 1 finger breadth, intercostal indrawing on inspiration and poor air entry and expiratory wheeze on auscultation.
4. A 22-year-old man with decreased expansion, decreased air entry and hyper-resonance on the right side of his chest. His trachea is central.

5. A 56-year-old woman with decreased expansion, dull percussion note and decreased air entry on the right side of her chest. Her trachea is deviated to the right.

---

3 History

a. Asthma
b. Bronchopneumonia
c. COPD
d. Cystic fibrosis
e. Idiopathic pulmonary fibrosis
f. Lobar pneumonia
g. Lung cancer
h. Non-tension pneumothorax
i. Obstructive sleep apnoea
j. Pleural effusion
k. Pulmonary collapse
l. Pulmonary embolus
m. Pulmonary tuberculosis
n. Sarcoidosis
o. Tension pneumothorax

For each of the patients whose history is described below choose the most likely diagnosis from the list above. Each diagnosis may be chosen once, more than once or not at all.

1. A 31-year-old woman who has had a productive cough for 3 months. On further questioning she admits to weight loss and night sweats. She has never smoked.
2. A 45-year-old woman complains of a painful rash on her shins. She also has had a dry cough for the past 4 months.
3. A 67-year-old man complains of a drooping left eyelid. His wife has noticed his left pupil is smaller than his right.
4. A 38-year-old man complains of sudden onset of pain on the right side of his chest. It is worse on taking a deep breath. He otherwise feels well, but has coughed up some clear sputum streaked with bright red blood.
5. A 27-year-old man complains of waking at night with a dry cough for the past 4 weeks. He has recurrent attacks of sneezing and eye irritation.

---

4 Chest X-ray interpretation

a. Asthma
b. Bronchopneumonia
c. COPD
d. Cystic fibrosis
e. Idiopathic pulmonary fibrosis
f. Lobar pneumonia
g. Lung cancer
h. Non-tension pneumothorax
i. Obstructive sleep apnoea
j. Pleural effusion
k. Pulmonary collapse
l. Pulmonary embolus
m. Sarcoidosis
n. Tension pneumothorax

For each of the patients whose chest X-rays are shown below choose the most likely diagnosis from the list above. Each diagnosis may be chosen once, more than once or not at all.

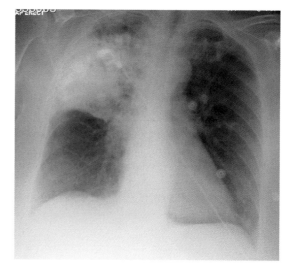

EMQ 4 X-ray 1.

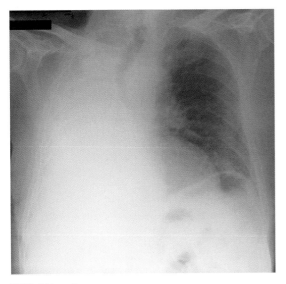

EMQ 4 X-ray 2.

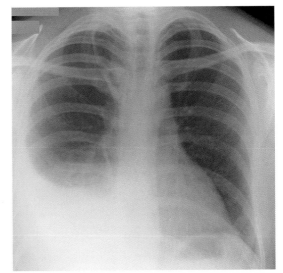

EMQ 4 X-ray 4.

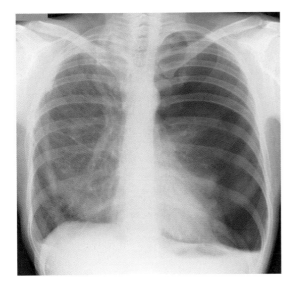

EMQ 4 X-ray 3.

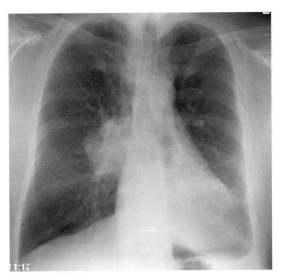

EMQ 4 X-ray 5.

5 Interpretation of investigations
a. Aspiration pneumonia
b. Asthma
c. Bronchiectasis
d. Cardiac failure
e. COPD
f. Empyema
g. HIV-related lung disease
h. Lobar pneumonia
i. Lung cancer
j. Mesothelioma
k. Non-tension pneumothorax
l. Obstructive sleep apnoea
m. Pulmonary embolus
n. Pulmonary fibrosis
o. Pulmonary tuberculosis

6 Choice of investigations
a. Avian precipitins
b. Bronchoalveolar lavage
c. Chest X-ray
d. D-dimers
e. Echocardiogram
f. Endobronchial biopsy
g. Fine needle aspirate
h. High-resolution CT scan
i. IgE level
j. Pleural biopsy
k. Skin prick allergy testing
l. Sweat test
m. Transbronchial biopsy
n. Ventilation–perfusion scan
o. Video-assisted thoracoscopy

For each of the patients whose investigation results are shown below choose the most likely diagnosis from the list above. Each diagnosis may be chosen once, more than once or not at all.

1. A 65-year-old man who has the following spirometry results:

	Before broncho-dilatators (L)	After broncho-dilatators (L)	Predicted (L)
FEV_1	1.6	1.7	3.2
FVC	3.2	3.3	4.1

2. A 72-year-old woman who has the following spirometry results:
    FEV_1 0.9 L (46% predicted)
    FVC   1.0 L (42% predicted)
3. A 46-year-old woman with a ventilation perfusion scan reported as showing multiple unmatched perfusion defects.
4. A 72-year-old woman with the following pleural aspirate results:
    Protein   22 g/L
    pH   7.58 (normal 7.60)
    Glucose   4.7 mmol/L (normal >3.3 mmol/L)
    Microbiology – no cells or organisms seen
5. A 25-year-old man with the following pleural aspirate results:
    Protein   48 g/L
    pH   7.31 (normal 7.60)
    Glucose   1.8 mmol/L (normal >3.3 mmol/L)
    Microbiology – neutrophils ++++

For each of the patients described below choose the single investigation that will be most useful in confirming the suspected diagnosis from the list above. Each test may be used once, more than once or not at all.

1. A 28-year-old man who has collapsed and has a provisional diagnosis of a massive pulmonary embolus.
2. A 56-year-old man with a pleural effusion suspected to be caused by *Mycobacterium tuberculosis*.
3. A 2-year-old girl with failure to thrive thought to be caused by cystic fibrosis.
4. A 73-year-old woman with a dry cough and reduced gas transfer thought to be caused by diffuse parenchymal lung disease.
5. A 17-year-old man with sudden onset shortness of breath who is thought to have a spontaneous pneumothorax.

7 Treatment of respiratory infection

a. Amoxicillin and clavulinic acid
b. Benzyl penicillin and flucloxacillin
c. Cefuroxime and metronidazole
d. Ciprofloxacin
e. Erythromycin and amoxicillin
f. Flucloxacillin and cefotaxime
g. Isoniazid and pyridoxine
h. Itraconazole
i. Metronidazole
j. Phenoxymethyl penicillin
k. Pyrazinamide and ethambutol
l. Pyridoxine, rifampicin and ethambutol
m. Rifampicin and isoniazid
n. Rifampicin, isoniazid, pyrazinamide and ethambutol
o. Trimethoprim and sulfamethoxazole

8 Treatment

a. Adrenaline, chlorphenamine and hydrocortisone
b. Ambulatory home oxygen
c. As required home oxygen by cylinder
d. Bilevel positive airways pressure (BiPAP)
e. Breathe into a paper bag
f. Continuous home oxygen by concentrator
g. Continuous positive airways pressure (CPAP)
h. High-dose inhaled steroids
i. High flow oxygen by mask
j. Intravenous magnesium
k. Intubation and ventilation
l. Mandibular advancement device
m. Nebulized salbutamol
n. No treatment
o. Short-term oxygen 28% via nasal cannulae

For each of the patients described below choose the most appropriate first treatment from the list above. Each treatment may be used once, more than once or not at all.

1. A 66-year-old man with a mild infective exacerbation of COPD caused by a β-lactamase producing strain of *Haemophilus influenzae*.
2. A 32-year-old woman with community acquired pneumonia who is confused, has respiratory rate of 34 breaths/min, urea 9.6 mmol/L and blood pressure 86/44 mmHg.
3. A 92-year-old woman on day 4 of cefotaxime treatment for respiratory infection who now has profuse diarrhoea.
4. A 48-year-old man with pulmonary tuberculosis who has completed 2 months of treatment and now requires continuation treatment for 4 months.
5. A 17-year-old man with cystic fibrosis with his first episode of infection with *Pseudomonas aeruginosa*.

Normal ranges: pH 7.35–7.45, PaO$_2$ 10–13.1 kPa, PaCO$_2$ 4.9–6.1 kPa

For each of the patients described below choose the most appropriate next treatment from the list above. Each treatment may be used once, more than once or not at all.

1. A 21-year-old girl with acute shortness of breath who has the following blood gases on air:
   pH   7.62
   PaO$_2$ 12 kPa
   PaCO$_2$ 2.2 kPa
2. A 23-year-old man with acute asthma who has the following blood gases on 60% oxygen:
   pH   7.20
   PaO$_2$ 6.4 kPa
   PaCO$_2$ 8.5 kPa
3. A 64-year-old man with an Epworth Sleepiness Score of 19/24 and nocturnal apnoea/hypopnoea rate of 40 per hour.
4. A 66-year-old woman with stable COPD who has the following blood gases on air:
   pH   7.41
   PaO$_2$ 6.6 kPa
   PaCO$_2$ 5.7 kPa
5. A 78-year-old man with an exacerbation of COPD on 28% oxygen:
   pH   7.24
   PaO$_2$ 5.3 kPa
   PaCO$_2$ 10.6 kPa

9 Treatment
a. Adrenaline (IM)
b. Beclometasone (inhaler)
c. Loratidine (O)
d. Low molecular weight heparin (SC)
e. Magnesium (IV)
f. Morphine (O)
g. Oxygen (inhaled)
h. Prednisolone (O)
i. Salbutamol (inhaler)
j. Salmeterol (inhaler)
k. Streptokinase (IV)
l. Tiotropium (inhaler)
m. Theophylline (O)
n. Unfractionated heparin (SC)
o. Warfarin (O)

10 Epidemiology
a. African/Caribbean parents
b. Asbestos exposure
c. Atopic phenotype
d. Caucasian parents
e. Cigarette smoking
f. Coal mining
g. Intravenous drug abuse
h. Keeps pigeons
i. Male gender
j. Obesity
k. Positive family history
l. Previous chickenpox
m. Recent immigration from Eastern Europe
n. South Asian parents
o. Whooping cough as child

Routes of administration are given in brackets. IM, intramuscular; IV, intravenous; O, oral (by mouth); SC, subcutaneous.

For each of the patients described below choose the most appropriate next treatment from the list given. Each treatment may be used once, more than once or not at all.

1. A 77-year-old woman with COPD who has ankle swelling. Echocardiography shows a pulmonary artery systolic pressure of 43 mmHg (normal <25 mmHg)
2. A 22-year-old man with asthma who is waking at night with a cough. He is using his salbutamol inhaler 2–3 times daily for wheeze.
3. A 43-year-old woman admitted acutely with a pulmonary embolus. Her blood pressure is 120/82 mmHg and her echocardiogram shows normal right ventricular size and function.
4. A 16-year-old girl who has collapsed after eating peanuts. She has blood pressure 88/56 mmHg, stridor and oxygen saturation 91%.
5. A 77-year-old man with terminal lung cancer who is extremely distressed by shortness of breath.

For each of the patients described below choose the risk factor most likely to have caused their condition from the list above. Each risk factor can be chosen once, more than once or not at all.

1. A patient with sarcoidosis causing bilateral hilar lymphadenopathy.
2. A patient with a cavitating lung lesion suggestive of tuberculosis.
3. A patient with a chronic cough productive of large volumes of sputum as a result of bronchiectasis.
4. A patient with severe hypoxia resulting from pneumocystis pneumonia.
5. A patient with pleural plaques on their chest X-ray.

SAQs

1 *A 25-year-old woman with known asthma comes to accident and emergency complaining of increasing shortness of breath. On examination she is able to complete sentences; her respiratory rate is 20 breaths/min, pulse 96 beats/min, oxygen saturations of 93% on air and peak flow 250 L/min (best 420 L/min). She has a widespread expiratory wheeze on auscultation.*

a. How severe is her asthma attack? Explain your assessment *(2 marks)*

b. Outline your immediate management of this patient *(4 marks)*

c. Which two investigations would be most useful in this patient. Explain why *(2 marks)*

d. Give two measures that could be taken after discharge to reduce the risk of further exacerbations *(2 marks)*

2 *A 56-year-old man is admitted through accident and emergency coughing up blood. He is worried that he may have lung cancer.*

a. State four other causes of haemoptysis *(4 marks)*

b. Give two risk factors for lung cancer that you would ask about when taking a history *(2 marks)*

c. Give two histological types of lung cancer *(2 marks)* and for each give one type of treatment that may cause remission or be curative *(2 marks)*

3 *A 59-year-old man with COPD comes into hospital with an exacerbation causing respiratory failure. On admission his blood gases are:*

pH	7.26	
PaO$_2$	6.7 kPa	(10–13.1 kPa)
PaCO$_2$	8.9 kPa	(4.9–6.1 kPa)
HCO$_3^-$	26 mmol/L	(22–28 mmol/L)

a. Give a pathophysiological explanation for each abnormality shown on arterial blood gas testing *(3 marks)*

b. Describe your immediate management of his respiratory failure and explain your answer *(4 marks)*. In outpatients when stable his blood gases are:

pH	7.39	
PaO$_2$	7.0 kPa	(10–13.1 kPa)
PaCO$_2$	8.1 kPa	(4.9–6.1 kPa)
HCO$_3^-$	38 mmol/L	(22–28 mmol/L)

c. How do you account for the change in pH? *(1 mark)*

d. Give two possible long-term complications of his condition based on these results and explain why each occurs *(2 marks)*

4 *A 53-year-old woman presents to the chest clinic complaining of a cough which has been present for 3 months. Her cough is embarrassing and restricting her social activities.*

a. How would you classify her cough? *(1 mark)*

b. Give three causes of cough other than lung disease? *(3 marks)*

c. What features in her history would be consistent with lung disease rather than other causes (b) as the cause of her cough? *(4 marks)*

d. Give two investigations you would perform and explain why you would do each *(2 marks)*

5 *A 48-year-old man is seen in accident and emergency, complaining of a sharp pain in his right side which is preventing him from taking a deep breath. He has no previous history of lung disease and has never smoked.*
Examination findings: oxygen saturations 96% on air, pulse 88 beats/min, blood pressure (BP) 114/76 mmHg, trachea – midline, expansion left > right, percussion – resonant right > left, breath sounds vesicular but reduced on the right, vocal resonance reduced at the right base.

a. What type of pain is he complaining of? *(1 mark)*

b. Interpret his examination findings *(3 marks)* and state the most likely diagnosis *(1 mark)*

c. Outline the management of this condition *(4 marks)*

d. Give two other possible causes of this type of pain *(1 mark)*

---

6 *A 76-year-old woman who was living independently is admitted with community acquired pneumonia. On examination her Glasgow Coma Score is 14/15, oxygen saturations are 88% on air, pulse 120 beats/min, BP 80/50 mmHg and respiratory rate 32 breaths/min. Blood tests show:*

		Normal range
Sodium	*141 mmol/L*	*(135–145 mmol/L)*
Potassium	*3.7 mmol/L*	*(3.5–5.0 mmol/L)*
Urea	*10.8 mmol/L*	*(2.5–8 mmol/L)*
Creatinine	*92 μmol/L*	*(60–110 μmol/L)*

a. How severe is her pneumonia? Explain your answer *(3 marks)*

b. What factors will you take into consideration when deciding which antibiotics to prescribe? *(4 marks)*

c. Outline the management of her condition in addition to the use of antibiotics *(3 marks)*

---

7 *A 26-year-old woman is referred to the medical team by accident and emergency with a suspected pulmonary embolus. She presents with a 2-day history of pleuritic chest pain, worse on inspiration. She is on the oral contraceptive pill and has sprained her left ankle 2 weeks ago. Examination findings are: pulse 94 beats/min, jugular venous pressure (JVP) +1 cm, BP 114/76 mmHg, chest examination normal, calf diameters left 34 cm, right 32 cm. D-dimer 0.6 mg/L (normal <0.3 mg/L)*

a. How likely is it that she has had a pulmonary embolus? *(2 marks)*

b. What are D-dimers? *(1 mark)* How does her D-dimer result help in her assessment? *(2 marks)*

c. Explain how you would confirm the diagnosis and treat her pulmonary embolus *(5 marks)*

---

8 *A 54-year-old woman with a cough has the following investigation results:*
FEV$_1$ 1.2 L (48% predicted), FVC 1.47 L (49% predicted), FEV$_1$/FVC 82%
Gas transfer 54% predicted
Transbronchial biopsy – non-caseating granulomas

a. How do you interpret her lung function results? *(3 marks)*

b. What is the most likely diagnosis? *(1 mark)* Explain how you made this diagnosis *(1 mark)*

c. What extrapulmonary abnormalities would you look for? *(4 marks)*

d. Outline the treatment of her condition *(1 mark)*

---

9 *A 42-year-old man, known to be living on the streets, is admitted with alcohol withdrawal. On examination his body mass index is 18 kg/m^2 and his temperature is 37.8°C. His chest X-ray shows a large cavity in the apex of the left lung.*

a. Give three possible causes for these X-ray findings *(3 marks)*

b. What is the most important step that should be taken in the immediate management of his respiratory condition? *(1 mark)*

c. How would you investigate his respiratory condition? *(4 marks)*

d. How might his social circumstances affect the treatment of his respiratory disease? *(2 marks)*

---

10 *A 27-year-old man sees his GP with a sore throat. He has no significant past medical history. He has been unwell for 3 days and is unable to eat, although he can take oral fluids. On examination his tonsils are enlarged and covered with a white exudate. He has tender cervical lymphadenopathy.*

a. Give two organisms most likely to be causing his sore throat *(2 marks)*

b. Would you prescribe antibiotics? *(1 mark)* Justify your answer *(3 marks)*

c. If antibiotics are prescribed, give one that would be suitable and one that would be contraindicated for the treatment of his condition *(2 marks)*

d. Give two complications that may arise following upper respiratory tract infection *(2 marks)*

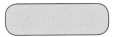

MCQs Answers

1. a	11. d	21. d
2. d	12. b	22. c
3. d	13. c	23. a
4. c	14. b	24. b
5. b	15. c	25. b
6. b	16. b	26. d
7. e	17. a	27. c
8. a	18. e	28. a
9. e	19. c	29. e
10. d	20. d	30. b

EMQs Answers

1
1. d
2. l
3. n
4. i
5. k

2
1. e
2. d
3. c
4. h
5. k

3
1. m
2. n
3. g
4. l
5. a

4
1. f

2. k
3. h
4. j
5. g

5
1. e
2. n
3. m
4. d
5. f

6
1. e
2. j
3. l
4. h
5. c

7
1. a
2. e
3. i

4. m
5. d

8
1. e
2. k
3. g
4. f
5. d

9
1. g
2. b
3. d
4. a
5. f

10
1. a
2. m
3. o
4. g
5. b

SAQs Answers

1

a. She is having a moderate asthma exacerbation *(1 mark)* as she has no clinical features of severe asthma and peak flow is >50% predicted *(1 mark)*.

b. *(1 mark for each correct answer, maximum 4 marks).* The first part of the management should be to establish whether the patient needs basic life support or not (ABC) *(1 mark)*. As this patient does not, the next step should be general supportive measures including administration of high flow oxygen *(1 mark)* and specific asthma treatment with nebulized salbutamol *(1 mark)* and systemic corticosteroids *(1 mark)*. Other immediate measures would include securing intravenous access *(1 mark)* and regular cardiorespiratory monitoring *(1 mark)*.

c. *(1 mark for each correct answer, maximum 2 marks).*
• Chest X-ray to establish whether or not she has a pneumothora**x**. This is important because it is a recognized complication of asthma and can be easily reversed. Chest X-ray will also provide information about other pathologies that can exacerbate asthma such as pneumonia *(1 mark)*.
• Inflammatory blood markers such as white cell count and C-reactive protein, which may indicate infection underlying the exacerbation *(1 mark)*.
• Also allow arterial blood gases to quantify hypoxia and look for hypercapnia or acid–base disturbances *(1 mark)*.

d. *(1 mark per correct answer, maximum 2 marks).*
• Regular inhaled steroids
• Self-management plan including regular peak flow monitoring and adjustment of medication
• Allergen avoidance

2

a. *(1 mark for each correct answer, maximum 4 marks).* Tuberculosis, bronchiectasis, pulmonary embolus, Goodpasture's syndrome, pneumonia, aspergilloma.

b. *(1 mark for each correct answer, maximum 2 marks).* Smoking, asbestos exposure (Box 62, p. 101).

c. Non-small cell such as squamous cell, adenocarcinoma, large cell *(1 mark)*. Curative treatment could be surgery *(1 mark)*.
Small cell *(1 mark)*. Treatment that may cause remission is chemotherapy *(1 mark)*.

3

a. • He is hypoxic. COPD causes a severe reduction in alveolar ventilation by obstructing the airways, preventing air entry, and by alveolar destruction (emphysema). This can be worse during an exacerbation. Poor alveolar ventilation results in V/Q mismatch and reduction in oxygen uptake *(1 mark)*
• He is hypercapnic. Excretion of CO_2 depends on adequacy of alveolar ventilation. Good ventilation blows off CO_2 and ensures a large diffusion gradient for CO_2 from blood to air. Hypercapnia indicates alveolar hypoventilation *(1 mark)* either because of severe lung damage (in his case) or neuromuscular disease (Fig. 7, p. 7)
• He is acidotic. The Henderson–Hasselbach equation describes the relationship between CO_2 and H^+.

$$H^+ + HCO_3^- \rightleftarrows H_2CO_3 \rightleftarrows H_2O + CO_2$$

His acidosis is caused by his hypercapnia which is driving the equation to the left, increasing generation of H^+ ions *(1 mark)*

b. • He needs oxygen as without this he is at risk of hypoxic damage especially to the brain and heart. However, as he is retaining CO_2 he is likely to have lost his central drive to breathe so too much oxygen could make things worse *(1 mark)*
• He therefore should receive oxygen at 24–28% initially. His blood gases should be checked around 30 min after starting *(1 mark)*
• If adequate oxygenation cannot be achieved without an increase in $PaCO_2$ and worsening of

acidosis, he will need non-invasive ventilation/BiPAP *(1 mark)*

- Treatment of his COPD exacerbation should be commenced immediately as improvement in his lung disease will help his respiratory failure *(1 mark)*. This should include salbutamol and ipratropium nebulizers, oral prednisolone and antibiotics

c. Renal retention of bicarbonate has occurred in response to respiratory acidosis. This has buffered the acidosis, with a return of pH to normal (respiratory acidosis with metabolic compensation) *(1 mark)*.

d. 1 mark per each *explained* answer. Chronic hypoxia will cause:

- Cor pulmonale *(0.5 mark)*. Hypoxia causes pulmonary arterial vasoconstriction, contributing to pulmonary hypertension and right heart dysfunction.

- Polycythaemia *(0.5 mark)* occurs because chronic hypoxia stimulates erythropoietin production, which in turn stimulates red blood cell production by the bone marrow *(0.5 mark)*.

4

a. This is a chronic cough as it has lasted longer than 8 weeks *(1 mark)*.

b. Nasal/sinus disease – postnasal drip *(1 mark)*; gastro-oesophageal reflux *(1 mark)*; drugs, e.g. ACE inhibitors *(1 mark)*; impaired swallow with aspiration *(1 mark)*.

c. *(1 mark for each correct answer, maximum 4 marks)*. Breathlessness *(1 mark)*, pleuritic chest pain *(1 mark)*, weight loss/night sweats indicative of TB/lung cancer *(1 mark)*, night cough and wheeze – may indicate asthma, significant smoking history *(1 mark)*, sputum production (although may see mucus with postnasal drip) *(1 mark)*.

d. *(1 mark for each correct answer, maximum 2 marks)*. Chest X-ray to look for lung disease, e.g. tuberculosis/lung cancer *(1 mark)*, spirometry/peak flow recording to look for airflow obstruction of asthma/COPD *(1 mark)*, sputum cultures (if produced) to look for bacterial infection/acid-fast bacilli *(1 mark)*, eosinophil count/IgE to look for atopy *(1 mark)*.

5

a. Pleuritic chest pain *(1 mark)*.

b. ABC are intact and he is stable from a cardiorespiratory point of view (normal oxygen

saturations, pulse and blood pressure) *(1 mark)*. Chest findings are asymmetrical and abnormal on the right *(1 mark)* indicating a *right-sided pneumothorax (1 mark)*. The mediastinum is not displaced, so this is *not* a tension pneumothorax *(1 mark)*.

c. *(1 mark per correct answer, maximum 4 marks)*. A chest X-ray should be performed to confirm the diagnosis *(1 mark)*. He should be started on high flow oxygen to speed reabsorption of the pneumothorax *(1 mark)*. If the pneumothorax is small (<2 cm visible rim of air on chest X-ray) it can be observed *(1 mark)*. If the pneumothorax is large (≥2 cm air rim) it should be aspirated *(1 mark)*. If unsuccessful a chest drain should be inserted *(1 mark)*.

d. *(0.5 mark per correct answer, maximum 1 mark)*. Pneumonia, pulmonary embolus, viral pleurisy.

6

a. Pneumonia severity is assessed using the CURB-65 score *(1 mark)*. Her CURB-65 score is 5 (Box 88, p. 151) *(1 mark)*. She thus has severe pneumonia and is at high risk of death *(1 mark)*.

b. *(1 mark per correct answer, maximum 4 marks)*. Best guess as to causative organism *(1 mark)* and likely microbial antibiotic resistance *(1 mark)*, patient antibiotic allergy *(1 mark)*, risk of side-effects (e.g. *Clostridium difficile* diarrhoea) *(1 mark)*, indications for intravenous therapy (severe illness, inability to swallow) *(1 mark)*.

c. *(1 mark per correct answer, maximum 3 marks)*. She requires oxygen to treat hypoxia *(1 mark)* and IV fluids to maintain blood pressure *(1 mark)*. She should be referred to intensive care (ICU) to consider admission *(1 mark)*. She needs careful monitoring (oxygen saturations, respiratory rate, blood pressure, Glasgow Coma Score, urinary output, electrolytes) *(1 mark)* and may need other supportive care on ICU including ventilation and inotropic support.

7

a. By Wells criteria (Table 6, p. 130) she scores 7.5 (i.e. swollen left calf –3, other diagnoses less likely –3, some immobilization from sprained ankle –1.5) *(1 mark)*, which indicates a high probability of her having had a pulmonary embolus (PE).

b. D-dimers are cross-linked fibrin degradation products formed by clot breakdown *(1 mark)*.

Elevated D-dimers are unhelpful as they can be produced by clot anywhere in the body *(1 mark)* and so do not add useful information to the clinical risk assessment *(1 mark)*. A normal D-dimer result would have been useful in ruling out thromboembolic disease as it has >90% negative predictive value for pulmonary embolus.

c. *(1 mark per correct answer, maximum 5 marks).* She should be started on low molecular weight heparin to prevent further clot on the presumption that she has had a PE *(1 mark)*. Imaging (V/Q scan or CTPA) should be performed to confirm the diagnosis *(1 mark)*. Once confirmed she should be commenced on warfarin *(1 mark)*. Low molecular weight heparin can be stopped when she is fully anticoagulated with warfarin *(1 mark)*. She should stay on warfarin for 6 months *(1 mark)*. She needs investigation for a predisposing cause (pelvic ultrasound, thrombophilia screen).

8

a. A proportionate reduction in FEV_1 and FVC (ratio >70%) *(1 mark)* indicates restrictive lung disease *(1 mark)*. She also has reduced gas transfer indicating probable involvement of the lung parenchyma *(1 mark)*.

b. Non-caseating granulomas are the pathological hallmark *(1 mark)* of sarcoidosis *(1 mark)*.

c. *(1 mark per correct answer, maximum 4 marks).* Extrapulmonary manifestations of sarcoidosis are given in Box 121, p. 210.

d. As she has significant impairment of pulmonary function *(0.5 mark)* immunosuppression with prednisolone should be tried *(0.5 mark)*.

9

a. Tuberculosis should be considered to be the diagnosis until proven otherwise *(1 mark)*. Other causes of cavitating lung disease include primary *(1 mark)* and secondary *(1 mark)* lung cancer, pulmonary embolus *(1 mark)* and bacterial pneumonia *(1 mark)* (Box 108, p. 190).

b. You should presume he has tuberculosis. Infection control is a priority and he should be isolated in a side room to prevent spread to staff and patients *(1 mark)*.

c. *(1 mark per correct answer, maximum 4 marks).* Three sputum samples should be examined microscopically *(1 mark)* with Ziehl–Neelsen staining to look for acid-fast bacilli, then cultured to look for *Mycobacterium tuberculosis (1 mark)*. Tuberculin skin test *(1 mark)* (Mantoux, Heaf) will detect an immune response to TB antigen. HIV testing may indicate underlying immunodeficiency *(1 mark)*. A thoracic CT scan will help to clarify nature of the cavity and look for other causes *(1 mark)*.

d. *(1 mark per correct answer, maximum 2 marks).* He is living on the streets and appears to be alcohol-dependent. This may make it difficult for him to adhere to therapy and attend for follow-up *(1 mark)*. Additionally, he is unlikely to have regular health care from his GP *(1 mark)*. His general health and nutrition appears poor (low body mass index), which may make it difficult for him to heal *(1 mark)*. Assuming that he has TB he will need directly observed therapy. Contact tracing will also be difficult.

10

a. His infection is most likely to be caused by a virus, e.g. rhinovirus *(1 mark)* or group A β-haemolytic streptococcus (Box 98, p. 170) *(1 mark)*.

b. No *(1 mark)*.
(1 mark for each correct answer, maximum 3 marks). The infection is more likely to be viral (unresponsive to antibiotics) than bacterial *(1 mark)* and these aetiologies cannot be distinguished using clinical features *(1 mark)*. Also, sore throats are usually self-limiting, whatever the organism *(1 mark)*. He does not meet NICE criteria for prescription of antibiotics (Box 103, p. 171) *(1 mark)*.

c. Suitable – penicillin or erythromycin *(1 mark)*. Contraindicated – amoxicillin or ampicillin (cause rash in patients with Epstein–Barr virus) *(1 mark)*.

d. *(1 mark for each correct answer, maximum 2 marks).* Complications of upper respiratory tract infections depend on the organism and include: common cold – exacerbation of underlying lung disease, e.g. COPD *(1 mark)*; group A streptococci (Box 101, p. 171) *(1 mark for any correct complication)*; diphtheria (Box 100, p. 171) *(1 mark for any correct complication)*.

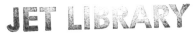

Index of cases by diagnosis

Index

Note: page numbers in *italics* refer to figures, those in **bold** refer to tables